Review of
PSYCHIATRY

Review of PSYCHIATRY

8th Edition

Praveen Tripathi MBBS MD
Director
The Renowa Care
Noida, Gautam Buddha Nagar
Uttar Pradesh, India

Foreword
Kailash Kedia

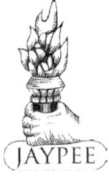

JAYPEE BROTHERS MEDICAL PUBLISHERS
The Health Sciences Publisher
New Delhi | London

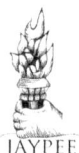
Jaypee Brothers Medical Publishers (P) Ltd

Headquarters
Jaypee Brothers Medical Publishers (P) Ltd
EMCA House, 23/23-B
Ansari Road, Daryaganj
New Delhi 110 002, India
Landline: +91-11-23272143, +91-11-23272703
+91-11-23282021, +91-11-23245672
Email: jaypee@jaypeebrothers.com

Corporate Office
Jaypee Brothers Medical Publishers (P) Ltd
4838/24, Ansari Road, Daryaganj
New Delhi 110 002, India
Phone: +91-11-43574357
Fax: +91-11-43574314
Email: jaypee@jaypeebrothers.com

Overseas Office
JP Medical Ltd
83 Victoria Street, London
SW1H 0HW (UK)
Phone: +44 20 3170 8910
Fax: +44 (0)20 3008 6180
Email: info@jpmedpub.com

Website: www.jaypeebrothers.com

Website: www.jaypeedigital.com

© 2023, Jaypee Brothers Medical Publishers

The views and opinions expressed in this book are solely those of the original contributor(s)/author(s) and do not necessarily represent those of editor(s) or publisher of the book.

All rights reserved. No part of this publication may be reproduced, stored or transmitted in any form or by any means, electronic, mechanical, photocopying, recording or otherwise, without the prior permission in writing of the publishers.

All brand names and product names used in this book are trade names, service marks, trademarks or registered trademarks of their respective owners. The publisher is not associated with any product or vendor mentioned in this book.

Medical knowledge and practice change constantly. This book is designed to provide accurate, authoritative information about the subject matter in question. However, readers are advised to check the most current information available on procedures included and check information from the manufacturer of each product to be administered, to verify the recommended dose, formula, method and duration of administration, adverse effects and contraindications. It is the responsibility of the practitioner to take all appropriate safety precautions. Neither the publisher nor the author(s)/editor(s) assume any liability for any injury and/ or damage to persons or property arising from or related to use of material in this book.

This book is sold on the understanding that the publisher is not engaged in providing professional medical services. If such advice or services are required, the services of a competent medical professional should be sought.

Every effort has been made where necessary to contact holders of copyright to obtain permission to reproduce copyright material. If any have been inadvertently overlooked, the publisher will be pleased to make the necessary arrangements at the first opportunity.

Inquiries for bulk sales may be solicited at: jaypee@jaypeebrothers.com

Review of Psychiatry

First Edition: 2016
Second Edition: 2017
Third Edition: 2018
Fourth Edition: 2019
Fifth Edition: 2020
Sixth Edition: 2021
Seventh Edition: 2022
Eighth Edition: 2023
ISBN: 978-93-5696-366-5

Dedicated to
My Parents

Foreword

Psychiatry is quite different from mainstream medical specialties and poses unique challenges when the novice medical graduate is attempting to understand these concepts. Psychiatry is also a fast-evolving science and the recent introduction of DSM-5 has led to several diagnostic revisions. Most of the textbooks on psychiatry are fairly exhaustive and can be difficult to read for students preparing for entrance examinations who are hard-pressed for time.

Keeping these aspects in mind, Dr Praveen Tripathi has made enthusiastic efforts to compile the exhaustive literature on mental health into a simple format that is highly readable and easy to understand. He has also included MCQs from past examinations for practice and to adapt to the examinations questions. I recommend this book as a powerful and time-efficient tool to prepare for psychiatry section of postgraduate entrance examinations.

I wish all the readers good luck and congratulate Dr Tripathi for his efforts in writing this book.

Kailash Kedia MBBS MD
Staff Specialist
Princess Alexandra Hospital
Woolloongabba, Queensland, Australia
Associate Lecturer
University of Queensland, Australia

Preface

Psychiatry is a complex subject and the students have minimal exposure to the cases with psychiatric disorders during their MBBS training. The terminology used in psychiatry is quite different from other medical specialties and makes the subject tough to understand. Most of the students resort to rote memorization and struggle with the conceptual aspects. In this book, an attempt has been made to explain the concepts in a simple language and without using the psychiatry jargons. A large number of examples have been included in the text to explain the concepts and help in learning.

Another important aspect of the book is that it has been fully updated with Diagnostic and Statistical Manual of Mental Disorders-5 (DSM-5). In DSM-5, a large number of new diagnoses have been introduced and diagnostic criteria of many existing disorders have been changed. All these changes have been incorporated in the book.

This book has been written keeping in mind the needs of students preparing for various postgraduate entrance examinations and MCI screening test. Nowadays, mastery over short subjects has become key to get a good rank. In most of the examinations (including INI-CET and NEET), at least 5–6 questions are being asked from psychiatry. If students can spare 5–6 days for psychiatry, they would easily be able to get those questions correct and that will make a real difference in the final ranks achieved.

Finally, a word of advice for the students—If you keep yourself motivated for the entire duration of preparation, cracking the entrance becomes a child's play. You should remain in regular touch with your seniors and take both tips and inspiration from them. Appearing regularly for mock tests and discussion with peers is a good way of assessing your strengths and weaknesses. It also motivates you to work harder and get better results next time. Remember that you need to win many small battles before you can win a war.

So, buckle up, get ready to bring your best to the table, work so hard that you surprise even yourself and achieve what you rightly deserve.

My best wishes and blessings are always with you.

November 2023

Praveen Tripathi MBBS MD
Director
The Renowa Care
Noida, Gautam Buddha Nagar
Uttar Pradesh, India
Website: www.therenowacare.com
Facebook group: Dr Praveen's Psychiatry Discussion Group
Facebook page: www.facebook.com/drpraveentripathipsychiatrist

Acknowledgments

Every endeavor, however big or small, needs contribution from many. This book is no exception. A large number of people have contributed directly or indirectly in the completion of this book.

At the outset, I would like to thank my parents who have backed all the decisions I have ever taken in my life and have supported me even when they did not agree with me. I am thankful to my elder brother, Dr Anurag Tripathi, who gave me a lot of suggestions while I was writing this book and pushed me to put more and better efforts. I want to convey special thanks to my wife, Dr Priyanka Goyal, for bearing with me for the long months during which this book was written and helping me with the content as well as editing of the book. Without her help, this book would not have seen the light of the day.

I am extremely thankful to Dr Apurv Mehra, who brought me into the field of teaching and is like a friend and teacher to me. I am also grateful to Dr Pritesh Singh, who taught me the art of writing a book and who has made important contributions in formatting the book.

I would also like to thank Shri Jitendar P Vij (Group Chairman), Mr Ankit Vij (Managing Director), Ms Chetna Malhotra (Senior Director—Professional Publishing, Marketing, and Business Development), Ms Pooja Bhandari (Director—Production), Ms Ruby Sharma (Business Manager) and the complete production team of M/s Jaypee Brothers Medical Publishers (P) Ltd, New Delhi, India.

Finally, I would like to thank my patients and my students. They have taught me a lot and continue to be my favorite teachers.

How to Use This Book

The book is meant to act as one stop solution for your preparation of postgraduate entrance examination. Every chapter starts with theory written in a simple language to build the concepts. In the theory itself, important points have been highlighted and the superscript 'Q' has been added after the points that have been asked in the examinations.

After reading the theory, the MCQs should be attempted. If theory has been read properly, more than 95% MCQs should get solved easily. The 'controversial questions' have been marked separately, and detailed explanations have also been added.

The book should preferably be used along with the lectures, that have been uploaded in the app *'Psychiatry by Dr Praveen Tripathi'*, which is available on Google play store and Apple store. App and book combined, should be enough for the detailed preparation of entrance examinations.

Unique Features of This Edition

- Latest MCQs for year 2020-2023
- Includes recently asked topics on POCSO Act, ICD-11 and Mental Health Care Act
- Concise theory
- Genuine questions with explanations
- Controversial questions fully explained.

Contents

1. Basics 1–11

2. Schizophrenia Spectrum or Other Primary Psychotic Disorders ★★★ 12–32

3. Mood Disorders 33–53

4. Neurotic, Stress-related and Somatoform Disorders ★★★ 54–75

5. Substance-related and Addictive Disorders 76–91

6. Neurocognitive Disorders (Organic Mental Disorders) 92–104

7. Personality Disorders ★★★ 105–110

8. Eating Disorders 111–114

9. Sleep Disorders 115–120

10. Sexual Disorders 121–125

11. Child Psychiatry ★★★ 126–134

12. Psychoanalysis 135–142

13. Miscellaneous ★★★ 143–158

    Recent Questions and Answer *159–172*

Most Important ★★★

CHAPTER 1: Basics

Psychiatry is the branch of medicine, which deals with morbid psychological processes. The term 'Psychiatry' was coined by a German physician, **Johann Christian Reil**. To establish the diagnosis of a psychiatric disorder, both history and clinical examination are required. History taking involves taking information from both the patient as well as the informant. Informant may be a relative or someone close to the patient. An informant is considered 'reliable'^{Q}, if the following five parameters are fulfilled (5 C's):

1. *Consistency*: Whether the informant provides the same information across the interviews (Is he consistent ?).
2. *Coherence*: Whether the different parts of information provided are logically connected to each other (Is he coherent?).
3. *Chronological information*: Whether the information follows a chronological sequence?
4. *Closeness with patient*: Whether the informant was close enough with patient to have an accurate account of information?
5. *Concern with patient*: Whether the informant is genuinely concerned for patient or is there a possibility of any malafide intention?

The clinical examination in psychiatry, wherein the clinician records the psychiatric signs and symptoms, is known as **Mental Status Examination (MSE)**^{Q}.

MENTAL STATUS EXAMINATION

In the mental status examination, following areas of mental functioning are assessed:

A. *General appearance and behavior*: The appearance of patient is described along with any gross abnormalities (such as abnormalities of dressing, etc.).
B. *Speech*: Various aspects of speech such as rate, tone, volume, spontaneity of speech are described.
C. *Mood and affect*: Both the terms "affect" and "mood" are both used to describe the emotions or emotional state.
   Mood is the sustained (longterm) and internal emotional state, which influences the way world is perceived, e.g. a person who is feeling low internally for a long time and hence finds everything in his surrounding dull and boring, would be described as having 'depressed mood'.
   Affect^Q is the short lived and external expression of internal emotions which can be observed, e.g. the above-mentioned person, during the interview avoided looking into the eyes of examiner and started crying. The facial expression and crying is the external expression of the underlying depressed mood.

The term affect and mood are at times used interchangeably. Affect and mood are further described under the following three subheads:

1. *Quality*: It refers to the predominant affective (or mood) state. Common disturbances in the quality of mood, common ones include:
   a. *Euphoric mood (elevation of mood)*: A state of excessive happiness, without any reason. It is usually seen in mania or hypomania.
   b. *Depressed mood*: Persistent and pervasive sadness of mood. The term 'persistent' means that person remains sad all the time, and the term 'pervasive' means that the person remains sad during all the activities (work, leisure activities, etc.). It is a feature of depression.
2. *Fluctuations*: It refers to the changes in mood/affect. The common disturbances of fluctuations include:
   a. *Labile mood*: Excessive variations in mood without any apparent reason. It is also known as **emotional lability**^{Q}. For example, a man starts crying and then starts laughing the next moment, without any apparent reason. It is usually seen in mania.
   b. *Affective flattening (flat affect, emotional bluting, blunt affect)*: Lack of emotional expressions. In this condition, patient does not experience any emotions hence his affect remains the same. For example, a patient with schizophrenia who had affective flattening, would not look happy during festivals and did not appear sad when his mother died. His affect remained the same irrespective of the situation.

3. *Appropriateness and congruency*:
   Appropriateness of affect is described in relation to the social situation. For example, in a funeral, the expected emotional state is sadness. Hence, being sad in a funeral is an appropriate affect. If a man starts laughing and looks extremely happy in a funeral, it would be diagnosed as inappropriate affect.

   Congruency of affect is described in relation to the thought content of the person. Congruency describes whether the emotional state of the person is in sync with his thought/speech or not. For example, if a man is thinking about or talking about the events which led to his mother's death, he is expected to be sad. Hence, appearing sad while talking about mother's death is a congruent affect. If a person, looks very happy and smiles while describing his mother's death, it would be considered as 'incongruent affect'. It must be stressed that while "appropriateness" of affect is described after comparing the current affect with expected affect in a given social situation, the congruence is described after comparing the current affect with the expected affect in the context of patients thoughts.

Few other important disturbances of emotions include:
a. *Alexithymia*: It refers to inability to understand emotions of others and inability to express emotions of self. Although alexithymia is closely related to affective flattening, **alexithymia**^{Q} is "lack of words to describe emotions" rather than the absence of emotions.
b. *Anhedonia*: It refers to the loss of capacity to experience pleasure in activities that were previously pleasurable

   Neuroanatomical substrate of emotions: **Limbic system**^{Q} (which includes hippocampus, amygdala, hypothalamus, cingulate gyrus and related thalamic and cortical areas) is the neural substrate for emotional experiences. The regulation of emotions is a function of frontal lobe^Q.

D. *Perception*: Perception is receiving of information using one of the sensory modalities (i.e. auditory, visual, tactile, olfactory and gustatory). Two most important disturbances of perception are:
   - *Illusions*^{Q}: Illusion is false perception of a real object. For example, a man mistakes a rope for snake in night.
   - *Hallucinations*: Hallucination is a false perception in the absence of any object or stimulus. For example, a patient with delirium reported seeing snakes on the ground of his room, when in reality there was nothing there. Hallucinations have the following criteria and all of these must be present to diagnose a perception as "hallucination".

Criterions of hallucinations:
a. Hallucinations occur in the absence of any sensory or perceptual stimulus.
b. Hallucinations are as vivid (clear or detailed) as true perceptions. It means that the person who experiences hallucinations is able to give a detailed description of what he is experiencing.
c. Hallucinations are experienced in **outer objective space**^{Q}. It means that patient experiences that the source of hallucinations is in outer world. For example, a patient who is having auditory hallucinations will report that the voices are coming from the wall or from outside the house. (**Pseudohallucinations**^{Q} are experienced in the inner subjective space, or originating from within the mind. For example, a patient with auditory pseudohallucinations will report that the voices are originating within his mind and not from outside).
d. Hallucinations are not under **willful control**^{Q} of the patient. It means that patient can neither start the hallucinations nor can he stop them.

Hallucinations can occur in any modality.

Few important points must be remembered:
a. The most common type of hallucinations in psychiatric disorders are **auditory hallucinations**^{Q}.
b. The most common hallucinations in organic psychiatric disorders (such as delirium) are **visual hallucinations**^{Q}.
c. In patients with **temporal lobe epilepsy**^{Q} all kinds of hallucinations can be present including olfactory and tactile hallucinations.
d. Tactile hallucinations are a typical feature of cocaine intoxication.

Few specific hallucinations:
a. *Hypnagogic hallucinations*^{Q}: These hallucinations occur while falling asleep or while going to sleep. Since hypnagogic has the word "go" in it, hence it's easy to remember that they occur while "going" to sleep. Hypnagogic hallucinations are seen in narcolepsy.
b. *Hypnopompic hallucinations*^{Q}: These hallucinations occur while getting up from the sleep. They too are a feature of narcolepsy.
c. *Reflex hallucinations (Synesthesia*^{Q}): In reflex hallucinations, stimulus in one sensory modality produces hallucinations in another sensory modality. For example, a patient reports that whenever he sees a white bulb (stimulus in visual modality), he starts hearing voices of god (hallucination in auditory modality). Reflex hallucinations are a feature of **cannabis and LSD**^{Q} (and other hallucinogens) **intoxication**.
d. *Functional hallucinations*: Here, stimulus in one sensory modality, produces hallucinations in the same sensory modality. For example, a patient reported that whenever he heard the sound of a ticking clock (stimulus in auditory modality), he would also start hearing voices of god (hallucinations in auditory modality).

E. *Thought (Cognition)*: The terms "thought" and "**cognition**"^{Q} are at times used interchangeably. However, in a stricter sense, cognition is the mental process of acquiring knowledge which not only includes thoughts but also experiences and sensations.

The thought disturbances are primary in many psychiatric disorders like schizophrenia. Thought and its disturbances can be described under the following subheads.

1. **Stream (Flow of thought)**: It refers to the speed with which thoughts follow each other. The disturbances of stream includes:
   a. **Flight of ideas**[Q]: Here, the thoughts follow each other very rapidly, and connection between different thoughts appears to be due to chance factors such as rhyming. It is usually seen in mania. For example, a manic patient when asked about his hometown said "I live in Delhi...my cat has a big belly.....I like to eat Jelly.....lilly lilly lilly". Some authors describe "flight of ideas" as an abnormality of form of thought.
   b. **Inhibition of thinking**: Here thoughts come in mind very slowly and thought progresses with a slow rate.

2. **Form of thought**: Form refers to the "organization" of thinking or "association" between the consecutive thoughts. Normally, the thoughts are well organized and there is a connection between various components of a single thought and between the consecutive thoughts. In formal thought disorders, there are disturbance in the organization, associations and connections of the thoughts. The important formal thought disorders include:
   a. **Derailment**: In derailment, the association between two successive thoughts is disturbed. For example, a patient said Jawahar Lal Nehru was the first prime minister of India and he was a congress leader. "Sachin Tendulkar scored 100 international hundreds". In this example, there is no link between the first thought about Nehru and second thought about Tendulkar.
   b. **Loosening of association**[Q]: Here, the connection is lost between components of a single thought. For example, a patient said "I thought that it will rain today, its going to be a blockbuster movie". In this example the phrase before the comma is totally disconnected from the phrase after the comma and hence this represents loosening of association.
   c. **Incoherence**: It is total lack of organization so that the thought is incomprehensible and does not convey any meaning. For example, a patient says "India me churchgate pulses cricket computer".
   d. **Circumstantiality**[Q]: It is a pattern of thought/speech which progresses with inclusion of lots of unnecessary details and progresses slowly however, **finally the goal of thought is reached**. For example, a medical student was asked about his preferred branch in postgraduation and he replied by saying "Sir, in the first year I was very interested in physiology, however in the second year I started liking pathology. In the third year, I started liking ophthalmology however in the final year I realized that I have a lot of liking for orthopaedics too and I liked putting casts and working with POP. I also think that after MBBS one should get married as soon as possible and that no one should have more than two kids... Well..you see i like pediatrics as a subject and I want to do my postgraduation in the pediatrics". In this example the thought process progressed with inclusion of lots of irrelevant details however in the end, the goal was reached and the student said that he wants to become a pediatrician.
   e. **Tangentiality**[Q]: In tangentiality, the answer is related to the question in some distant way and the goal of thought is never reached. For example, a patient was asked about his favourite Indian actor and he replied "Well, you see Indian movies are mostly hero centric and usually deal with relationship issues whereas the Hollywood movies have lots of action and science fiction. I think the Indian Film Industry is growing rapidly and it's a good medium for entertainment of masses". In this example, the patients answer was distantly related to the question, however the exact answer was never given.
   f. **Neologism**: **Neologism**[Q] is coining of a new word, whose derivation cannot be understood. For example, a patient would use the word "tintin tapa" for a pen. Neologism is highly suggestive of schizophrenia.
   g. **Word approximations (metonyms)**: Here, old words are used in a new or unconventional way. The meaning will be easily evident, though the word in itself might appear strange. For example, a patient would use the word "time vessel" for watch, and use the word "handshoes" for gloves.
   h. **Clanging (Clang associations)**: Here, the words are associated with each other as they sound similar, and there may be lack of any meaningful connection between the words. For example, a patient said 'I make sense out of nonsense and nonsense is the essence of the turbulence of life. In 'flight of ideas', clanging is frequently observed.
   i. **Perseveration**: It is repetition of the same response, beyond point of relevance. For example, a patient was asked the following questions. Q: What is

your name. Ans. Mahesh kumar.... Q: Where do you live. Ans: Mahesh Kumar..... Q: How many children do you have... A: Mahesh Kumar. It must be noted that the perseveration is in response to a question and is not spontaneous.

3. **Content of thought**: Content refers to what person is actually thinking about.

   Delusion^Q is a disorder of content of thought. It is defined as a:
   i. False belief, that is
   ii. Unshakeable (doesnt not change if there is evidence against the belief), and
   iii. Cannot be explained on the basis of person's social and cultural background.

   Following are the types of delusion:
   a. **Delusion of persecution**: It is the **most common^Q** type of delusion. The patient believes that someone wants to harm him. For example, a patient claimed that Indian police along with CBI is hatching a conspiracy to kill him.
   b. **Delusion of reference**: The patient believes that neutral events happening around him are somehow related to him. For example, a patient claimed that the tubelight of his apartment was flickering as there was a camera fitted inside through which his movements were being recorded.
   c. **Delusion of grandeur or grandiosity**: The patient believes that he has some exceptional identity or power. For example, a patient claimed that he is the reincarnation of Lord Hanuman and that he can carry the mountains on his shoulders.
   d. **Delusion of love (erotomania^Q, fantasy lover syndrome)**: Patient may have a false belief that someone is in love with them. This 'lover' is someone who is usually from a higher socio - economic status than the patient. It is also known as de Clerambault syndrome. For example, a rickshaw puller claimed that Katrina Kaif is in love with him though he admitted that he has never met her.
   e. **Nihilistic delusion (delusion of negation, Cotard's syndrome^Q)**: Here, the patients may deny existence of their body, their mind, or the world in general. They may claim that everybody is dead, the world has stopped, etc. The basic theme of delusion is the "end of existence".
   f. **Delusion of enormity^Q**: Sometimes nihilistic delusions are associated with 'delusions of enormity', in which patient may believe that some of their action may cause a catastrophe (e.g. A patient refused to 'sneeze' as he believed that his 'sneeze' will blow away the world).
   g. **Delusion of infidelity (delusion of jealousy)**: The patient has a false belief that his partner/spouse is having an affair. It is also known as **morbid jealousy (Pathological jealousy^Q)** or **Othello syndrome^Q**.
   h. **Delusion of guilt**: Here, the patients may develop a delusion that they are bad or evil person and may claim that they have committed unpardonable sins. It is usually seen in severe depression.

    Bizarre Vs Nonbizarre Delusions

   Bizarre delusions: The term bizarre is used for delusions which are scientifically impossible and culturally implausible (ununderstandable). For example, if a patient says that aliens have stolen his heart, it would be an example of bizarre delusion. Its scientifically impossible that anyone's heart can be stolen, and it's also ununderstandable that how can someone start believing that their heart has been stolen.

   Nonbizarre delusions: These are delusions which are false but are possible, i.e. they can happen. For example, if a patient develops a delusion that his family members want to take away his property, it would be an example of nonbizarre delusion, since it is not impossible for a family member to take away property of another family member.

4. **Possession of thought**: Normally one experiences that his thoughts belong to himself and no one else can influence his thinking process, also there is a sense of control over one's thought. In disturbances of possession of thought patient either experiences that others are tampering with his thoughts or that he has lost control over his thoughts. The disorders of possession include the following:
   a. **Obsessions^Q**: Here, a thought comes repeatedly into the mind of patient against his will. The patient recognizes the thought as his own, however is distressed by the repetitive and intrusive nature of thought and tries to stop it. The patient feels that he has lost control over his thoughts. Patient also understands that the thoughts that are coming in his mind are 'senseless' and irrational and experience obsessions as 'ego dystonic' (i.e. unwanted and unacceptable). Obsessions are explained in more details, in chapter 4.
   b. **Thought alienation**: Here, the patient feels that his thoughts are under the control of an outside agency or that others are interfering with his thought process. Thought alienation phenomenon is of following types:
   – Thought insertion: Patient feels that some external agency is inserting foreign thoughts into his mind. (E.g. A patient complained, 'doctor, something weird is happening. I was

sitting and thinking about a cricket match, and suddenly a thought about terrorists entered my mind. This thought about terrorists was not my thought, my neighbour used some technology, to force that thought into my mind. Its scary'

- *Thought withdrawal*: Patient experiences that his thoughts are being withdrawn from his mind by an external agency. (e.g. A patient complained, 'doctor, something weird is happening. I was sitting and thinking about a cricket match, and suddenly my mind went blank, I could not think of anything. My neighbour is using some technology and stealing away all my thoughts. Its scary'

- *Thought broadcast*: Patient experiences that thoughts are escaping from his minds and other people are able to access them, (e.g. A patient complained, 'doctor, something weird is happening. I was sitting and thinking about a cricket match, and suddenly my neighbour entered my house carrying a cricket bat. My thoughts escaped from my mind and my neighbour already knew what I was thinking'

F. *Higher mental functions*: In this component of MSE, various higher mental functions are assessed. These include:

a. *Attention*: Attention is the ability to attend to a specific stimulus without getting distracted. In clinical practice, attention is tested using **Digit Repetition Test (Digit Span Test),** in which examiner says some numbers and patient is asked to repeat them. The examiner starts with a single number and gradually increases to two number sequence, three number sequence and so on and so forth, till patient fails to repeat.

e.g. 2, 25, 387, 4980, 132587

An inability to repeat more than five digits indicates defective attention.

b. *Concentration*: Concentration is basically the ability to sustain attention for longer duration. It is usually tested by **Serial Sevens Subtraction Test**, in which patient is asked to serially decrease 7s from 100 (100, 93, 86, 79....).

1. *Memory*: Memory is clinically divided into following three types:*Immediate memory*: It is the ability to recall a material after interval of few seconds. At times the term "working memory" is used as a synonymous for immediate memory, though there are finer differences. Immediate memory is tested by **Digit Repetition Test**^{Q} or Serial Seven Subtraction Tests.

2. *Recent memory*: It is the ability to recall material after an interval of minutes, hours or days. A common test is "24 hour recall" in which patient is asked simple questions like what he had in meal last night, how did he reach the hospital, etc. Questions on patients orientation to time, place and person, also test recent memory.

3. *Remote memory*: It is ability to recall the material after an interval of years. It includes recall of both personal events and historical events. The example of questions asked are: Where did you go to school? When was your first child born? Name four prime ministers of India?

c. *Intelligence*: It is usually tested by asking questions about general information and assessing calculation skills.

d. *Abstract thinking*: Abstract thinking is the ability to form concepts and make generalizations. It can be assessed by (a) Proverb testing: Here, the patient is asked to explain the meaning of proverbs, (b) Similarities testing: Here, patient is asked similarities between objects, e.g. similarity is asked between chair and table. If the patient answers that both are pieces of furniture, it would show that patient has abstract thinking and is able to conceptualize at a higher level. On the other hand, if patient answers that both are kept on the floor, it would show an absence of higher level of thinking, also known as concrete thinking.

e. *Judgement*: It is the ability to respond appropriately in a particular situation. There are three types of judgement (1) **Test judgement**^{Q}: Here, a test situation is given and patient is asked to respond. The commonly asked question is: What would the patient do if he sees a "house on fire" or "an addressed envelope lying on the ground". If the patient responds that he will 'call the fire brigade" or "drop it in the letterbox" respectively, it will suggest normal judgement. (2) Personal judgement: Here, patients plans for his future life are asked and his response is assessed. (3) Social judgement: Here, patients ability to interact properly in social situations is assessed.

f. *Insight*^{Q}: Insight is defined as awareness and understanding about the illness. Insight can be rated on 6 point scale as described below:

1. Complete denial of insight (Absent insight).
2. Some awareness of being sick but denying it at the same time.
3. Awareness of being sick but attributing symptoms to external or physical factors. (e.g. patient says that symptoms are because of black magic).
4. Awareness of being sick, but not knowing the cause.
5. Awareness of illness but no change in behavior on the basis of this awareness (known as Intellectual Insight).
6. Awareness of illness and change in behavior on the basis of this awareness (known as **Emotional Insight**^{Q}, which is the **highest level**^{Q} of insight).

CLASSIFICATION

At present, there are two major classificatory systems in psychiatry.
1. ***ICD-11 (International classification of diseases, 11th edition)***: It was published by WHO in 2018, and provides classification for all medical disorders (including psychiatric disorders). The psychiatric disorders have been classified in Chapter 6 of ICD-11.
2. ***DSM-5 (Diagnostic and statistical manual of mental disorders)***: It is published by American Psychiatric Association. The fifth edition of DSM (DSM-5) was published in 2013. In DSM-IV, a multiaxial system was used for making a comprehensive clinical diagnosis, according to which any diagnosis would be given on the following axes:

   Axis I: Clinical psychiatry diagnosis (Here, the psychiatry diagnoses would be mentioned)

   Axis II: Personality disorders and Mental Retardation (Here, if patient had any personality disorder or mental retardation, that would be mentioned)

   Axis III: Medical conditions (Here, any accompanying medical illness would be mentioned)

   Axis IV: Psychosocial problems (Here psychosocial problems such as poor relationship with spouse, etc. would be mentioned)

   Axis V: Global Assessment of Functioning (It is a measure of patients functioning in last one year)

   In DSM-5, the concept of multiaxial diagnoses was removed. In DSM-5, Axis I, II and III of DSMIV have been combined, and Axis IV and Axis V are described separately.

3. ***Research Domain Criteria***^{Q}: The existing classificatory systems (DSM and ICD) have been criticised for being symptom based and not having a sound biological validity. **National Institute of Mental Health (NIMH)**, USA, has started a new project called **Research Domain Criteria (RDoC)**, which aims to develop a new experimental classification of mental illnesses, based on dimensions of behaviours and neurobiology.

Other Classifications

Psychiatric disorders have been classified in multiple ways. The most important classifications include organic vs functional psychiatric disorders and psychosis vs neurosis.

Organic vs Functional (Nonorganic) mental disorders: This was the first major classification of psychiatric/mental disorders.

A. ***Organic mental disorders***: These disorders are caused by demonstrable disturbances of brain (primary brain disturbances or systemic disturbances which are known to affect brain parenchyma). For example, delirium, dementia, etc.

B. ***Functional (Nonorganic) mental disorders***: These disorders do not have any demonstrable disturbance of brain parenchyma. For example, schizophrenia, mania, etc.

This classification is at best arbitrary, since with the advent of science its possible to demonstrate brain parenchyma disturbances even in socalled "functional" mental disorders.

Psychoses vs neuroses: The functional disorders can be further classified into psychotic disorders (psychoses) and neurotic disorders (neuroses).

A. ***Psychoses***: Psychotic disorders are characterized by **lack of awareness** of **illness (also known as lack of insight)**^{Q} and impaired reality testing (i.e. the patients loses contact with reality and starts living in a fantasy world created by their ill mind). For example, schizophrenia, bipolar disorder. Delusions and hallucinations are the prototype psychotic symptoms.

B. ***Neuroses***: Neurotic disorders are characterized by awareness of the illness (insight is present) and reality contact is also intact. For example, anxiety disorders, depression, etc.

	Psychosis	Neurosis
Insight	Absent	Present
Reality testing	Absent	Present
Delusions/Hallucinations	Present	Absent

Multiple Choice Questions

1. **Which of the following are sections of Mental State Examination?** *(DNB NEET 2014-15)*
   A. Mood and affect
   B. Speech and language
   C. Cognition
   D. All of the above

2. **Who coined the term 'Psychiatry'?** *(DNB 2013)*
   A. Johann Christian Reil
   B. Sigmund Freud
   C. Erik Erikson
   D. Carl Jung

3. **Which of the following is not asked in personal history in a psychiatric disorder?** *(AIIMS May 2016)*
   A. Occupational history
   B. Academic history
   C. Food preferences
   D. Marital History

4. **Reliability of information about patient provided by informants depend on all except:** *(AIIMS Nov, 2017)*
   A. Biological relationship
   B. Educational status
   C. Consistency of information
   D. Duration of stay with patient

5. **National Institute of Mental Health (NIMH, USA) uses which of the following to classify the behavioural disorders:** *(NIMHANS 2019)*
   A. International classification of diseases-11th edition (ICD-11)
   B. International classification of diseases- 10th edition (ICD-10)
   C. Diagnostic and statistical manual of mental disorders - 5th edition (DSM-5)
   D. Research domain criterion (RDoC)

Affect and Mood

6. **A 25-year-old woman complaints of intense depressed mood for last 6 months. She also reports inability to enjoy previously pleasurable activities. This symptom is known as:** *(AIIMS Nov 2005)*
   A. Anhedonia
   B. Avolition
   C. Apathy
   D. Amotivation

7. **Alexithymia is:** *(Kerala 2000, DNB 2004)*
   A. A feeling of intense rapture
   B. Pathological sadness
   C. Affective flattening
   D. Inability to recognize and describe feelings
   E. Inappropriate mood

8. **A person who laughs at one minute and cries the next minute without any clear stimulus is said to have:** *(AIIMS Nov 2005)*
   A. Incongruent affect
   B. Euphoria
   C. Labile affect
   D. Split personality

9. **Emotion is controlled by:** *(PGI 1997)*
   A. Limbic system
   B. Frontal lobe
   C. Temporal lobe
   D. Occipital lobe

Perception

10. **Phantom limb is an example of disorder of:** *(DNB NEET 2014-15)*
    A. Thought
    B. Perception
    C. Cognition
    D. None of the above

11. **A patient wanting to scratch for itching in his amputated limb is an example of:** *(DNB NEET 2014-15)*
    A. Illusion
    B. Pseudohallucination
    C. Phantom limb hallucination
    D. Autoscopic hallucination

12. **A patient sees a rope and gets afraid that it is a snake. This sign is known as:** *(DNB NEET 2014-15, PGI 2002)*
    A. Illusion
    B. Hallucination
    C. Delusion
    D. Depersonalization
    E. Derealization

13. **Which statement is not true about hallucinations?** *(AIIMS 2009)*
    A. It is as vivid as a real perception
    B. It occurs in inner subjective space
    C. It is independent of will of observer
    D. It occurs in the absence of any perceptual stimulus

14. **False statement about hallucinations is:** *(NIMHANS 2015)*
    A. Perceived as not real
    B. Appears to be coming from external world
    C. Sensory organs are not involved
    D. Occurs in absence of any stimulus

Controversial Question

15. **All of the following are features of hallucinations, except:** *(AI 2003)*
    A. It is independent of will of observer
    B. Sensory organs are not involved
    C. It is as vivid as a real perception
    D. It occurs in the absence of any perceptual stimulus

16. **All of the following are true about pseudohallucinations except:** *(DNB NEET 2014-15)*
    A. It arises in inner subjective self
    B. Patient describes that the sensations are being perceived by 'mind's eyes'
    C. They are under the voluntary control of patient
    D. Distressing flashbacks of PTSD is an example

17. **Formed visual hallucinations are seen in lesions of:** *(PGI 2006, 2000)*
    A. Frontal lobe
    B. Temporal lobe
    C. Occipital lobe
    D. Parietal lobe

18. **The following is suggestive of an organic cause of behavioral symptoms:** *(AI 2002)*
    A. Formal thought disorder
    B. Auditory hallucinations
    C. Delusion of guilt
    D. Prominent visual hallucinations

19. Which of the following is not an example of disorder of perception? *(NEET 2016)*
    A. Illusion
    B. Hallucination
    C. Pseudohallucination
    D. Delusion

20. Hallucinations which occur at the "start" of sleep are known as: *(JIPMER 2002, DNB 2005)*
    A. Hypnagogic hallucinations
    B. Hypnopompic hallucinations
    C. Jactatio capitis nocturna
    D. Extracampine hallucinations

21. Hallucinations are seen in all except: *(MP 1999, DNB 2001)*
    A. Schizophrenia
    B. Seizures due to intracerebral space occupying lesions
    C. Lysergic acid diethyl amide intoxication (LSD intoxication)
    D. Anxiety

22. Olfactory hallucinations are seen in: *(PGI May 2011)*
    A. Schizophrenia
    B. Alzheimer's disease
    C. Mesial temporal sclerosis
    D. Body dysmorphic disorder
    E. Temporal lobe epilepsy

23. Visual hallucinations are seen in: *(PGI June 2009)*
    A. Hebephrenic schizophrenia
    B. Residual schizophrenia
    C. Simple schizophrenia
    D. Delirium
    E. Temporal lobe epilepsy

24. Reflex hallucinations is a morbid variety of: *(AIIMS May 2009, 2011)*
    A. Kinesthesia
    B. Paresthesia
    C. Hyperesthesia
    D. Synesthesia

Thought

25. The term "cognition" is used to imply about: *(AI 1997, Jharkhand 2003, DNB 1998)*
    A. Affect
    B. Perception
    C. Thought
    D. Speech

26. True about thought is all except: *(PGI Feb 2007)*
    A. Perseveration is out of context repetition
    B. Circumstantiality is over inclusion of irrelevant details while eventually getting back to the original point
    C. Verbigeration is senseless repetition
    D. Vorbeireden is skirting around the end point but never reaching it
    E. Loosening of association is logically connected thoughts with loss of goal

27. Perseveration is: *(AI 2005)*
    A. Persistent and inappropriate repetition of the same thoughts
    B. Feeling of distress in a patient with schizophrenia
    C. Characteristic of schizophrenia
    D. Characteristic of obsessive compulsive disorder

28. In schizophrenia, characteristic feature is: *(PGI 1997)*
    A. Formal thought disorder
    B. Delusion
    C. Hallucination
    D. Apathy

29. When a person is asked about his blood sugar level, he answers "Diabetics have sweet urine... urine and faeces are excreta"... Before finally telling his blood sugar level. It is an example of? *(DNB 2017)*
    A. Tangentiality
    B. Circumstantiality
    C. Flight of ideas
    D. Loosening of association

30. Not a disorder of form of thought is: *(AIIMS May 2012)*
    A. Tangentiality
    B. Derailment
    C. Thought block
    D. Loosening of association

31. Which of the following is/are thought disorder? *(DNB NEET 2014-15)*
    A. Circumstantiality
    B. Tangentiality
    C. Prolixity
    D. All of the above

32. Schizophrenia and depression both have the following features except: *(PGI 2002)*
    A. Formal thought disorder
    B. Social withdrawal
    C. Poor personal care
    D. Decreased interest in sex
    E. Suicidal tendency

33. Delusion is a disorder of: *(DNB NEET 2014-15, AIIMS Nov 2006, AI 2007)*
    A. Perception
    B. Flow of thought
    C. Content of thought
    D. Affect

34. A false belief which is unexplained by reality and is shared by a number of people is: *(AIIMS 2003, 2004 Jipmer 1998)*
    A. Illusion
    B. Delusion
    C. Obsession
    D. Superstition

35. Which of the following is the most common type of delusion? *(NEET 2016)*
    A. Delusion of Persecution
    B. Delusion of Love
    C. Delusion of Reference
    D. Delusion of Infidelity

36. Delusions are not likely to be seen in: *(AI 2012)*
    A. Dementia
    B. Depression
    C. Schizophrenia
    D. Conversion disorder

37. Delusions can be seen in all of the following except: *(SGPGI 2002, DNB 2001)*
    A. OCD
    B. Depression
    C. Mania
    D. Schizophrenia

38. Delusion of persecution can be seen in: *(PGI June 2009)*
    A. Schizophrenia
    B. Delusional disorder
    C. Manic episode
    D. Melancholic depression

39. Delusion of grandiosity can be seen in: *(PGI Nov 2010, May 2011)*
    A. Hypomania
    B. Paranoid schizophrenia
    C. Schizoaffective disorder
    D. Kleptomania/Pyromania
    E. Cyclothymia

40. Erotomania is seen in: *(DNB NEET 2014-15)*
    A. Schizophrenia
    B. Mania
    C. Neurosis
    D. OCD

41. A depressed patient thinks her intestines are rotten. It is an example of? *(DNB 2017)*
    A. Hallucination
    B. Illusion
    C. Ekbom syndrome
    D. Nihilistic delusion

42. Nihilistic ideas are seen in: *(PGI Dec 2008)*
    A. Simple schizophrenia
    B. Paranoid schizophrenia
    C. Cotard's syndrome
    D. Depression
    E. Body dysmorphic disorder

43. A 25-year-old university student had a fight with the neighboring boy. On the next day while out, he started feeling that two men in police uniform were observing his movements. When he reached home in the evening he was frightened and told his family members that police was after him and would arrest him. Despite reassurances by family members, he remained afraid that he is about to be arrested. The history is suggestive of which psychiatric sign/symptom: *(AIIMS Nov 2003)*
    A. Delusion of persecution
    B. Delusion of reference
    C. Somatic passivity
    D. Thought insertion

44. A man is brought to psychiatry OPD. He believes that he is the richest person in the world and that his family members and neighbours are plotting against him and planning to harm him. The family members disagree with him. Which disorder of content of thought is the patient suffering from: *(AIIMS Nov 2017)*
    A. Delusion of grandeur
    B. Delusion of grandeur and persecution
    C. Delusion of grandeur, persecution and reference
    D. Delusion of persecution

45. A man had a fight with his neighbor. The next day he started feeling that police is following him and his brain is being controlled by radio waves by his neighbor. The history is suggestive of which psychiatric sign/symptom:
    A. Thought insertion   B. Passivity   *(AIIMS 1999)*
    C. Delusion of persecution   D. Obsession

46. Healthy thinking includes all of the following except: *(AIIMS 2011)*
    A. Continuity   B. Constancy
    C. Organization   D. Clarity

47. An example for a bizarre delusion: *(JIPMER 2017)*
    A. Delusion of infidelity (My wife has an affair with another person)
    B. Delusion of control (My brain is being controlled by a microchip)
    C. Delusion of grandiosity (I am the greatest person in the world)
    D. Delusion of reference (Neighbours are talking about me)

Controversial Question
48. All are true about obsessions except: *(AIIMS May 2016)*
    A. Obsession persists despite resistance by the patient
    B. Obsessions are Ego dystonic
    C. Disorder of thought content
    D. Can be seen in schizophrenia

Higher Mental Functions

49. The awareness regarding the disease in mental status examination is known as: *(AIIMS Nov 2012, May 2013)*
    A. Insight   B. Orientation
    C. Judgment   D. Rapport

50. Serial 7 subtraction is used to test: *(DNB NEET 2014-15)*
    A. Working memory
    B. Long-term memory
    C. Mathematical ability
    D. Recall power

51. Immediate memory is tested by: *(AIIMS NOV 2017)*
    A. Digit span forward
    B. Digit span backward
    C. Subtraction test 20–1
    D. Subtraction test 100–7

52. Highest level of insight is: *(DNB NEET 2014-15)*
    A. Intellectual insight
    B. Emotional insight
    C. Affective insight
    D. Intellectual insight

53. Impaired insight is found in: *(PGI 1997)*
    A. Acute psychosis
    B. Schizophrenia
    C. Anxiety disorder
    D. Obsessive compulsive disorder

54. If a person is asked, "what will he do if he sees a house on fire"? Then what is being tested in that person? *(DNB NEET 2014-15)*
    A. Social Judgment   B. Test Judgment
    C. Response Judgment   D. None

AIIMS New Pattern Question

55. Match the abnormalities mentioned in column A with MSE (mental status examination) component in column B

Column A	Column B
a. Delusions	1. Stream of thought
b. Flight of ideas	2. Content of thought
c. Derailment	3. Perception
d. Illusions	4. Affect
	5. Form of thought
	6. Possession of thought

   A. a-2, b-1, c-4, d-4   B. a-3, b-2, c-5, c-6
   C. a-2, b-1, c-5, d-3   D. a-3, b-1, c-5, d-3

Answers With Explanations

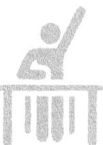

1. D. All of the above.
2. A. The term 'Psychiatry' was given by Johann Christian Reil.
3. C. Food preferences is not a standard component of psychiatric history.
4. B. The reliability does not depend on the educational status of the informant. Biological relationship and duration of stay with patient indicate 'closeness' with the patient.
5. D. Research domain criterion

Affect and Mood

6. A. Anhedonia. Anhedonia is seen in depression as well as schizophrenia.
7. D. Inability to recognize and describe feelings.
8. C. Labile affect.
9. B. Frontal lobe. The neuroanatomical substrate for generation of emotions is limbic system however the regulation/control of emotions is a function of frontal lobe.

Perception

10. B. Perception. In phantom limb, the patient feels sensations in the amputated limb. Hence, its a disorder of perception.
11. C. Phantom limb hallucination. Since, patient experiences sensation in the absence of any stimulus, it is a hallucination. In autoscopic hallucination, patient sees himself in the mirror and feels that "he" is the "image" i.e. what he is seeing is not only an image but him.
12. A. Illusion.
13. B. It occurs in inner subjective space. Hallucinations occur in outer and objective space; pseudohallucinations occur in inner and subjective space.
14. A. Halluicnations are perceived as 'real' by patients. Patients are not able to differentiate between real perception and hallucinations.
15. None > B.
    All the statements are correct. However, if one has to chose, the best answer would be B (sensory organs are not involved) as rest three options form the criterion of hallucinations.
16. C. Pseudohallucinations are not under the voluntary control of patient
17. B. Temporal lobe. The lesions of temporal lobe can cause all types of hallucinations and formed visual hallucinations (elaborate visual hallucinations) should raise a strong doubt of an organic cause, specifically a temporal lobe pathology.
18. D. Prominent visual hallucinations. The presence of prominent visual hallucinations is a strong pointer towards an organic cause (i.e. a disturbance of brain parenchyma such as tumors).
19. D. Delusion is not a disorder of perception, it is a disorder of thought.
20. A. Hypnagogic hallucinations. These occur while "going" to sleep. Jactatio capitis nocturna, or rhythmic movement disorder is a neurological disorder characterized by involuntary movements, usually of head and neck, before and during the sleep.
21. D. Anxiety.
22. A, B, C, E.
    Olfactory hallucinations can be seen in temporal lobe epilepsy, medial temporal sclerosis (which is a common cause of epilepsy). Though rare, olfactory hallucinations can also be present in schizophrenia and Alzheimer's disease.
23. A, D, E.
    Visual hallucinations are the most common type of hallucinations in delirium. Temporal lobe epilepsy can present with all types of hallucinations including visual hallucinations. In hebephrenic schizophrenia, the primary symptom is disorganized behavior and formal though disorders however hallucinations can also be seen.
24. D. Synesthesia.

Thought

25. C. Thought.
26. E. Loosening of association is logically connected thoughts with loss of goal. In loosening of association, the connections between the thought is lost. The rest of the statements are true. Verbigeration is a senseless repetition of one or several sentences or phrases. For example, a patient continued to repeat the following sentences for hours "Life is great. The lord is great. Summer will come soon". Its an example of verbigeration. Vorbeireden or vorbeigehen is seen in Ganser's syndrome (described in later chapters) and is another name for approximate answers in which patient reaches close to the right answer, but never gives the right answer.
27. A. Persistent and inappropriate repetition of the same thoughts.
28. A. Formal thought disorders are characteristic abnormalities in schizophrenia. In schizophrenia, the abnormalities of affect, perception, motor system as well as thought are present, however the characteristic abnormality in schizophrenia is that of thought, and more specifically the form of thought (known as formal thought disorder).
29. B. The patient is giving unnecessary information but finally is able to tell the answer. Hence, it is an example circumstantiality.
30. C. Thought block.
31. D. All of the above. Prolixity is a milder form of "flight of ideas". As mentioned in the text, flight of ideas can be

considered as both a disorder of stream of thought and form of thought.

32. A. Formal thought disorder is seen only in schizophrenia and not in depression. Rest all options can be present in either of the illnesses.
33. C. Delusion is a disorder of content of thought.
34. D. Superstition. There are many beliefs which are false and are shared by whole communities e.g. black magic, witches, etc. These beliefs are considered as superstitions. In comparison, delusions are not shared by members of the same sociocultural background. For example, if a villager starts claiming that he is lord Hanuman, no one in his village will share his belief.
35. A. Delusion of persecution.
36. D. Conversion disorder. Conversion disorder is a neurotic disorder (described in later chapters). Delusion is not a feature of conversion disorder.
37. None > A.
    Delusion can be seen in schizophrenia, mania, depression as well as OCD. However the best answer here would be OCD, as delusions are rarely seen in OCD.
38. A, B, C, D.
    Delusions can be seen in all of these disorders. Melancholic depression is usually seen in elderlies.
39. B, C.
    Delusion of grandiosity can be seen in paranoid schizophrenia and schizoaffective disorders. Delusion of grandiosity can be seen in mania but not in hypomania. Hypomania can never present with delusions or hallucinations.
40. A. Schizophrenia. Erotomania (Delusion of Love) is usually seen in schizophrenia and delusional disorder.
41. D. Nihilistic delusion
42. B, C, D.
    Nihilistic delusions can be seen in paranoid schizophrenia, Cotard's syndrome and de-pression.
43. A. Delusion of persecution.
44. B. Delusion of grandeur and persecution
45. B. Passivity. This question is controversial. 'Passivity' experiences are those in which patient experiences that his thoughts, emotions, actions or sensations are controlled/influenced by others. Passivity of thought is described as thought insertion, withdrawal and broadcast. Here the description that "brain is being controlled by radio waves by neighbor" is indicative of 'passivity'. In the question the history for delusion of persecution (i.e. police is following) is also present. Given that passivity experiences are more important diagnostically, a better answer would be passivity.
46. D. Clarity. Healthy thinking has three characteristics (1) Continuity (2) Organization and (3) Constancy.
47. B. Out of the given options, belief that brain is being controlled by a microchip is both scientifically impossible and ununderstandable. Hence, it's a bizzare delusion.
48. C. This question is slightly controversial. Option A and B are of course true. Also remember that obsessions can be seen in schizophrenia. Strictly speaking, Obsessions are disorders of "possession" of thought and not "content" of thought, although some books wrongly tend to club obsessions as a part of content of thought. This question is from the topic of "psychopatholgy" for which the standard book is Fish's clinical psychopathology, which clearly says that "obsessions are disturbances of 'possession' of thought."

Higher Mental Functions

49. A. Insight.
50. A. Working memory.
51. A. Immediate memory is usually tested by digit repetition test (digit span test). Usually digit repetition forward is used however digit repetition backward (here if examiner says 2..5..9, patient has to respond by saying 9..5..2) is also used by some examiners, though it's not the preferred technique. (Reference Strub and Black's The Mental status examination in neurology)
52. B Emotional insight.
53. A, B.
    Only first two options are psychotic illnesses in which insight is impaired.
54. B. Test Judgment.

AIIMS New Pattern Answer

55. C.

2 Schizophrenia Spectrum or Other Primary Psychotic Disorders

Schizophrenia is the prototype of psychotic disorders. It is one of the most common serious mental disorders.

HISTORY

Emil Kraepelin

Kraepelin classified psychotic illnesses into two clinical types: **Dementia Praecox**^Q and **Manic Depressive Illness**^Q. The basis of this classification was the course of illness and the cognitive decline, as the illness progressed.

According to Kraepelin, dementia praecox was characterized by a **chronic and deteriorating course** along with a **gradual decline of cognitive functions** (i.e. gradual decline of memory, attention and goal directed behavior).

	Dementia Praecox	Manic Depressive Illness (manic depressive psychosis)
Course	Chronic and deteriorating	Episodic
Cognitive decline	Gradual and progressive	None

The term "dementia" was used to indicate gradual decline in cognitive functions and the term "praecox" was added since the onset of illness was in young age (praecox means early onset).

In contrast manic depressive illness was characterized by **distinct**^Q **episodes of illness alternating with period of normal functioning**. Also, there was **no cognitive decline**.

Eugene Bleuler

Bleuler **coined** the term **"schizophrenia"**^Q, and changed the name of 'dementia praecox' to 'schizophrenia'. Bleuler proposed that diagnosis of schizophrenia should be based on the presence of characteristic symptoms. He proposed four symptoms, which he called as **fundamental (or primary) symptoms of schizophrenia**. These symptoms are also known as 4 **A's of Bleuler**^Q. They include:

A. ***Autistic thinking and behavior (Autism)***^Q: Excessive fantasy thinking which is irrational and withdrawn behavior.
B. ***Ambivalence***: Marked inability to take a decision.
C. ***Affect disturbances***: Disturbances of emotions such as inappropriate affect.
D. ***Association disturbances***: Disturbances of association of thoughts such as formal thought disorders.

Kurt Schneider

Schneider described a group of symptoms, popularly known as **Schneiderian First Rank Symptoms (SFRS)**^Q which were frequently seen in patients with schizophrenia and were characteristic of the illness. It must be however remembered that these symptoms can also be present in other illnesses and hence are not specific or pathognomonic of schizophrenia. There are 11 Schneiderian First Rank Symptoms and include:

A. ***Three thought phenomenon***: In the three thought phenomenon (or thought alienation phenomenon), the patient experiences that 'someone is tampering with his mind and thoughts.' The thought alienation includes the following:
   - **Thought insertion** (patient reports that someone is putting thoughts in his mind)
   - **Thought withdrawal** (patient experiences that thoughts are being taken out of his mind)
   - **Thought broadcast** (patient experiences that thoughts are leaving his mind and that others are able to access his thoughts, e.g. a patient said that "everybody understands my thoughts, though I never say anything)".

B. ***Three made phenomenon***: Here the patient experiences that his emotions, actions and drives are being influenced by others. It includes the following:
   - ***Made volition***: The patient experiences that his actions are being controlled by an external agency and not by himself. For example, a patient would repeatedly put his hand in the ceiling fan, and on

asking the reason reported, "I don't want to do it myself but I am being controlled by aliens who control my actions, I am a robot for them and they have my remote control".

- *Made affect*: The patient experiences that someone is changing his affect (emotions). For example, a patient reported "at times I start laughing loudly and at times I cry. The neighbors control my emotions, they can change it whenever they want to. I feel helpless".
- *Made impulses*: The patient experiences that someone is putting certain "drives" in his mind. For example, a patient suddenly threw his coffee mug onto a nurse. On asking about it he reported "a sudden impulse came over me, this impulse was sent by CBI officers who wanted me to throw the mug. I tried to resist the impulse, but could not control it".

C. **Three auditory hallucinations**: *Three specific types of auditory hallucinations are included in SFRS:*

- *Voices arguing or discussing*: The patient reports hearing of two or more 'voices' (auditory hallucinations) which argue or discuss about the patient. The patient is usually referred to in third person (hence also called **third person auditory hallucinations**[Q]). For example, the first voice would say "he is a strange man, he doesn't have any good qualities". The second voice would respond "yes, also look how fat he has become". In this example, the patient is hearing two voices and the voices are using the word "he" to refer to the patient, hence patient is being referred to in third person.
- *Voices commenting on patient's action*: The patient hears voices which give a running commentary on the patient's activities. For example, a patient who was working in the kitchen heard the following voice "she has peeled the potato and now she is about to switch on the gas. Now, she has started to wash the potatoes". The voice usually refers to the patient in the third person, hence this can again be an example of third person auditory hallucinations.
- *Audible thoughts*: Here the patient hears a voice, which would say aloud whatever patient would think. For example, a patient had a thought that "I will have dinner at a restaurant tonight". Immediately he heard a voice of a middle-aged women who said "I will have dinner at a restaurant tonight".
  The German word "**Gedankenlautwerden**" or the French word "**echo de pensees**" are occasionally used to describe these audible thoughts.

D. **Somatic passivity**: In somatic passivity, patient experiences certain somatic hallucinations (e.g. tactile hallucinations) which he believes are being imposed by some external agent. For example, a patient reported that he feels intense burning sensation inside his right knee and claimed that it is because of UV rays sent by FBI agents from New York".

E. **Delusional perception**: In Delusional perception, a delusion is attached to a normal perception. For example, a patient with schizophrenia looked at the ceiling fan and immediately understood that "all the people in the city consider him a homosexual". In this example, there was a normal perception in the first step (i.e. the patient saw a ceiling fan) and in the second step a delusion was attached to this normal perception (i.e. the delusion that everybody in city considers patient a homosexual). Delusional perception is a type of "**primary delusion**"[Q].

Primary and Secondary Delusions

- *Primary delusions*: These delusions arise as a direct result of morbid psychological process, caused by the underlying disorder
- *Secondary delusions*: These develop secondarily to some other psychopathological phenomenon. For example, a patient who had continuous auditory hallucinations and heard a voice which said "you will be killed", started believing that "somebody wants to harm me". Now, this "delusion of persecution" which developed is a secondary delusion as it developed secondarily to the auditory hallucinations.

EPIDEMIOLOGY

1. Lifetime prevalence - **1%**
2. Point prevalence - **0.5–1%**
3. Incidence rate - **0.15–0.25 per thousand**.
4. *Prevalence in specific population*: Schizophrenia has **high heritability**[Q] and the prevalence in relatives of patients is higher. Table 1 mentions the rates for specific population groups.

Table 1: Prevalence of Schizophrenia in specific populations.
• General: 1%
• Non twin sibling of a schizophrenia patient: 8%
• Dizygotic twin of a schizophrenic patient: 12%
• Monozygotic twin of a schizophrenic patient: 47%
• Child with one parent with schizophrenia: 12%
• Child with both parents with schizophrenia: 40%

5. *Age of onset*: The usual age of onset of schizophrenia is **adolescence**^{Q} **and young adulthood**. When the onset occurs after age of **45 years**, the disorder is called as **late-onset schizophrenia**^{Q}.
6. *Sex ratio*: It is equally prevalent in men and women, however the onset is earlier in men.
7. Schizophrenia is more prevalent in lower socioeconomic status.
8. *Body type*: It was earlier believed that different body types were related to different personalities and also had different vulnerability to some disorders. Three types of body types were described:
   a. **Asthenic (thin and weak)**,
   b. **Athletic (muscular)** and
   c. **Pyknic (short and fat)**.

   The **asthenic**^{Q} and to a lesser extent athletic persons were believed to be predisposed to development of **schizophrenia** whereas the **pyknic** were believed to be predisposed to development of manic depressive illness (**bipolar disorder**).

ETIOLOGY AND PATHOGENESIS

A. *Genetic factors*:
   - Schizophrenia has a genetic contribution as reflected by higher monozygotic concordance rate than dizygotic concordance rate. Several genes appear to make a contribution to schizophrenia and nine linkage sites have been identified: 1q, 5q, 6p, 6q, 8p, 10p, 13q, 15q and 22q. Deletions at chromosome 22q11.2 (22q11 deletion syndrome, velocardiofacial syndrome, **DiGeorge syndrome**^{Q}) have been associated with development of schizophrenia in around 30% cases.
   - Several candidate genes contributing to schizophrenia have been identified, and they include α 7 nicotinic receptor, DISC 1 (Disrupted in schizophrenia), COMT (catechol-o-methyl transferase), NRG 1 (Neuregulin 1), GRM3 (Glutamate receptor metabotropic), RGS4 (Regulator of G protein signaling) and DAOA (or G72) (DAmino acid oxidase activator).
   - There is increased risk of development of schizophrenia in family members of patients with schizophrenia. Also, family members of patients with bipolar disorders too have a slightly increased risk of development of schizophrenia^Q.

B. *Biochemical factors*:
   - **Dopamine hypothesis**: This hypothesis proposes that **excess** of **dopaminergic activity**^{Q} is responsible for schizophrenia.
   - **Serotonin**: Currently, along with dopamine, an excess of serotonin is also considered to be responsible for development of schizophrenia.
   - Other neurotransmitters like GABA, glutamate, norepinephrine, acetylcholine, nicotine have also been implicated in pathogenesis of schizophrenia.

C. *Neuropathological factors*: The neuropathology of schizophrenia is still not clear. Abnormalities have been found in various structures, such as:
   - **Cerebral ventricles**: Reduction in cortical gray matter volume and enlargement of lateral and third ventricles has been consistently observed.
   - **Limbic system**: Abnormalities in limbic system components such as hippocampus (smaller in size and functionally abnormal), amygdala (smaller size) and parahippocampal gyrus (smaller size) have been observed.
   - **Prefrontal cortex**: Anatomical abnormalities have been found.
   - **Thalamus**: Neuronal loss especially in medial dorsal nucleus of thalamus.
   - **Basal ganglia and cerebellum**: Abnormalities have been reported but findings are not consistent.

D. *Environmental factors*: Apart from genetic factors, the following environmental factors have also been associated with development of schizophrenia.
   - **Obstetric complications and abnormalities in development**: Patients with schizophrenia are more likely to have history of obstetric complications in comparison to general population. Similarly they *more* often have abnormal development such as delayed milestones, poor motor coordination, etc.
   - **Stressful life events**: Early childhood trauma (including sexual abuse) is a risk factor. Furthermore, studies have shown an excess of stressful life events in few weeks prior to onset of schizophrenia.
   - **Season of birth and maternal exposure to infection**: Studies have shown that people who are born in **winters**^{Q} and early spring are more likely to develop schizophrenia. Also prenatal exposure to influenza virus and prenatal malnutrition also increase the risk.
   - **Advanced paternal age**: Advanced paternal age has been found to be strongly associated with the risk of development of schizophrenia.
   - **Immigration**: Migrants have higher chances of developing schizophrenia than natives. The risk is especially higher for the second generation, who are born in the new homeland (the country of migration).

- **Drug abuse**: Studies have shown that cannabis use increases the risk of development of schizophrenia.
- **Urban birth and upbringing**: Birth and upbringing in urban areas have been associated with increase in risk for schizophrenia, in comparison to rural settings.

SYMPTOMS

The symptoms of schizophrenia can be divided into various symptom complexes, described as follows:

A. *Positive symptoms (or psychotic symptoms)*: The two positive symptoms include **delusions** and **hallucinations**.

They respond **well to medications** and the presence of positive symptoms is **a good prognostic factor**[Q] in schizophrenia.

Delusions: The most common delusion in schizophrenia is **delusion of persecution**[Q].
- *Hallucinations*: The most common hallucinations in schizophrenia are **auditory hallucinations**[Q]. Visual hallucinations are the second most common, however the presence of visual hallucination should always raise the suspicion of an organic mental disorder.
- The positive symptoms of schizophrenia are due to **dopamine excess** in **mesolimbic tract**[Q] (neural pathway from ventral segmental area to nucleus accumbens)[Q].

B. *Negative symptoms*: Negative symptoms represent "loss of normal functions" in patients with schizophrenia. These symptoms **respond poorly to medications** and their presence is **a bad prognostic factor**[Q] in schizophrenia. Following are the negative symptoms:
- *Avolition*: Loss of will or drive to indulge in goal directed activities (such as grooming and hygiene, educational and occupational activities).
- *Apathy*: Loss of concern for an idea or task or results. For example, a student who had developed schizophrenia failed in exams. However, he appeared unconcerned with his results.
- *Anhedonia*: Loss of ability to derive pleasure from activities or relationships.
- *Asociality*: Indifference to social relationships and decrease in the drive to socialize.
- *Affective flattening (or blunting*[Q]*)*: Inability of patient to understand emotions of others and inability to express own emotions.
- *Alogia*: Decrease in verbal communication. The negative symptoms are due to decreased dopamine activity in **mesocortical pathway** (neural pathway from ventral segmental area to prefrontal cortex).

C. *Disorganization symptoms*: This symptom complex includes the following symptoms:
- *Formal thought disorder*: These are the disturbances in the form of thought characterized by loss of organization of thought.
- *Disorganized behavior*: It is the odd and **inappropriate behavior** which may break the social norms. For example, a hospitalized schizophrenic patient would masturbate in front of the nursing staff, another patient of schizophrenia would wear sweaters and coats in hot summer season.
- *Inappropriate affect*: Affect which is not in sync with the social situation.

D. *Motor symptoms (catatonic symptoms or symptoms of conation)*: The term "**catatonia**[Q]" was given by **Karl Kahlbaum**[Q] who described these motor symptoms for the first time. These symptoms are sometimes described along with disorganization symptoms. For more clarity, they have been described separately here. These include:
- *Stupor*[Q]: **Extreme hypoactivity** or **immobility (akinesis)** and minimal responsiveness to stimuli.
- *Excitement*: Extreme hyperactivity which is usually non goal directed (i.e. the patient is very active but does not do any meaningful work).
- *Posturing*: Spontaneous maintenance of posture for long periods of time.
- *Waxy flexibility*: When examiner makes a passive movement on patient, there is a feeling of plastic resistance which resembles bending of a soft wax candle.
- *Catalepsy*: When examiner makes a passive movement (e.g. say abduction at shoulder joint) on the patient, no resistance is experienced. But as the examiner stops the movement, whatever position the patient had reached, that position is maintained (e.g. say the examiner had taken the shoulder to 45 degree abduction, and after that he stops, now 45 degree abduction position at the shoulder joint will be maintained by the patient).
- *Automatic obedience*: Excessive cooperation with examiner's commands despite unpleasant consequences. For example, a patient kept on protruding his tongue in response to examiner's commands, despite the fact that his tongue would be pricked by a pin every time he protruded it.
- *Echolalia*: Mimicking of **examiner's speech**.
- *Echopraxia*: Mimicking of **examiner's movements**.

- *Negativism*: Patient refuses to accept examiner's instructions or any attempts to move him.
- *Grimacing*^Q: **Maintenance of odd facial expressions**.
- *Stereotypy*^Q: Spontaneous repetition of **odd, purposeless movements**. For example, making strange movements of fingers repeatedly^Q.
- *Gegenhalten*: Resistance to passive movement, which is directly proportional to the strength of force applied.
- *Mannerisms*: Spontaneous repetition of **odd, purposeful movements**. For example, repeatedly saluting the passerby.
- *Perseveration*: It is an induced movement which is senselessly repeated. For example, a patient takes his tongue out and in, when asked however then keeps on repeating the out and in movement, even when he is no longer asked. It must be noted that perseveration occurs in response to an instruction, whereas stereotypy and mannerisms are spontaneous. Perseveration is also a sign of brain damage (**organic brain disorders**)^Q.

  When perseveration, affects speech, the patient may keep on repeating the same word or phrase. Logoclonia and palilalia are special forms of perseveration.

  Logoclonia: In logoclonia, the last syllable of last word is repeated. E.g. A patient may say 'tomorrow is Monday-ay-ay-ay-ay'. Here, the last syllable 'ay' is being repeated again and again.

  Palilalia: In palilalia, the patient repeats the perseverated word with increasing frequency.
- *Ambitendency*: Inability to decide the desired motor movement. For example, when offered a hand for handshake, patient may repeatedly bring his hand forward and backward as he is not able to decide whether he wants to shake the hand or not. It is **ambivalence in motor movements**^Q.

E. *Violence, homicide and suicide*: Violent behavior (excluding homicide) may be seen commonly in untreated patients with schizophrenia although schizophrenia patients are much more commonly the victims of violence rather than being the perpetrators. Also contrary to the common belief, the rate of homicide by patients with schizophrenia is no more than a member of general population. Suicide is the most common cause of premature death in patients with schizophrenia^Q. Traditionally the suicide rate in schizophrenia was put at **10%**. However, according to newer studies and DSM5, the suicide rate is around 5 to 6% (around 20% patients attempt suicide). The risk factors for suicide in a patient with schizophrenia include:

a. The most important factor associated with suicide is presence of a major depressive episode, feeling of helplessness
b. Also periods of increased symptoms^Q (especially presence of delusion of persecution, command hallucinations in which the hallucinatory voices give certain commands to the patient) are associated with increased risk.
c. At times, patients with better prognosis (such as lesser negative symptoms, absence of affect disturbances) have a paradoxically higher suicide risk. This may be because these patients are better able to understand the devastating effects of schizophrenia on their health and may become hopeless about future.
d. It has been found that there is increased risk of suicide early in course of illness, immediately after admission and also immediately after discharge.
e. Young males with comorbid substance use, and being unemployed.

DIAGNOSIS

According to DSM5, two or more of the following symptoms should be present for the duration of 1 month period and at least one of these must be either (1), (2) or (3).
1. Delusions
2. Hallucinations
3. Disorganized speech (or formal thought disorder)
4. Disorganized or catatonic behavior
5. Negative symptoms.

The total duration of illness should be at least 6 months, and the 6 months period must include at least one month of above mentioned symptoms.

The ICD-11 also uses similar criterion for diagnosis of schizophrenia however the total duration of symptoms should be more than **one month** unlike DSM5 which requires a total duration more than **six months**.

 DSM-5 Update

In DSM-4, only one of the above symptoms was required if the delusions were bizarre or hallucinations were one of Schneiderian first rank symptoms (either voices discussing about the patient or voices giving a running commentary). However in DSM-5, this special attribution to bizarre delusions and schneiderian auditory hallucinations has been removed.

TYPES

According to ICD-10, the following are types of schizophrenia:

A. *Paranoid schizophrenia*: This type is dominated by hallucinations and delusions. This is the **most common type**^{Q} of schizophrenia. It has a **late onset** and a **good prognosis**^{Q}. The **personality** is **usually preserved** (the person is able to maintain daily activities and social interaction is normal).

B. *Catatonic schizophrenia*: This type is dominated by catatonic (motor) symptoms. It has the **best prognosis**^{Q} of all types. The first line treatment for catatonic schizophrenia includes **intravenous lorazepam** and **electroconvulsive therapy**.

C. *Hebephrenic (disorganized) schizophrenia*: This type is dominated by prominent disorganization symptoms and negative symptoms. It has an **early onset** and **bad prognosis**^{Q}. There is **severe deterioration of personality** (patient is not able to maintain hygiene, social interaction is inappropriate, odd behaviors are present).

D. *Undifferentiated schizophrenia*: The schizophrenia not conforming to any of the above subtypes or exhibiting features of more than one of them.

E. *Residual schizophrenia*: Residual schizophrenia is characterized by progression from an early stage (with prominent delusions and hallucinations) to a later stage where the delusions and hallucinations have become minimal and mostly negative symptoms are present.

F. *Simple schizophrenia*: There are prominent negative symptoms without any history of positive symptoms like delusion and hallucinations. It has the **worst prognosis**.

G. *Postschizophrenic depression*: A depressive episode which develops after the resolution of schizophrenic symptoms. This disorder is associated with an **increased risk of suicide**.

> **DSM-5 & ICD-11 Update**
>
> Both DSM-IV and ICD-10, divided schizophrenia into types (e.g. paranoid, catatonic, etc.) on the basis of symptoms. DSM-5 and ICD-11 have removed these symptoms based subtypes. The types of schizophrenia that have been described in ICD-11 are according to the course of illness and include:
> a. *Schizophrenia, first episode*: If patient meets diagnostic criterion of schizophrenia and there have been no past episodes
> b. *Schizophrenia, multiple episodes*: If patient meets diagnostic criterion of schizophrenia, and there has been at least one episode in the past. Between the last and current episode, there was significant remission of symptoms
> c. *Schizophrenia, continuous*: If patient has been fulfilling the diagnostic criterions of schizophrenia for almost the entire duration of illness (duration should be more than one year)

> **ICD-11 Update**
>
> In ICD-11, Catatonia has been made a separate diagnostic category. It has been further divided into following groups:
> a. Catatonia associated with another mental disorder (e.g. catatonia associated with schizophrenia, mood disorders or autism spectrum disorder)
> b. Catatonia induced by use of psychoactive substances (drugs of abuse) and medications

Other Classifications

Apart from ICD10 and DSM5, various other classifications have been proposed.

A. TJ Crow divided schizophrenia into two subtypes, namely Type I and Type II schizophrenia:
   - *Type I*: Mostly positive symptoms with normal ventricles, good response **to medications** and **better prognosis**.

   > Substances which can cause schizophrenia like symptoms: Amphetamines, cocaine, phencyclidine and other hallucinogens, cannabis.

   - *Type II*: Mostly **negative symptoms** with **dilated ventricles**, **poor response** to medications and **poor prognosis**.

B. *Pfropf-schizophrenia*: Schizophrenia in a patient with mental retardation.

C. *Van Gogh syndrome:* Self-mutilation (injuring self) occurring in schizophrenia has also been called as **Van Gogh syndrome**.

TREATMENT

Antipsychotics (also known as neuroleptics) are the main stay of treatment for psychotic disorders like schizophrenia, schizoaffective disorders, delusional disorders and others. Antipsychotics have been divided into two classes:

(1) Typical antipsychotics and (2) Atypical antipsychotics

1. *Typical antipsychotics or first generation antipsychotics or dopamine receptor antagonists (DRAs)*: These drugs mainly act through dopamine, **D2 receptor antagonism**. They were the first antipsychotics that were used in the clinical practice. They are **effective** against **positive symptoms** but have **minimal effect** on **negative symptoms**. The therapeutic effect of improvement in psychotic symptoms is mediated by D2 receptor antagonism in mesolimbic tract. The typical antipsychotics can further be classified according to their chemical groups, as described here:

- *Phenothiazines*: Chlorpromazine, thioridazine, trifluoperazine, prochlorperazine, triflupromazine, fluphenazine, perphenazine

- ***Thioxanthenes***: Thiothixene, flupenthixol
- ***Butyrophenones***: Haloperidol, droperidol, penfluridol
- ***Miscellaneous***: Pimozide, loxapine, molindone.

The typical antipsychotics can further be classified as **low potency (like chlorpromazine, thioridazine)** and **high potency (like haloperidol and fluphenazine)**. Apart from differing in potency, the low potency and high potency antipsychotics also differ in their side effects profile. The common side effects of typical antipsychotics are as follows:

A. *Movement disorders*: The antipsychotics can cause various movement disorders, which collectively are often referred as **extrapyramidal symptoms** (or **extrapyramidal side effects**). These side effects are caused by blockade of dopamine receptors in **nigrostriatal tract** (neural pathway from substantia nigra to striatum). The movement disorders are **more commonly** seen with typical antipsychotics in comparison to atypical antipsychotics and amongst typical antipsychotics, high potency typical antipsychotics are **more likely to** cause this side effect. The movement disorders can be of the following types:

- *Acute dystonia*: It is the **earliest side effect**^{Q} of antipsychotics and can be seen within minutes of receiving an injectable antipsychotic (also with oral antipsychotic). It is characterized by **sudden contraction** of a muscle group and can result in symptoms like **torticollis**^{Q}, trismus (contraction of jaw muscles),^{Q} **deviation of eye balls** (oculogyric crisis due to contraction of extraocular muscles), laryngospasm, etc. The management includes immediate administration of parenteral **anticholinergics**^{Q} like benztropine, promethazine or **diphenhydramine**^{Q}. To prevent acute dystonia, prophylactic use of oral anticholinergics is suggested while prescribing typical antipsychotics.

- *Acute akathisia*: It is the **commonest side** effect of antipsychotics and is characterized by an **inner sense of restlessness** along with **objective, observable movements** such as **fidgeting**^{Q} of legs, **pacing around, inability to sit** or **stand** in one place for a long time. The treatment options include β **blockers**^{Q} such as propranolol (**drug of choice**), **anticholinergics** and **benzodiazepines**. The antipsychotic can also be changed to a second generation or low potency first generation antipsychotics, which have lesser incidence of akathisia.

- *Drug induced parkinsonism*: It is characterized by the triad of rigidity, bradykinesia and resting tremors. The treatment options include use of anticholinergics or change of antipsychotics to second generation or low potency first generation antipsychotics. The dose reduction can also be tried. Often, use of prophylactic anticholinergics prevents the development of drug induced parkinsonism.

- *Tardive dyskinesia*: The term "tardive" refers to features which develop after prolonged exposure. Tardive dyskinesia develops after long-term treatment with antipsychotics and can present as involuntary movements of the tongue (e.g. twisting, protrusion), jaw (e.g. chewing), lips (e.g. smacking, puckering), trunk or extremities. Patient may also have rapid, jerky movements (choreiform movements) or slow, sinusoid movements (athetoid movements). The management usually includes shifting to a second generation medication.

- *Neuroleptic malignant syndrome*: It is a fatal side effect of antipsychotic use. It is characterized by **muscle rigidity**, **elevated temperature (greater than 38°C)**, and **increased CPK (creatine phosphokinase) levels**. The other symptoms include diaphoresis, tremors, confusion, autonomic disturbances, liver enzyme elevation and **leukocytosis**. The pathophysiology involves D2 antagonism at various levels. The D2 receptors blockade in corpus striatum causes muscle contraction and rigidity that initiates heat generation, whereas blockade of dopamine receptors in hypothalamus interferes with heat regulation. The autonomic disturbances are caused by dopamine blockade of spinal neurons. The increased CPK indicates muscle injury. The early recognition of symptoms and prompt withdrawal of antipsychotics is of paramount importance, otherwise the continuing muscle damage can cause **myoglobinuria** and **renal failure**. The treatment includes skeletal muscle relaxants like **dantrolene**^{Q}, dopamine agonists such as amantadine and bromocriptine are also useful. Supportive measures including adequate hydration are also important in the management. When drug treatment with antipsychotics is restarted, second generation antipsychotics should be used.

B. *Endocrine side effects*: The blockage of dopamine receptors in **tuberoinfundibular tract** results in **hyperprolactinemia** (remember dopamine inhibits prolactin secretion and hence dopamine blockade causes hyperprolactinemia) and can cause galactorrhea, menstrual disturbances in females and impotence in males.

C. Sedation, orthostatic hypotension and anticholinergic side effects are usually see with low potency typical antipsychotics.

2. *Atypical antipsychotics or second generation antipsychotics or serotonin dopamine antagonists*: These drugs act through **antagonism** of **5-HT2 receptors** as well of **D2 receptors**. These drugs have a higher ratio of 5 HT2 to D2 blockade, in contrast the typical antipsychotics primarily act on D2 receptors. Due to lesser D2 blockade, atypical antipsychotics have lesser risk of causing extrapyramidal side effects as well as hyperprolactinemia. Atypical antipsychotics are effective in treatment of **both** positive and negative symptoms. The following drugs are classified as atypical antipsychotics:

- Clozapine
- Olanzapine
- Risperidone
- Paliperidone
- Iloperidone
- Quetiapine
- Ziprasidone
- Aripiprazole
- Sertindole
- Zotepine
- Lurasidone
- Asenapine
- Amisulpride
- Brexpiprazole
- Cariprazine
- Pimavanserin

Newer Antipsychotics

Brexpiprazole: It is an atypical antipsychotic that acts as a partial agonist at D2 and 5HT1A receptors, and an antagonist at 5HT2A receptor.
Cariprazine: It is an atypical antipsychotics that acts as a partial agonist at D2, D3 and 5HT1A receptors and an antagonist at 5HT2A receptor. However, unlike aripiprazole and brexpiprazole, cariprazine exhibits higher affinity for the D3 versus the D2 receptor.
Pimavanserin: It is the first FDA approved drug for treatment of delusions and hallucinations in Parkinson's disease associated psychosis. Pimavanserin has a combination of inverse agonist and antagonist activity at 5HT2A receptors (and to a lesser extent 5HT2C receptors). It does not bind to D2 receptors. It can increase QT interval.

The side effect profile of atypical antipsychotics is as follows:

A. *Movement disorders*: Atypical antipsychotics can cause all kind of extrapyramidal side effects described earlier, however the incidence is lesser in comparison to the typical antipsychotics.

B. *Endocrine side effects*: The incidence of hyperprolactinemia is also lesser with atypical antipsychotics (except **risperidone**^{Q} and amisulpride which have a higher incidence).

C. Weight gain and increased risk of dyslipidemia, diabetes and cardiovascular disease is more commonly seen with atypical antipsychotics in comparison to typical antipsychotics.

D. Other side effects include sedation, **QTc prolongation (especially with ziprasidone)** and seizures.

Clozapine

It was the first atypical antipsychotic to be synthesized. Clozapine is the drug of choice in treatment resistance schizophrenia, **TRS**^{Q} (TRS is defined as a lack of response to two different antipsychotic given at adequate dosages for adequate duration of 4 to 6 weeks). Clozapine is a unique drug as unlike other antipsychotics, it has a relatively low affinity for D2 receptors. This low affinity for D2 receptor explains lack of extrapyramidal side effects on clozapine. Clozapine has a strong affinity for D4 receptors and also acts as an antagonist at 5 HT2A, D1, D3 and α (alpha) adrenergic receptors. The lack of extrapyramidal symptoms, makes clozapine a preferred antipsychotic in patients who are intolerant to other antipsychotics because of extrapyramidal side effects including tardive dyskinesia. Clozapine is the only antipsychotic that decreases the suicidal ideation in patients with schizophrenia who have been previously hospitalized for suicidality^Q.

Side effects: The common side effects of clozapine include sedation, syncope, hypotension, tachycardia, nausea and vomiting. Other side effects include weight gain (**clozapine causes highest** weight gain **amongst all antipsychotics**^{Q}), constipation, anticholinergic side effects. A particularly problematic side effect is **sialorrhea** or hypersalivation. Clozapine can also cause life-threatening side effects which include **agranulocytosis, seizures and myocarditis**. In view of possibility of agranulocytosis, during the first six months of clozapine treatment, WBC and neutrophil counts should be measured every week. Also, if during the therapy, WBC counts fall below 3000/mm^3 or neutrophil counts fall below 1500/mm^3, the clozapine therapy should be stopped. The agranulocytosis and myocarditis are dose independent side effects of clozapine whereas seizures are dose dependent^Q (seen only at higher dosages).

The only contraindication to clozapine use is a **WBC count of less than 3500/dL** at the time of starting clozapine, a history of agranulocytosis during clozapine treatment or use of other drug that is known to suppress the bone marrow (e.g. clozapine and carbamazepine cannot be given together as both are bone marrow suppressants).

Specific Points about Antipsychotics

A. **Long-acting injectable antipsychotics (Depot antipsychotics)**: In patients who have **poor compliance**[Q] with medications (i.e. who refuse to take medications) long-acting injectable antipsychotics can be used. The patients typically receive the **intramuscular injections** of antipsychotics once a month or once a fortnight. Long-acting injectable preparations are available for following antipsychotics:
   - Flupenthixol
   - Fluphenazine
   - Haloperidol
   - Pipotiazine
   - Zuclopenthixol
   - Risperidone
   - Olanzapine
   - Paliperidone
   - Aripiprazole

B. Thioridazine can cause irreversible **retinal pigmentation**[Q]. Thioridazine can also cause **cardiac arrhythmias**[Q] (prolongation of QT interval). It is also the drug with **least extrapyramidal side effects**[Q] amongst typical antipsychotics, overall clozapine is the antipsychotic with least extrapyramidal side effect.

C. Chlorpromazine can cause **corneal** and **lenticular deposits**[Q].

D. Penfluridol is the **longest acting antipsychotic**[Q].

E. Ziprasidone is known to cause **cardiac arrhythmias** (prolongation of QT interval).

F. Aripiprazole is a partial agonist at **D2 receptors** (all other antipsychotics are D2 antagonists).

Psychosocial Treatment[Q]: Apart from medications, psychological and social interventions have been found to be effective in treatment of schizophrenia, especially after the acute phase is treated with medications. The following psychosocial treatments can be used:

a. *Family interventions*: The family of patient is involved with focus on illness education, coping with the illness and providing emotional support to the entire family.

b. *Supported employment*: An attempt is made to provide employment to patient while giving ongoing support.

c. *Assertive community treatment*: It involves reaching out to the patient in community and providing necessary support.

d. *Skills training*: The focus is on improving skills, especially social skills of the patient.

e. *Cognitive behavioral therapy*: It involves use of cognitive behavioral therapy (explained in next chapter in detail) for management of residual symptoms (the symptoms that have not responded to medicine).

Another therapy, called **cognitive remediation therapy**[Q] (or cognitive enhancement therapy) focuses on improvement of cognitive functions (such as attention and concentration, working memory, etc.) and has shown promising results in patients with schizophrenia.

f. *Token economy*: Mostly used in inpatient settings, it involves use of tokens, which are given to patients, when they indulge in desirable behaviors (like remaining calm, taking medicines regularly, etc.). Patients can redeem the tokens to get material items or privileges.

PROGNOSIS

Good prognostic factors:
1. Acute or abrupt onset
2. **Advanced age at onset (age > 35 years)**[Q]
3. Catatonic subtype and paranoid subtype
4. Female sex
5. Prominent positive symptoms
6. Presence of **affective symptoms** (such **as depression**[Q])
7. **Family history**[Q] of mood disorder.

Bad prognostic factors:
1. Insidious onset
2. Early onset (age < 20 years)
3. Simple, disorganized, undifferentiated subtype
4. Male sex
5. Prominent negative symptoms
6. Absence of affective symptoms
7. **Family history** of schizophrenia.

OTHER PSYCHOTIC DISORDERS

A. *Acute psychotic disorders*: There are disorders which have symptoms (e.g. delusions, hallucinations and disorganization symptoms) similar to schizophrenia, however do not meet the duration criterion. These disorders have been classified separately in DSM-5 and ICD-11. These disorders frequently are preceded by a **stressor** (stressful life event), have an acute onset and often resolve completely. These disorders may also be precipitated by **fever**[Q].

In ICD-11, if the symptoms (delusions, hallucinations, disorganization) are present for less than one month, a diagnosis of **acute and transient psychotic disorder** is made.

In DSM-5, if symptoms (delusions, hallucinations, disorganization) are present for less than one month, a diagnosis **of brief psychotic disorder** is made; and if symptoms last between **1–6 months**, a diagnosis of **schizophreniform disorder** is made.

Treatment: Antipsychotics and benzodiazepines are used for the treatment of acute psychotic disorders.

B. *Schizoaffective disorder*: Schizoaffective disorder has features of both schizophrenia and mood disorders concurrently. Depending on whether manic episode or depressive episode is present along with schizophrenia symptoms, there are two subtypes:
- *Schizoaffective disorder (Bipolar type or manic type)*: With manic symptoms
- *Schizoaffective disorder (Depressive type)*: With depressive symptoms.

    Treatment: It involves combination of mood stabilizers, antipsychotics and antidepressants depending on the presentation. In schizoaffective (manic type episodes) a combination of antipsychotics and mood stabilizer is commonly used. In schizoaffective (depressive type episodes) a combination of antipsychotics, and antidepressants is often used.

C. *Delusional disorder*: These disorders are characterized by development of either a **single delusion** or a **set of related delusions**, which are usually persistent and sometimes are life long. Other psychotic symptoms like hallucinations, disorganization, negative symptoms are usually absent. If hallucinations occur they are for a very short duration, presence of frequent hallucinations goes against the diagnosis of delusional disorder. The following are the risk factors for development of delusional disorders:
   a. Advanced age
   b. Social isolation
   c. Sensory impairment or isolation (e.g. auditory or visual disturbances)
   d. Family history of delusional disorder
   e. Recent immigration
   f. Certain personality features, like excessive interpersonal sensitivity (even trivial interpersonal problems cause lot of negative emotions)

   The following are the types of delusional disorder:
   - *Persecutory type*: Delusion of persecution.
   - *Jealous type*: Delusion of infidelity.
   - *Erotomanic type*: Delusion of love.
   - *Somatic type*: Patient may have delusion that he is infested by parasites (**delusional parasitosis**), that he has misshaped body parts (delusion of dysmorphophobia) or that his body has a foul odor (**delusion of halitosis**).
   - *Grandiose type*: Delusion of grandiosity.
   - *Unspecified type*: In patients where the above-mentioned categories are not applicable. Delusion of misidentification is an example of unspecified type. Delusion of misidentification can be of many types like:

Capgras syndrome: Patient believes that a familiar person has been replaced by an impostor. For example, a patient believed that his wife has been replaced by a stranger who looks exactly like his wife.
- *Fregoli syndrome*[Q]: Patient believes that a familiar persons are can change his physical appearance and disguise as a stranger, and that he can take multiple different appearances. For example, a patient saw a beggar, and claimed that his brother is following him in the guise of the beggar.
- *Syndrome of intermetamorphosis:* Patient believes that people can undergo changes in physical and psychological identity and become a different person altogether.
- *Syndrome of subjective doubles*: Patient believes that he has many doubles who are living life of their own.

The patients of delusional disorder are usually able to **function normally in domains which are unaffected by the delusion**. For example, a patient with delusion of infidelity may incessantly doubt his wife and fight with her, however he may be perfectly normal at work place.

Treatment: Antipsychotics are the drug of choice.

D. *Shared psychotic disorders (or induced delusional disorder)*: This disorder is characterized by spread of delusions from one person to another. The individual who has the delusion (the primary case) is typically the influential member of close relationship with a more suggestible person (the secondary case) who also develops the delusion. When two people are involved, the term **"folie a deux"** is used. Occasionally more than two individuals are involved (known as **folie a trois, folie a quatre**, etc.).

E. *Attenuated psychosis syndrome*: Attenuated Psychosis Syndrome has been included in DSM-5 as a condition that needs further study before it can be included as an official diagnosis. The proposed criterion for this condition include, the following:
1. At least one of the following symptoms is present in attenuated (less severe and transient) form, with relatively intact insight,—a. delusions b. hallucinations, c. Disorganized speech. [Here attenuated means that, for example, if delusions are present patient may appear suspicious at times (transient) but not always and he may be made to question his beliefs (less severe, not fixed)].
2. Symptom(s) must have been present at least once per week for the past month.
3. Symptom(s) must have begun or worsened in the past year.
4. Symptom(s) is sufficiently distressing and disabling to the individual to warrant clinical attention.

Multiple Choice Questions

History

1. The term "Dementia praecox" was coined by: *(AI 2008)*
   A. Freud
   B. Bleuler
   C. Kraepelin
   D. Schneider

2. The term "schizophrenia" was coined by:
   (DNB NEET 2014-15)
   A. Eugen Bleuler
   B. Emil Kraepelin
   C. Hecker
   D. Kurt Schneider

3. The term "catatonia" was coined by:
   A. Kahlbaum
   B. Freud
   C. Maxwell
   D. Adler

4. Not a fundamental symptom of schizophrenia:
   (FMGE 2018, NIMHANS 2018)
   A. Autism
   B. Automatism
   C. Association disturbances
   D. Ambivalence

5. Schneiderian First Rank Symptoms are found in:
   A. Schizophrenia *(PGI Nov 2011)*
   B. Organic mental disorders
   C. Schizoaffective disorder
   D. Mood disorder
   E. Delusional disorder

6. The American mathematician who got a Noble prize for game theory and also was a known case paranoid schizophrenia? *(NIMHANS 2018)*
   A. John Nash
   B. Reinhard Selten
   C. John Harsanyi
   D. Sylvia Nasar

Epidemiology

7. Schizophrenia is associated with which of the following personalities? *(AIIMS 1997)*
   A. Athletic
   B. Pyknic
   C. Asthenic
   D. All of the above

8. True about late onset schizophrenia: *(AIIMS Nov 2010)*
   A. Onset is after 45 years
   B. Onset is between 25-30 years
   C. Prognosis is poor
   D. Olfactory hallucinations are common

9. Maximum heritability is seen in which of the following illness? *(DNB 2005, MP 2004, WB 2003, UP 2001)*
   A. Depression
   B. Mania
   C. Schizophrenia
   D. Panic disorder

Etiology and Pathogenesis

10. Neurotransmitter related to the pathology of schizophrenia are: *(PGI 1997)*
    A. Acetylcholine
    B. Dopamine
    C. Serotonin
    D. Norepinephrine

11. Which of the following is not an environmental risk factor for schizophrenia? *(NIMHANS 2014)*
    A. Cannabis use
    B. Migration
    C. Higher socioeconomic status
    D. Obstetric complications

12. Schizophrenia is a common presentation in which genetic disease? *(NIMHANS 2013)*
    A. Down's syndrome
    B. DiGeorge syndrome
    C. Klinefelter's syndrome
    D. Neurofibromatosis

Controversial Question

13. Blood sample of a 45-year-old male shows increased levels of homovanillic acid (HVA). This patient is most likely suffering from: *(AIIMS Nov 2008)*
    A. Dementia
    B. Schizophrenia
    C. Depression
    D. Parkinson's disease

14. Schizophrenia is caused by overactivity in which of the following dopaminergic systems?
    (NIMHANS 2014, DNB 2007)
    A. Nigrostriatal pathway
    B. Tuberoinfundibular pathway
    C. Mesolimbic/Mesocortical pathway
    D. None of the above

15. True about schizophrenia is all except: *(NIMHANS 2016)*
    A. Ambivalence
    B. Hypodopaminergic state
    C. Hyperdopaminergic state
    D. Autism

Symptoms and Diagnosis

16. Which of the following is a first rank symptom in schizophrenia? *(JIPMER Nov, 2018)*
    A. Delusions
    B. Thought insertion
    C. Hallucinations
    D. Word salad

17. Which of the following is not a paranoid symptom?
    A. Delusion of persecution *(NIMHANS 2017)*
    B. Delusion of reference
    C. Delusion of grandiosity
    D. Thought alienation

18. Mutism and akinesia in a person in awake state is a feature of: *(AIIMS May 2017)*
    A. Oneiroid state
    B. Stupor
    C. Twilight state
    D. Delirium

19. Schizophrenia is characterized by all of the following symptoms except: *(AI 1993)*
    A. Delusion of reference
    B. Delusion of control
    C. Waxy flexibility
    D. Altered sensorium

20. The characteristic clinical manifestation of schizophrenia is: *(PGI 1998)*
    A. Confusion
    B. Anxiety
    C. Auditory hallucinations
    D. Visual hallucinations

21. Which of the following hallucinations is pathognomonic of schizophrenia? *(AIIMS 2K, Delhi 2003)*
    A. Auditory hallucinations commanding the patient
    B. Auditory hallucinations giving running commentary
    C. Auditory hallucinations criticising the patient
    D. Auditory hallucinations talking to the patient

22. Which of the following is not a risk factor for development of schizophrenia? *(NIMHANS 2019)*
    A. Family history of bipolar disorder
    B. History of childhood sexual abuse
    C. Child born to a younger mother
    D. Winter birth

23. Hallucinations in schizophrenia are characterized by all of the following except:
    A. Hallucinations commanding and controlling action of the person
    B. Hallucinations of voices, singing songs
    C. Hallucinations are almost always continuous
    D. Hallucinations commenting on action of the person

24. Which of the following sign is not a part of catatonia? *(AIIMS May 2015)*
    A. Akathisia
    B. Ambivalence
    C. Ambitendency
    D. Akinesia

25. All of the following are features of catatonia except: *(DNB NEET 2014-15)*
    A. Automatic obedience
    B. Cataplexy
    C. Catalepsy
    D. Negativism

26. Which of the following is the surest sign of schizophrenia? *(NEET 2016)*
    A. Auditory hallucinations
    B. Delusion of persecution
    C. Thought broadcast
    D. Visual hallucinations

27. The following are features of catatonic schizophrenia, except: *(MP 2000)*
    A. Mutism
    B. Echolalia
    C. Waxy flexibility
    D. Deep tendon reflexes are increased

28. In catatonic schizophrenia, which of the following sign is not found: *(PGI Dec 2008)*
    A. Waxy flexibility
    B. Automatic obedience
    C. Somatic passivity
    D. Gegenhalten
    E. Hallucinations

29. True about schizophrenia: *(PGI 2003)*
    A. Thought broadcasting
    B. Third person hallucinations
    C. Violent behavior
    D. Elated mood
    E. Good self care

30. All of the following are true about paranoid schizophrenia except: *(MP 1997)*
    A. Most common type of schizophrenia
    B. Onset in 3rd/4th decade
    C. Delusion of grandeur is a symptom
    D. Rapid deterioration of personality

31. Defect of conation is typically seen in: *(PGI 1997, AIIMS 1996, UP 2006)*
    A. Simple schizophrenia
    B. Hebephrenic schizophrenia
    C. Catatonic schizophrenia
    D. Paranoid schizophrenia

32. Stereotypic movements are: *(NEET 2018)*
    A. Sustained posture against gravity
    B. Passive inducible movements
    C. Repetitive, spontaneous nonfunctional movements
    D. Resistance to passive movements

33. Waxy flexibility is a characteristic sign of: *(NIMHANS 2013, Orissa 2004, Jharkhand 2006)*
    A. Excitatory catatonia
    B. Stuporous catatonia
    C. Obsessive compulsive disorder
    D. All of the above

34. Early onset and bad prognosis is seen in: *(NIMHANS 2012, AIIMS 1991)*
    A. Catatonic schizophrenia
    B. Hebephrenic schizophrenia
    C. Paranoid schizophrenia
    D. Undifferentiated schizophrenia

35. Schizophrenia with late onset and best prognosis: *(NEET 2016, DNB NEET 2014-15)*
    A. Simple schizophrenia
    B. Hebephrenic schizophrenia
    C. Catatonic schizophrenia
    D. Paranoid schizophrenia

36. Good prognosis in schizophrenia is indicated by: *(PGI 1998)*
    A. Soft neurological signs
    B. Affective symptoms
    C. Emotional blunting
    D. Insidious onset

37. A 30-year-old female was diagnosed with paranoid schizophrenia. Her father wanted to know about the poor prognostic factors. Which of the following is a poor prognostic factor? *(NIMHANS 2018)*
    A. Married
    B. Female gender
    C. Insidious onset
    D. Concomitant mood disorder

38. Prognosis of schizophrenia is less favorable in the following clinical scenario: *(MCI Screening)*
    A. Occurring in women
    B. Anxiety is prominent
    C. Emotional blunting is present
    D. In presence of rapid onset of psychosis

39. Type two schizophrenia is characterized by all of the following features except: *(AIIMS Nov 2008)*
   A. Negative symptoms
   B. Poor response to treatment
   C. Disorganized behavior
   D. CT scan abnormalities

40. Van Gogh syndrome is seen in: *(PGI 2003)*
   A. Mania
   B. Depression
   C. Schizophrenia
   D. OCD

41. Which of the following is the most common cause of premature death in schizophrenia? *(AI 2011)*
   A. Homicide
   B. Suicide
   C. Toxicity of antipsychotic drugs
   D. Hospital acquired infections

42. Expressed emotionality is related to which of the following illnesses? *(MH 2010)*
   A. Depression
   B. Schizophrenia
   C. Mania
   D. Somatoform disorder

43. In which of the following stages, a patient with schizophrenia is most likely to commit suicide? *(NEET 2016)*
   A. During worsening of symptoms
   B. Immediately after discharge
   C. Both
   D. None

44. The following picture describes what sign of schizophrenia?
   A. Posturing
   B. Cataplexy
   C. Waxy flexibility
   D. Negativism

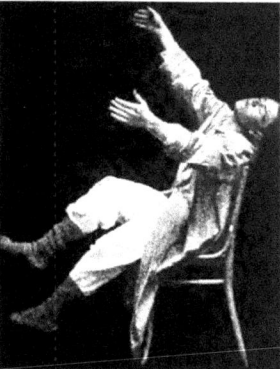

Clinical Vignettes

45. A patient of Schizophrenia was started on neuroleptics, his psychotic symptoms began to improve however he developed sadness, would talks less to others, would mostly remain on bed. This presentation could be caused by all of following except: *(AIIMS 2000)*
   A. Parkinsonism
   B. Major depression
   C. Negative symptoms are still persisting
   D. He is reacting to external stimuli

46. Kallu, a 24-year-old occasional alcoholic was brought to psychiatry OPD with a history of behavioral changes. According to family members, he has become suspicious that people are trying to conspire against him, though his father states that there is no reason for his fears. Kallu also reports of hearing voices that comment on his actions. What is the most probable diagnosis? *(AIIMS 2000)*
   A. Delirium tremens
   B. Alcohol induced psychosis
   C. Schizophrenia
   D. Delusional disorder

Controversial Question

47. A 70-year-old male, Babulal was brought to the hospital with the history of third person auditory hallucinations. He has no history of similar problems previously. What is the most likely diagnosis? *(AIIMS 2001)*
   A. Dementia
   B. Delusional disorder
   C. Schizophrenia
   D. Acute psychosis

48. A 60-year-old man is brought to a psychiatrist with a 10-year history, that he suspects his neighbors and he feels that whenever he passes by they sneeze and plan against him behind his back. He feels that his wife has been replaced by a double and calls police for help. He is quite well-groomed, alert, occasionally consumes alcohol, likely diagnosis is: *(AIIMS May 2002)*
   A. Paranoid personality disorder
   B. Paranoid schizophrenia
   C. Alcohol withdrawal
   D. Conversion disorder

49. Lallo, a 40-year-old male has recently started writing books. But the matter in his book could not be understood by anybody since it contained words which were never there in any dictionary and the theme was very disjoint. Nowadays he has become very shy and self absorbed. When he addresses people he speaks about metaphilosophical ideas. What is the likely diagnosis? *(AIIMS 2000)*
   A. Mania
   B. Schizophrenia
   C. A genius writer
   D. Delusional disorder

50. A patient is brought with 6 months history of odd behavior. There is history of a family member having disappeared some years back. He seems to be talking to himself and sometimes laughing loudly. The likely diagnosis is: *(AIIMS May 2002)*
   A. Schizophrenia
   B. Conversion disorder
   C. Major depression
   D. Delusional disorder

Controversial Question

51. A 16-year-old boy does not attend school because of the fear of being harmed by school mates. He thinks that his classmates laugh at him and talk about him. He is even scared of going out to the market. He is most likely suffering from: *(AI 2004)*
   A. Anxiety disorder
   B. Manic depressive psychosis (bipolar disorder)
   C. Adjustment reaction
   D. Schizophrenia

52. **True about schizophrenia is:** *(PGI May 2016)*
    A. Onset is most common in fourth decade
    B. Severe depression is most common association
    C. Cognitive deficit are present in the prodromal stage
    D. Shows characteristic changes on Q-EEG
    E. Psychosurgery can be done in resistant cases

53. **A patient with paranoid schizophrenia talks about 'omni micro', but he is unable to explain it in detail and reach a conclusion. He often repeats last syllable of last word of last sentence. This can be related to:** *(PGI May 2018)*
    A. Circumstantiality
    B. Neologism
    C. Perseveration
    D. Knight's move thinking
    E. Logoclonia

Treatment

54. **Depot preparations are available for:** *(PGI Nov 2010)*
    A. Haloperidol
    B. Risperidone
    C. Olanzapine
    D. Imipramine
    E. Fluphenazine

55. **A 23-year-old boy with schizophrenia is well-maintained on risperidone for the last 2 months. He has no family history of the disease. For how long will you continue treatment in this patient?** *(AIIMS Nov 2015)*
    A. 5 years
    B. 6 months
    C. 2 years
    D. 12 months

56. **A person with violent behavior and agitation was diagnosed to have schizophrenia and was started on haloperidol. Following this he developed rigidity and inability to move his eyes. Which of the following drugs should be added to his treatment intravenously for this condition?** *(AIIMS May 2015)*
    A. Promethazine
    B. Haloperidol
    C. Risperidone
    D. Diazepam

57. **Antipsychotic drug with least incidence of extrapyramidal side effects and maximum incidence of weight gain is:** *(DNB NEET 2014-15)*
    A. Pimozide
    B. Thioridazine
    C. Clozapine
    D. Chlorpromazine

58. **Not true about clozapine is:** *(AI 2012)*
    A. Should be discontinued, if WBC counts < 3000/mm^3
    B. Blood levels should be maintained < 350 ng/mL to avoid agranulocytosis
    C. Should not be used along with carbamazepine
    D. The action is more on D4 receptors than D2 receptors

59. **Which of the following is the most common side effect of clozapine?**
    A. Tachycardia
    B. Sialorrhea
    C. Sedation
    D. Constipation

60. **Which of the following is the drug of choice in treatment resistant schizophrenia?** *(NIMHANS 2016, AI 2000)*
    A. Olanzapine
    B. Clozapine
    C. Amisulpride
    D. Risperidone

61. **A patient with acute psychosis, who is on haloperidol 20 mg/day for last 2 days, has an episode characterized by tongue protrusion, oculogyric crisis, stiffness and abnormal posture of limbs and trunk without loss of consciousness for last 20 minutes before presenting to casualty. This improved within a few minutes after administration of diphenhydramine HCl. The most likely diagnosis is:** *(AIIMS 2011, May 2006)*
    A. Acute dystonia
    B. Akathisia
    C. Tardive dyskinesia
    D. Neuroleptic malignant syndrome

62. **Side effect of clozapine include:** *(PGI Nov 2017)*
    A. Seizures
    B. Sedation
    C. Dry mouth
    D. Hypothermia
    E. Constipation

63. **An elderly woman suffering from schizophrenia is on antipsychotic medication. She developed purposeless involuntary facial and limb movements, constant chewing and puffing of cheeks. Which of the following drugs is least likely to be involved in this side effect?** *(AIIMS Nov 2003)*
    A. Haloperidol
    B. Clozapine
    C. Fluphenazine
    D. Loxapine

64. **A 19-year-old boy suffering from chronic schizophrenia is put on haloperidol at the dose of 20 mg/day. A week after the initiation of medication the patient shows restlessness, fidgetiness, irritability and cannot sit still at one place. The most appropriate treatment strategy is:** *(AIIMS May 2004)*
    A. Increase in the dose of haloperidol
    B. Addition of anticholinergic drug
    C. Addition of beta blocker
    D. Adding another antipsychotic drug

65. **Incorrectly matched is:** *(NIMHANS 2019)*
    A. Haloperidol- EPS
    B. Chlorpromazine- orthostatic hypotension
    C. Clozapine-hyperprolactinemia
    D. Olanzapine- weight gain

66. **A psychotic patient on antipsychotic drugs develops torticollis within 4 days of starting therapy. What is the appropriate medication that should be added in the treatment regimen?** *(DNB NEET 2014-15)*
    A. Central anticholinergic
    B. Peripheral anticholinergic
    C. Beta-blocker
    D. Dantrolene

67. **A patient who is taking antipsychotics for 3 weeks, presents with high grade fever, raised CPK and myoglobinuria. What is the most probable diagnosis?** *(DNB NEET 2014-15)*
    A. Neuroleptic malignant syndrome
    B. Tardive dyskinesia
    C. Acute dystonia
    D. Akathisia

68. **A 31-year-old male, with mood disorder, on 30 mg of haloperidol and 100 mg of lithium, is brought to the hospital emergency room with history of acute onset of fever, excessive sweating, confusion, rigidity of limbs and decreased communication for a day. Examination reveals tachycardia and labile blood pressure and investigations

reveal increased CPK enzyme levels and leukocytosis. He is likely to have developed: *(AIIMS May 2004)*
   A. Lithium toxicity
   B. Tardive dyskinesia
   C. Neuroleptic malignant syndrome
   D. Hypertensive encephalopathy

69. A patient was on treatment with trifluoperazine for some time. He presents with complaint of hyperthermia, lethargy and sweating. Needed investigations are: *(AIIMS 2000)*
   A. CT scan brain and hemogram
   B. Hemogram, electrolyte level and creatinine
   C. ECG, chest X-ray and hemogram
   D. Hemogram, CPK and renal function test

70. Which of the following is NOT a symptom of neuroleptic malignant syndrome? *(NIMHANS 2016, DNB NEET 2014-15)*
   A. Autonomic dysregulation
   B. Hypothermia
   C. Muscle rigidity
   D. Catatonia and stupor

71. What is produced by the supersensitivity of dopamine receptors? *(DNB NEET 2014-15)*
   A. Dyskinesia
   B. Hyperphagia
   C. Hyperpathia
   D. Hypomania

72. Drug of choice for treatment of neuroleptic malignant syndrome is: *(DNB NEET 2014-15)*
   A. Dantrolene
   B. Beta blockers
   C. Central anticholinergics
   D. None of the above

73. A young patient of schizophrenia is intolerant to antipsychotic medications. Which drug is most preferred?
   A. Clozapine
   B. Olanzapine
   C. Risperidone
   D. Haloperidol

74. Antipsychotic drug causing retinal pigmentation disorder is: *(DNB NEET 2014-15)*
   A. Thioridazine
   B. Clozapine
   C. Chlorpromazine
   D. None of the above

75. Patients using which of the following drugs are at greatest risk of development of neuroleptic malignant syndrome? *(NIMHANS 2014)*
   A. Clozapine
   B. Olanzapine
   C. Ziprasidone
   D. Haloperidol

76. The antipsychotic with least incidence of extrapyramidal symptoms is: *(NIMHANS 2017)*
   A. Haloperidol
   B. Thiothixene
   C. Thioridazine
   D. Perphenazine

77. A 30-year-old patient of schizophrenia on antipsychotics presents with amenorrhea and galactorrhea. Which of the following antipsychotic should she be shifted to: *(NIMHANS 2012)*
   A. Haloperidol
   B. Olanzapine
   C. Risperidone
   D. Aripiprazole

78. Antipsychotic commonly associated with hyperprolactinemia is: *(NEET 2018)*
   A. Ziprasidone
   B. Clozapine
   C. Olanzapine
   D. Risperidone

79. In comparison to haloperidol, clozapine causes more: *(PGI May 2015)*
   A. Weight gain
   B. Agranulocytosis
   C. Sedation
   D. Severe extrapyramidal symptoms
   E. Less epileptogenic potential

80. Cognitive remediation is used for: *(AIIMS 2013)*
   A. Cognitive restructuring
   B. Memory improvement
   C. Correcting cognitive distortion
   D. Improving study habits

81. A 28-year-old patient presented with history of suspiciousness, hearing voices not heard by other, aggression, poor sleep and appetite for last 3 months. During investigations, his ECG was done and it showed QTc of 480 ms. Which of the following drugs should be avoided in this patient? *(NIMHANS 2018)*
   A. Ziprasidone
   B. Aripiprazole
   C. Clozapine
   D. Risperidone

82. Hyperprolactinemia is seen in all except: *(NIMHANS 2018)*
   A. Risperidone
   B. Metoclopramide
   C. Amisulpride
   D. Aripiprazole

83. A patient of schizophrenia was started on a new drug. Three months later she complains of weight gain and her HbA1c was 8. What is the most likely drug?
   A. Olanzapine *(NIMHANS 2018)*
   B. Amisulpride
   C. Risperidone
   D. Haloperidol

Other Psychotic Disorders

84. What is the content of most common type of persistent delusional disorder? *(DNB NEET 2014-15)*
   A. Delusion of persecution
   B. Somatic delusion
   C. Delusion of jealousy
   D. Delusion of grandeur

85. Alcoholic paranoia is associated with: *(AI 2010)*
   A. Fixed delusions
   B. Hallucinations
   C. Drowsiness
   D. Impulsivity

86. Delusion of doubles is seen in: *(AIIMS 1999)*
   A. Schizoaffective disorder
   B. Capgras syndrome
   C. Reactive psychosis
   D. Paranoid schizophrenia

87. Characteristic symptom in induced psychotic disorder is:
   A. Insomnia *(AIIMS 1992)*
   B. Profound mood disturbance
   C. Accepting delusions of other person
   D. Suicidal ideation

88. A person aged 35 years is having firm belief about infidelity involving the spouse. He never allows her to go out of home alone. He often locks his house, while going to the office. In spite of all this, he is persistently suspicious about the character of his wife. The probable diagnosis is: *(AIIMS 1999)*
    A. Schizophrenia
    B. Delusional parasitosis
    C. De Clerambault's syndrome
    D. Othello syndrome

89. Basanti, 27-year female thinks that her nose is ugly. Her idea is fixed and is not shared by anyone else. Whenever she goes out of the home, she hides her face? She visits a surgeon for plastic surgery. The appropriate next step would be: *(AI 2001)*
    A. Investigate and then operate
    B. Reassure the patient
    C. Immediate operation
    D. Refer to psychiatrist

90. A 41-year-old woman working as an executive in a company is convinced that the management has denied her promotion by preparing false reports about her competence and have forged her signature on sensitive documents so as to convict her. She files a complaint in the police station and requests for security. Despite all this she attends to her work and manages the household. What is the most likely diagnosis? *(AI 2004)*
    A. Paranoid schizophrenia
    B. Late onset psychosis
    C. Persistent delusional disorder
    D. Obsessive compulsive disorder

91. A 30-year-old unmarried woman from a low socioeconomic status family believes that a rich boy staying in her neighborhood is in deep love with her. The boy clearly denies his love towards this lady. Still the lady insists that his denial is a secret affirmation of his love towards her. She makes desperate attempts to meet the boy despite resistance from her family. She also develops sadness at times when her effort to meet the boy does not materialize. She is able to maintain her daily routine. She however, remains preoccupied with the thoughts of this boy. She is likely to be suffering from: *(AI 2004)*
    A. Delusional disorder   B. Depression
    C Mania   D. Schizophrenia

92. A 20-year-old boy complains of hearing of voices and aggressive behavior for last 2 days. He had fever before the onset of these symptoms. The family members report that he has been muttering to self and gesticulating as if he is talking to someone. There is no history of any past psychiatric illness. The likely diagnosis is: *(AIIMS Nov 2010)*
    A. Dementia   B. Acute psychosis
    C. Delirium   D. Delusional disorder

93. A 30-year-old man has become suspicious that his wife is having an affair with his boss. He thinks his friend is also involved from abroad and is providing technology support. He also thinks that people talk ill about him. His friends tried to convince him but failed to do so. The patient otherwise is normal, doesn't have any thought disorder or any other inappropriate behavior. The most likely diagnosis is: *(NIMHANS 2018, AI 2010)*
    A. Paranoid personality disorder
    B. Persistent delusional disorder
    C. Schizophrenia
    D. Obsessive compulsive disorder

94. In the image given below, what is the diagnosis of Person A? *(NEET 2016)*
    A. Capgras syndrome   B. Fregoli syndrome
    C. Ekbom syndrome   D. Othello syndrome

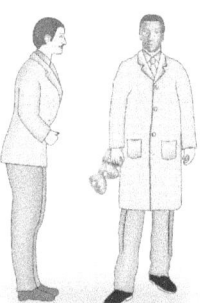

95. A patient with schizophrenia was admitted in psychiatry ward. When the nurse entered the room, he started beating the nurse and accused that actually this nurse is his real wife and accuses her of giving him wrong medication. What is the diagnosis? *(AIIMS Nov 17)*
    A. Syndrome of subjective double
    B. Othello syndrome
    C. Capgras syndrome
    D. Fregoli syndrome

96. All of the following statements about "attenuated psychosis syndrome" are true except: *(NIMHANS 2018)*
    A. Insight is absent
    B. Symptoms appeared or got aggravated in last one year
    C. No criterion for other psychotic disorder gets met
    D. Symptoms are distressing enough

AIIMS New Pattern Questions

97. Arrange the following subtypes of schizophrenia, in order of prognosis, with the best prognosis first and the worst prognosis last,
    1. Paranoid schizophrenia
    2. Catatonic schizophrenia
    3. Simple schizophrenia
    4. Disorganized schizophrenia
    A. 1-2-4-3
    B. 2-1-4-3
    C. 2-1-3-4
    D. 1-2-3-4

98. **Extended Matching Items/Questions (EMI/EMQ)**
    Theme and focus- Delusions
    Answer option list
    A. Schizophrenia
    B. Delusional disorder
    C. Acute and transient psychotic disorder

D. Schizoaffective disorder
E. Schizophreniform disorder
F. Severe depression with psychotic symptoms

Lead in question

For each of the following patients as described in the scenarios below, identify the cause from the above Answer Option List

Case 1: A 19-year-old male was brought to psychiatry emergency after he attacked one of the neighbors. At the time of presentation, he appeared agitated and aggressive. The family members revealed that 2 weeks back, he had an episode of fever, after which he started behaving abnormally. He started saying that the neighbors want to harm him and that they have fitted cameras in the house. He kept on searching for the cameras and removed all the lights from his room saying that one of the lights has camera fitted in it. He also said that the neighbors are talking obscenely with him with the help of microphones. He was not sleeping properly and today in the morning he started fighting with the neighbors and attacked them with the cricket bat. What is the diagnosis?

Case 2: A 29-year-old male presented to psychiatry outpatient department with complaints of suspiciousness towards the wife for last 7 months. The patient said that he knows that wife is having an affair with the security guard of his colony and he frequently visits her. The wife as well as the parents of patients who lived with them, denied that any such affair exists. On asking for proof, patient reported that whenever he comes home, the security guard smiles after looking at him and that wife is wearing new clothes now a days, because she wants to look pretty to the guard. What is the diagnosis?

Answers With Explanations

History

1. C. Kraepelin.
2. A. Eugen Bleuler.
3. A. Kahlbaum.
4. B. Automatisms are usually a feature of epilepsy. They are apparently meaningful behaviors, for which patient doesn't have any memory later on. They are not seen in schizophrenia.
5. A, B, C, D, E.
   Although, SFRS were described in relation to schizophrenia, however they are not specific to schizophrenia. They can be found in all the disorders mentioned in this question. However, if it was not a PGI question, and only option had to be chosen, it would be schizophrenia.
6. A. John Nash was a famous mathematician who later developed Paranoid Schizophrenia. A movie called 'A beautiful mind' was also made and was based on the life of John Nash.

Epidemiology

7. C. Asthenic.
8. A. Onset is after 45 years.
9. C. Schizophrenia. Amongst psychiatric disorders, highest heritability is seen in autism spectrum disorders. Schizophrenia and bipolar disorder too have high heritability.

Etiology and Pathogenesis

10. A, B, C, D.
11. C. Higher socioeconomic status is not a risk factor.
12. B. DiGeorge syndrome.
13. B. The HVA is a metabolite of dopamine and dopamine is usually increased in schizophrenia. A large number of studies have found that levels of HVA are increased in schizophrenia.
14. C. Strictly speaking, only positive symptoms are caused by dopaminergic excess in mesolimbic pathway.
15. B. Hypodopaminergic state. The best answer here is B. Although now we know that negative symptoms are caused by a hypodopaminergic state in mesocortical tract, however the traditional hypothesis that schizophrenia is caused by dopaminergic excess, should be given preference while answering such questions. Ambivalence and autism are of course symptoms of schizophrenia.

Symptoms and Diagnosis

16. B. Thought insertion.
17. D. The term 'paranoid' is often used as a substitute for the term 'persecutory' hence paranoid delusions usually means Delusion of persecution but strictly speaking the term 'paranoid' means 'delusional'. Hence all delusions are paranoid symptoms (Reference Fish's clinical psychopathology)
18. B. Stupor
    In stupor, patient is minimally responsive (including lack of speech output, i.e. mutism) and immobile (akinesis).
19. D. Please remember altered sensorium (or clouding of consciousness) is a sign of delirium. This is a frequently repeated question.
20. C. Auditory hallucinations are the most common type of hallucinations in schizophrenia and the third person auditory hallucinations are quite characteristic for schizophrenia.
21. B. Actually, the correct answer is none. No single symptom or sign is pathognomonic of schizophrenia. However, earlier, the Schneider's first rank symptoms were considered to be pathognomonic. Hence the best answer here is B.
22. C. Younger maternal age at time of birth is not a risk factor for development of schizophrenia.
23. C. Hallucinations in schizophrenia are usually not continuous.
24. A. Akathisia is a side effect of antipsychotics. Ambivalence might be confusing here, but please remember ambitendency is nothing but ambivalence of motor movements. Akinesia, which is lack of voluntary movements is another term for stupor.
25. B. Cataplexy is a feature of narcolepsy.
26. C. Thought broadcast. The language of this question is tricky. As such there is no pathognomonic or 'surest' sign of schizophrenia. However, if we have to choose, thought broadcast would be the best answer as presence of thought broadcast will be enough to diagnose schizophrenia if duration criterion is also met. Rest three options are not enough by themselves to make the diagnosis of schizophrenia.
27. D. Deep tendon reflexes are increased.
28. C, E.
    The other three options are classical catatonic signs. While in catatonic schizophrenia, hallucinations and delusions can be seen, however they are not prominent.
29. A, B, C.
    Schizophrenic patients are much more likely to engage in violent acts in comparison to those without schizophrenia.
30. D. Rapid deterioration of personality.
31. C. Catatonic schizophrenia.
32. C. Repetitive, spontaneous nonfunctional movements.
33. B. Stuporous catatonia has stupor as a prominent symptom. Waxy flexibility is seen in stuporous catatonia more commonly.
34. B. Hebephrenic schizophrenia.

35. D. The best prognosis is of catatonic schizophrenia. However in this question, the better answer is paranoid schizophrenia, as it is the one which has both late onset and good prognosis.
36. B. Presence of affective symptoms (manic or depressive) is a good prognostic sign.
37. C. Insidious onset is a poor prognostic factor.
38. C. Emotional blunting is quite similar to affective flattening and hence is a negative prognostic sign.
39. C. Disorganized behavior.
40. C. Schizophrenia.
41. B. Suicide is the most common cause of premature death. Around **5-10%** of patients with schizophrenia commit suicide.
42. B. "Expressed emotions" is a term which is used to describe certain attitudes of family members of patients with schizophrenia, which have an impact on the illness itself. These attitudes include over involvement, hostility, passing critical comments, etc.
43. C. Both.
44. A. This patient is maintaining an abnormal posture, hence its posturing.

Clinical Vignettes

45. D. Kindly remember that the negative symptoms of schizophrenia have a similar presentation as depression. Speaking less, staying on bed mostly can be due to either negative symptoms or depression. Further, the use of antipsychotics can cause drug induced parkinsonism which again looks quite similar to negative symptoms.
46. C. There is history of delusions and auditory hallucinations, (running commentary type). Hence, the diagnosis is most likely schizophrenia. Occasional alcohol use is unlikely to cause psychosis.
47. A. Third person auditory hallucination for the first time in a 70-year-old individual should strongly raise the suspicion of an organic mental disorder such as dementia. Although its an incomplete question, and information about duration of symptoms, any memory disturbances would have helped in making a more definitive diagnosis.
48. B. Kindly note that this patient also has Capgras syndrome (feeling that his wife has been replaced by a double) which is usually seen in patients with schizophrenia. Also the history is suggestive of delusion of persecution (neighbors are planning against him). Also, note that he is quite well groomed suggesting that personality is preserved as is seen in patients with paranoid schizophrenia.
49. B. The history is suggestive of neologisms (words which are not present in any dictionary) and formal thought disorders (theme is very disjoint). Further, there are negative symptoms (shy and self absorbed). All point towards the diagnosis of schizophrenia.
50. A. There is history of disorganized behavior (odd behavior), hallucinations (talking to self and laughing loudly is most likely a result of patient hearing some voices and communicating with the voices), the history of disappeared family member is again suggesting that some family member may have had a mental illness because of which either he got lost or committed suicide. All factors combined, the likely diagnosis is schizophrenia.
51. D. The history is suggestive of delusion of persecution (fear that schoolmates may "harm" him) and delusion of reference (belief that classmates laugh at him and talk about him). Had they not used the term "harm" and "scared" a diagnosis of social anxiety disorder could have been entertained.
52. C, E.

    The onset of schizophrenia is usually in second and third decade (option A is false).

    The most common comorbidities in schizophrenia are substance use disorders and anxiety disorders. DSM doesn't allow to diagnose major depressive episode in presence of schizophrenia, though its known that depressive symptoms are quite common and increase the suicide risk. Given that DSM-5, doesn't even include depression in the list of comorbidities in schizophrenia, the second option can be ruled out (option B is false).

    Cognitive symptoms are present in prodromal stages of schizophrenia. In fact many studies have found that presence of cognitive deficits can even predict individuals with high risk for schizophrenia (option C is correct). No consistent EEG changes have been found in schizophrenia (option D is false).

    Psychosurgery can definitely be done in cases with resistant schizophrenia however there use remains controversial and is not backed by any well designed study. The use of term "can be done" is the reason why i would mark this option E as correct. Had it been, "psychosurgery are done in resistant cases", I would have marked this option as incorrect.
53. B, C, E

    'Omni micro' is a new word and patient is not able to explain its meaning. It appears to be a 'neologism'. The question stem says 'he often repeats last syllable of last word of the last sentence', this is suggestive of logoclonia. In logoclonia, the last syllable of last word is repeated. E.g. A patient may say 'tomorrow is monday-ay-ay-ay-ay'. Here, the last syllable 'ay' is being repeated again and again. Logoclonia is special form of perseveration.

    Knight's move thinking is synonymous with derailment and loosening of association. The question stem doesn't give any indication about presence of it.

Treatment

54. A, B, C, D, E.

    There is a depot preparation available for imipramine, which is an antidepressant.
55. C. The history is suggesting that the patient had first episode of schizophrenia (i.e. he developed schizophrenia for the first time and no history of any relapse has been provided) and is now maintaining well for last two months. It is generally recommended that after first episode, the treatment with antipsychotics should be continued for at least two years. If there are more than one episodes (i.e. there is history of relapses)

the treatment should continue for at least 5 years. In patients with multiple relapses, indefinite treatment is given.

56. A. The symptoms are suggestive of acute dystonia (inability to move eyes is most likely due to oculogyric crisis) and drug induced parkinsonism (development of rigidity). For both, an anticholinergic needs to be added.
57. C. Clozapine.
58. B. Agranulocytosis is an idiosyncratic reaction and is not related to blood levels.
59. C. Sedation is the most common side effect of clozapine.
60. B. Clozapine.
61. A. Acute dystonia.
62. A, B, E. Clozapine is associated with sialorrhea and not dry mouth.
63. B. The history here is suggestive of tardive dyskinesia. Clozapine is the antipsychotic with minimum incidence of tardive dyskinesia.
64. C. The history here is suggestive of akathisia.
65. C. Clozapine is unlikely to cause hyperprolactinemia as it has low affinity for D2 receptors. Orthostatic hypotension is a common side effects of low potency typical antipsychotics like chlorpromazine.
66. A. Central anticholinergic.
67. A. Neuroleptic malignant syndrome.
68. C. Neuroleptic malignant syndrome.
69. D. Here, we need to rule out the neuroleptic malignant syndrome and also check the renal functions (as NMS can result in renal failure secondary to myoglobinuria).
70. A. Haloperidol belongs to the chemical group, buytyrophenone.
71. A. It is believed that long-term blockade of D2 receptors by antipsychotics causes supersensitivity of the receptors which results in tardive dyskinesia.
72. A. Dantrolene
73. A. In patients who are intolerant to the extrapyramidal side effects, clozapine is the preferred antipsychotic.
74. A. Thioridazine
75. D. Haloperidol. Typical antipsychotics are more commonly associated with neuroleptic malignant syndrome.
76. C. Amongst typical antipyshotics, thioridazine causes minimum EPS.
77. D. Aripiprazole. The history is suggestive of hyperprolactinemia. The drugs which are mostly associated with hyperprolactinemia include typical antipsychotics, risperidone, paliperidone, sulpiride and amisulpride. Olanzapine can occasionally cause hyperprolactinemia. Aripiprazole, due to partial dopamine agonism, usually decreases serum prolactin and hence should be used in this case.
78. D. Amongst the atypical antipsychotics, risperidone and amisulpride are frequently associated with hyperprolactinemia.
79. A, B, C.
80. B. Cognitive remediation is a therapy usually used in schizophrenia for improvement of cognitive functions such as attention, concentration, memory, planning and execution.
81. A. Ziprasidone is known to increase QTc interval and should be avoided in this case.
82. D. Aripiprazole, being a partial D2 agonist is not usually associated with hyperprolactinemia.
83. A. Olanzapine. After clozapine, olanzapine is associated with most weight gain and development of metabolic syndrome.

Other Psychotic Disorders

84. A. Delusion of persecution.
85. A. Alcoholic paranoia usually presents with delusion of infidelity (also known as morbid jealousy).
86. B. Please remember delusion of doubles is also known as Capgras syndrome and is usually seen in patients with schizophrenia.
87. C. In Induced psychotic disorder or shared psychotic disorder, one person who has the delusion (primary case) induces the delusion in another person (secondary case).
88. D. Here, there is only one delusion, i.e. delusion of infidelity, also known as Othello syndrome.
89. D. This appears to be a case of delusional disorder, somatic type. Its important to differentiate it from body dysmorphic disorder. Here, the question says that the idea is fixed (fixed means that the belief persists despite evidences to contrary and despite reassurances by others) and is not shared by anyone else and patient is further hiding her face when visiting outside (i.e. acting on her belief). In body dysmorphic disorder, the belief is not fixed and may be at least temporarily changed by reassurances of others. In body dysmorphic disorder, the problem is more of a preoccupation with the thought that a body part is deformed, this preoccupation is however not fixed (which means person can be reassured at least for some time).
90. C. In this question, there is a single delusion that management is against her (delusion of persecution) and her actions are according to that delusion. Please remember that in delusional disorders, the areas of functioning which does not involve the delusion, remain unaffected. In this patient also, the history that she is able to do her work and manage household is suggesting that she is able to manage the areas of her life which are not affected by the delusion. In questions of delusional disorder, this history is very important and should be looked for.
91. A. The diagnosis is delusional disorder, jealousy type.
92. B. The duration of symptoms is less than one month. Also please remember that in a large number of cases acute psychosis is preceded by fever, hence don't get confused. In this case if the history also mentioned disturbances of consciousness or history of disorientation, the likely diagnosis would be delirium.
93. B. Here again, there is a central delusion that wife is having an affair, and the rest of history is extension of that delusion (i.e. friend is providing support and people are talking ill). The question has mentioned the lack of any thought disorder and inappropriate behavior to provide evidence against the diagnosis of schizophrenia.

94. B. In this image person A believes that person B is wearing a mask or in other words he is disguising his face. Further, there are many more masks in the hands of person B, which he can use to change his physical appearance. These thoughts are consistent with the diagnosis of Fregoli syndrome, in which patient believes that a familiar person can change his physical appearance and disguise as a stranger and that he can take multiple different appearances.
95. D. Fregoli syndrome. The patient believes that his wife (a familiar person) is disguising as a nurse (stranger).
96. A. In Attenuated Psychosis Syndrome, insight is usually present.

AIIMS New Pattern Answers

97. B. The correct sequence is Catatonic schizophrenia followed by Paranoid schizophrenia followed by Disorganized schizophrenia followed by Simple Schizophrenia. Please remember in both DSM-5 and ICD-11, these subtypes have been removed.
98. Case 1- C. Acute and transient psychotic disorder. The history is suggestive of delusion of persecution (neighbour wants to harm) and delusion of reference (cameras have been fitted), auditory hallucinations (obscene words are being spoken using microphones), poor sleep, and aggression. The duration of episodes is 2 weeks (less than one month) and was triggered by fever. This is suggestive of the diagnosis of acute and transient psychotic disorder

    Case 2- B. Delusion disorder. The history is suggestive of delusion of infidelity. There is a central delusion that explains the entire presentation. No history of auditory hallucinations, any other delusion, negative symptoms, motor symptoms, has been given. The likely diagnosis is delusional disorder.

CHAPTER 3

Mood Disorders

Mood disorders are so called as their main feature is abnormality of mood. They are also sometimes referred to as affective disorders.

DEPRESSION

Various terms such as major depressive disorder, unipolar depression and depression have been used for the same illness. It is characterized by major depressive episodes (also known as depressive episodes) in the absence of any manic, mixed or hypomanic episodes.

According to WHO World Mental Health Survey, depression is the second most prevalent mental disorder (most prevalent mental disorder is specific phobias). According to National Mental Health Study (NMHS-2016), carried out by NIMHANS, Bangalore, Depression is the most common mental illness in India (excluding tobacco use disorders).

Following facts must be remembered about depression:
1. Lifetime prevalence - around 12% (5%-17% range)
2. **Male**: Female prevalence ratio is 1:2 (twice as prevalent in females in comparison to males)
3. Mean age of onset is around 40 years (so it's most commonly seen in **middle-aged females**[Q]).
4. It is more commonly seen in divorced and separated persons
5. Amongst psychiatric disorders, depression is associated with maximum DALYs (disability adjusted life years).
6. According to Global Burden of Disease Study, amongst all the medical disorders, depression would become the **second leading cause of DALYs**[Q] by 2020, with ischemic heart diseases being the leading cause.
7. Depression is the **most common**[Q] cause of suicide.

Symptoms

The symptoms of depression can be remembered, using the mnemonic, **SIGECAPSS**. According to DSM-5, to diagnose depression, **five out of the below nine symptoms** should be present, and at least **one symptom should be present out of the first two symptoms** (i.e. sadness of mood & loss of interest)

1. Sadness of mood (depressed mood).
2. *Interest (loss)*: Patient loses interest in the activities which he used to enjoy earlier (**anhedonia**).
3. *Guilt or feelings of worthlessness*: Patient has excessive **guilt feelings** and may blame himself for trivial matters.
4. *Energy (lack)*: Patient may have decreased energy levels and easy fatigability (gets tired easily).
5. *Concentration*: Patient may have poor concentration.
6. *Appetite*: Usually the appetite and weight are lost, in some patients appetite and weight gain may be present (significant weight change is more than 5% change in one month).
7. *Psychomotor agitation or retardation*: The term 'psychomotor' refers to the changes in motor activity secondary to psychological causes. It may be increased (e.g. in restless patients) or may be decreased (e.g. a patient who keeps on lying on the bed and rarely gets up).
8. **S**uicidal thoughts.
9. *Sleep disturbances*: Usually **insomnia** is seen, however hypersomnia can also be a symptom. The two characteristic sleep disturbances in depression are - a) **'early morning awakening**[Q] (patient gets awake more than 2 hours earlier than the usual) and b) **reduced latency of REM sleep**

Duration criterion - **2 weeks**[Q].

Physical Signs

Certain physical signs can be present in patients with depression. These include:

A. **Veraguth fold**[Q]: Otto veraguth described a triangular shape fold in the nasal corner of upper eyelid, called veraguth fold in patients with depression.
B. **Omega sign**: It is the omega shaped fold (like the Greek letter omega, Ω) in the forehead above the root of the nose, seen in patients with depression.

Apart from the above mentioned symptoms, the patient may have few other special features which must be mentioned along with the diagnosis, such as psychotic features, atypical features, melancholic features and catatonic features. These have been described below:

A. **With psychotic features**: Patients with moderate and severe depression may develop psychotic symptoms (delusions and hallucinations). These psychotic symptoms could be **mood congruent** (i.e. content of delusion/hallucination is consistent with the depressed mood, e.g. a severely depressed patient developed a delusion that the world is about to end, nihilistic delusion) or mood incongruent (i.e. content of delusion is inconsistent with the depressed mood, e.g. a severely depressed patient developed the delusion that he is the richest man on earth). The term "**psychotic depression^Q**" is used for depression with psychotic features.

> **ICD-11 Update**
>
> In ICD-10, the specifier 'psychotic symptoms' could be used only with severe depression. ICD-11 has allowed the use of the specifier 'psychotic symptoms' with moderate depression too.

B. **With atypical features (or atypical depression)**: Atypical depression is characterised by the presence of following features-
   a. Reversed biological symptoms: 1. hypersomnia 2. increased appetite and weight gain
   b. Leaden paralysis (feeling that limbs have become heavy and difficulty in moving the limbs)
   c. Presence of 'mood reactivity' (i.e. the patient's mood improves if some positive events occurs)
   d. Long standing pattern of interpersonal rejection sensitivity (i.e. person is extremely sensitive to events where he feels that he is being rejected/ disliked by others)

C. **With melancholic features (melancholic depression, involutional melancholia)**: Depression with melancholic features is usually seen in **old age, and is characterised by the following features:**
   a. Prominent biological symptoms- 1. early morning awakening (waking up at least 2 hours before usual time) 2. significant anorexia and weight loss
   b. Significant psychomotor agitation or retardation
   c. Anhedonia and lack of mood reactivity (i.e. the patient's mood doesn't improve even if some positive event occurs)
   d. A distinct quality of intensely depressed mood, often referred to as a state of despondency or despair, also called as empty mood. The patients feels miserable^Q.
   e. Depression is worse in the morning
   f. Excessive guilt.
   These patients have a higher suicide risk.

D. **With catatonic features**: Patient with depression may develop catatonic symptoms such as **stupor^Q**, negativism, etc.

Endogenous vs Exogenous (Reactive) Depression

In older classificatory system, two subtypes of depression were described.

a. **Endogenous depression**: It occurred in the absence of any precipitating negative life event, and was considered to be caused by biological factors. The symptoms described were early morning awakening, psychotic symptoms, psychomotor retardation and feelings of guilt and higher suicide risk. The symptoms of endogenous depression were quite similar to today's psychotic and melancholic depression.

b. Exogenous depression (reactive depression) was believed to occur in response to a negative life event and the symptoms which were described included initial insomnia (difficulty in falling asleep), absence of psychotic symptoms and multiple somatic complaints and lower suicide risk.

Etiology

A. *Biological factors*:
   - **Neurotransmitters disturbances**: **Decreased levels of serotonin and norepinephrineQ** are most important factors implicated in the pathophysiology of depression. Dopamine has also been found to be decreased in a subset of patients.
   - *Hormonal disturbances*: Around 50% of patients with depression have dysfunction of HPA axis, which manifests as **cortisol hyper secretion^Q** (as measured by urinary free cortisol levels, salivary cortisol levels, plasma cortisol levels) as well as more definitive **dexamethasone suppression test** (DST) indicating HPA overactivity (*In dexamethasone suppression test, a high potency glucocorticoid is administered in night and normally, it should suppress the release of CRH and ACTH and finally the next morning cortisol surge should also get suppressed. However in patients with depression, the cortisol surge doesn't get suppressed suggesting a HPA axis overactivity*).
   - **Hypothyroidism^Q** is a common cause of depression.
   - *Neuroanatomical considerations*: **Decreased activity** in dorsolateral **prefrontal cortex^Q** and

increased activity in amygdala (and other limbic tissue) has been found in depression.

B. *Genetic factors*: Gene mapping studies have found evidence of linkage to locus for cAMP response element binding protein (CREB 1) on chromosome 2. **Serotonin transporter gene** polymorphism has been show to influence susceptibilty to development of depression.

C. *Psychological theories*:
- *Cognitive theory*: It was proposed by **Aaron Beck**^{Q}. According to this theory negative thoughts have a central role in development of depression. Beck proposed that there are three central thoughts/ideas in depression, the so called **cognitive triad** of **depression**^{Q}. These include:
  1. Negative view of self (**ideas of worthlessness**^{Q})
  2. Negative views about environment—A tendency to experience world as hostile (**ideas of help-lessness**^{Q})
  3. Negative view about future (**ideas of hopelessness**).
- *Learned helplessness*: According to this theory, due to repeated adverse events, patient starts believing that he has no control over events happening around him and loses the motivation to act, which results in depression.

Treatment

1. *Pharmacotherapy*: The use of specific pharmacotherapy doubles the chances that a depressed patient will recover in 1 month. All the available antidepressants take up to **3-4 weeks** to exert significant therapeutic effects. The available antidepressants do not differ in the overall efficacy, speed of response or long term effectiveness and the choice of antidepressants is mostly determined by the **side effect profile**^{Q} of the drugs. Antidepressant treatment should be maintained for at least 6 months or equal to the duration of a previous episode, whichever is greater.

Prophylactic treatment with antidepressants is effective in reducing the number and severity of episodes. It should be given to patients who have had
   a. Three or more prior depressive episodes or
   b. Have chronic major depressive disorder (> 2 years duration is chronic depression). The following classes of medications can be used:
      A. ***Tricyclic and tetracyclic antidepressants (TCAs)***: These were the first class of antidepressants that were widely used in clinical practice. They act by blocking the transporters of **serotonin** and **norepinephrine** and hence increase the levels of these neurotransmitters in synapses. Secondary effects of TCAs include antagonism of muscarinic, histaminic H1, α1 and α2 adrenergic receptors and blockage of cardiac sodium channels. These secondary effects are responsible for the unfavorable side effect profile of these drugs.

TCA Toxicity

A patient with TCA toxicity (after unintentional or intentional over ingestion of tablets) presents with cardiovascular manifestations that include hypotension, chest pain, palpitations; CNS manifestations that may include **altered sensorium, respiratory depression and seizures**^{Q}; and peripheral autonomic manifestations such as dry mouth, blurred vision, urinary retention, etc. **Metabolic acidosis**^{Q} can be present secondary to tissue hypoxia caused by cardiovascular abnormality/TCA induced seizures. ECG findings may include sinus tachycardia, **prolongation of PR, QRS and QT interval**^{Q}, AV block and **right axis deviation**^{Q}. A QRS interval of more than **100 millisecond**^{Q} is the basis of treatment with **intravenous sodium bicarbonate**^{Q} (serum arlkalinization) which is the mainstay of treatment in TCA toxicity. Gastric lavage and use of activated charcoal is only beneficial if administered immediately after the overdosage

The class TCAs include the following drugs: Imipramine, desipramine, trimipramine, amitriptyline, nortriptyline, protriptyline, amoxapine, doxepin, maprotiline and clomipramine. The TCAs differ in their affinity for transporters, with clomipramine being the most serotonin selective and desipramine the most norepinephrine selective of TCAs. The side effects of TCAs include the following:

- **Anticholinergic side effects**^{Q} like **constipation, urinary retention**^{Q}, blurred vision, dry mouth, decreased sweating and delirium. Due to significant anticholinergic side effects TCAs should be avoided in **glaucoma**^{Q} and prostate hypertrophy.
- Side effects due to blockade of α (alpha) receptors like postural hypotension (rarely **hypertension**^{Q} can also be seen)
- Cardiac side effects- TCAs can cause tachycardia, fattened T waves, prolongation of QT interval and ST segment depression. Severe side effects like cardiac **arrhythmias**, and hypotension can occur due to blocking of cardiac sodium channels.
- Neurological side effects- Fine, rapid **tremor**^{Q} can occur. Excessive blockade of

serotonin and norepinephrine receptors can cause seizures.
- Sedation due to blockage of H1 histaminic receptors.
- Other side effects- Weight gain is common. TCAs (especially amoxapine) have also been found to be associated with hyperprolcatinemia and may cause amennorhea, **gynaecomastia**^{Q}, impotence, galactorrhea etc.

Important properties of individual drugs:
a. **Amoxapine**^{Q} has D2 blocking action and hence can cause extrapyramidal side effects like antipsychotics.
b. **Imipramine**^{Q} is used in the treatment of nocturnal enuresis (however the drug of choice is desmopressin; the treatment of choice is behavioral methods like night alarms).
c. Clomipramine is the first line therapy in OCD, however due to better side effect profile, SSRIs are preferred over clomipramine.

B. **Selective serotonin reuptake inhibitors (SSRIs):** These are the most commonly prescribed antidepressants. They act by blocking the reuptake of serotonin and do not have the problematic side effects, as seen with TCAs. The SSRIs include fluoxetine, fluvoxamine, citalopram, escitalopram, sertraline, paroxetine and **vilazodone**. The SSRIs are the first line drugs for depression, obsessive compulsive disorder, posttraumatic stress disorder, panic disorder, generalized anxiety disorder and phobias.

- *Side effects*: The side effects of the SSRIs include the following
- *GI side effects*: Gastrointestinal side effect are the most commonly reported side effects and include nausea (most common), diarrhoea, anorexia and constipation (constipation is seen with paroxetine). Gastrointestinal side effects are usually short lasting and improve with time.
- *Sexual dysfunction*: Sexual dysfunctions (including anorgasmia, decreased libido and inhibited orgasm) are the most common side effects associated with long term treatment with SSRIs
- QTc interval prolongation

- *CNS side effects*: Anxiety, insomnia, sedation, vivid dreams^Q, nightmares, emotional blunting, seizures, extrapyramidal symptoms, sweating^Q
- *Anticholinergic side effects*: Mostly associated with paroxetine
- *Hematologic adverse effects*: Functional impairment of platelet aggregation, hyponatremia
- *Miscellaneous*: Weight gain is a common side effect, rarely hyperprolactinemia and allergic rashes can be present.

Serotonin Syndrome^Q

Concurrent administration of an SSRI with MAO inhibitor, L-tryptophan or lithium can raise plasma serotonin concentration, resulting in serotonin syndrome. It is a potentially fatal syndrome and presents with the following features:
1. Diarrhoea, restlessness
2. **Hyperreflexia**, agitation and autonomic instability
3. **Myoclonus**, hyperthermia, rigidity, seizures
4. Delirium, coma and death

It is treated using cyproheptadine and supportive care.

Vortioxetine: A recently introduced antidepressant works as an inhibitor of serotonin reuptake, but also has other actions like agonism at 5HT1A receptor, partial agonism at 5HT1B receptor and antagonism at 5HT3, 5HT1D and 5HT7 receptors.

C. **SNRIs (Serotonin Norepinephrine Reuptake Inhibitors):** These drugs produce blockade of neuronal serotonin and norepinephrine uptake transporters and hence are also referred as dual reuptake inhibitors. They include venlafaxine, desvenlafaxine, duloxetine, milnacipran, levomilnacipran. The side effect profile is quite similar to SSRIs. In addition, SNRIs can cause hypertension at higher dosages.

Discontinuation Syndrome

Sudden discontinuation or rapid reduction of dosage of antidepressants can cause, a **discontinuation syndrome**. It is characterised by the following symptoms- (mnemonic FINISH)
a. Flu like symptoms (lethargy, fatigue, aches)
b. Insomnia
c. Nausea
d. Imbalance (dizziness, vertigo)
e. Sensory disturbances (paraesthesias)
f. Hyperarousal (anxiety, irritability)

All antidepressants can cause discontinuation syndrome. **Venlafaxine**^{Q} is most commonly associated with discontinuation syndrome. Short acting SSRIs (paroxetine and fluvoxamine) are also commonly associated with discontinuation syndrome.

D. ***Monoamine oxidase inhibitors***: These drugs act by inhibiting the metabolism of monoamines. There are two isoforms of the enzymes (MAO), MAO-A (involved in metabolism of serotonin, norepinephrine and dopamine) and MAO-B (preferential metabolism of dopamine). The nonselective MAO inhibitors which includes tranylcypromine, phenelzine and isocarboxazid inhibits both the isoforms irreversibly. These drugs are rarely used now as they can cause hypertensive crisis. MAOIs (and SSRIs) were found to be more effective than TCAs, in the treatment of atypical depression.

Cheese reaction: Cheese, red wine and beer contains tyramine (which is an indirectly acting sympathomimetic). Normally, when these items are consumed, the MAO-A present in the gastrointestinal tract degrades the tyramine. However when MAO inhibitors are used, the tyramine escapes degradation and gets absorbed resulting in dangerous elevation of blood pressure, causing hypertensive crisis (also called cheese reaction). Hence these food items are restricted in a patient who is on MAO inhibitors. **Phentolamine** is the drug of choice for cheese reaction.

E. ***Atypical antidepressants***: There are many other antidepressants which have novel mechanisms of actions. These include:
- ***Trazodone and nefazodone***: These drugs are classified as SARI (serotonin antagonist and reuptake inhibitors). The mechanism of action is weak inhibition of serotonin reuptake and strong antagonism at 5 HT2A and 5 HT2C receptors. Trazodone can cause **priapism**^{Q} as a side effect.
- ***Mirtazapine***: Mirtazapine belongs to a class called NSSA (nor adrenergic and specific serotonergic antidepressant). The mechanism of action is antagonism of central presynaptic α2 (alpha2) receptors which results in increased firing of norepinephrine and serotonin neurons. The other important action is antagonism of postsynaptic serotonin 5 HT2 and 5 HT3 receptors. Mirtazapine causes sedation and weight gain but doesn't have problematic sexual side effects. Other side effects include dry mouth, constipation, myalgia and disturbing dreams.
- ***Bupropion***: Bupropion belongs to a class called NDRI (norepinephrine dopamine reuptake inhibitors). The mechanism of action is inhibition of reuptake of both **norepinephrine and dopamine**^{Q}. The advantage of bupropion is a good side effect profile with low risk of sexual side effects, weight gain or sedation. The common side effects are insomnia, tremors, restlessness and nausea. A particular worrisome side effect is **seizures** (usually seen at higher dosages). Bupropion is also used for smoking cessation.
- ***Tianeptine and amineptine***: These antidepressants work by **enhancing**^{Q} the reuptake of serotonin (serotonin reuptake enhancer).
- ***Antipsychotics***: If patient has depression with psychotic symptoms, a combination of antidepressants and antipsychotics is used.

> **Esketamine**
>
> In 2019, FDA has approved use of **nasal spray of esketamine** (the senantiomer of ketamine) for treatment of treatment resistant depression. The important points to be noted are:
> a. Esketamine uses a novel mechanism of **glutamate receptors modulation**, and is claimed to have a much **faster onset of action** in comparison to the currently available antidepressants
> b. Esketamine is approved for use in patients with treatment resistant depression (defined as lack of response to two different antidepressants, given in adequate dosage and for adequate period)
> c. Esketamine would be used as a nasal spray and would be given along with an oral antidepressant.
> d. Because of risk of misuse, it would be administered in the office of a certified medical doctor. Patient would self administer the nasal spray under the supervision of doctor

2. *Psychotherapy*: It is the treatment using psychological techniques. The following psychotherapeutic techniques are effective in depression:
   A. **Cognitive behavioral therapy**: This therapy aims at correcting cognitive distortions (faulty ways of thinking) and faulty behaviors. It is the **most effective**^{Q} psychotherapeutic technique in depression.
   B. *Interpersonal therapy:* In interpersonal therapy, the focus is on management of patient's current interpersonal problems (e.g. relationship problems).
   C. Other less commonly used therapeutic techniques include behavior therapy, family therapy and psychoanalytically oriented therapy.

3. ***Other somatic treatments:***
   A. *Electroconvulsive therapy (ECTs):* The indications for ECT in depression includes:
   - Severe depression with **suicide risk**^{Q} (**If the patient is suicidal, ECT is the preferred treatment modality**)^Q.
   - Severe depression with **stupor**^{Q}.
   - Other indications include depression with psychotic symptoms, refractoriness to other treatment modalities.

B. **Transcranial magnetic stimulation**^{Q}: It is a newer modality which uses magnetic energy to stimulate nerve cells. It is nonconvulsive, requires no anesthesia, has a safe side effect profile and is not associated with cognitive side effects. Its use is yet not widespread.
C. **Vagal nerve stimulation**^{Q}: This modality involves stimulation of vagal nerve using an electrode.
D. **Deep brain stimulation**^{Q}: This modality involves implantation of leads into specific brain areas and has been used in patients with chronic and intractable depression. However, deep brain stimulation has yet not been approved by FDA (Food and drug administration, the licensing authority in USA) for treatment of depression^Q
E. **Sleep deprivation:** Sleep deprivation can produce significant benefits however these are transient and are typically reversed by next night of sleep. Research is ongoing to produce sustained benefits.
F. **Phototherapy**: It has been primarily used for **seasonal affective disorders (mood disorder with seasonal pattern**^{Q}**)**. In this disorder patients typically develop depressive symptoms during winter seasons which are associated with decreased day time. The phototherapy involves exposure to bright light in range of 1500–10,000 lux or more.

Usually a combination of pharmacotherapy and psychotherapy is used in management of depressed patients, in cases of suicide risk, ECT is the preferred treatment.

BIPOLAR DISORDER

Bipolar disorder is characterized by episodes of both mania and depression. Even if a patient has **only manic episodes**^{Q}, he would still be diagnosed with bipolar disorder, as in all likelihood he would develop a depressive episode in future. The lifetime prevalence of Bipolar disorder is 1%. The prevalence of bipolar I disorder is quite similar in men and women with the lifetime male to female prevalence ratio being 1.1:1. Manic episodes are more common in men and depressive episodes are more common in women.

The mean age of onset for bipolar I is around 18 years and for bipolar II is in mid 20s. It is more commonly seen in divorced and single persons. Bipolar disorder has multiple subtypes which have been illustrated in the following Table 1.

Table 1: Types of bipolar disorders.

Bipolar 1/2	Schizobipolar disorder (schizoaffective disorder)
Bipolar I	Mania with depression (or mania alone)
Bipolar I 1/2	Depression with protracted hypomania

Contd...

Contd...

Bipolar II	Depression with discrete hypomanic episodes
Bipolar II 1/2	Depression superimposed on cyclothymia
Bipolar III	Depression plus induced hypomania (e.g. hypomania occurring solely in association with antidepressants or other somatic treatment
Bipolar III 1/2	Bipolar disorder associated with substance use
Bipolar IV	Depression superimposed on hyperthymic temperament

 ICD-11 Update

In ICD-11, for the first time, the two types of Bipolar disorders (Bipolar type I disorder and Bipolar type II disorder) have been included in the formal classification

Symptoms

The symptoms of manic episode are as follows: Mnemonic- My Asia FAST GDP

According to DSM-5, to make a diagnosis of manic episode, Five out of the below nine symptoms should be present and both symptoms, 1 (mood elevation) and 2 (increased activity levels) should present:

1. Mood elevation (undue excessive happiness) or irritable mood
2. Activity levels are increased
3. Flight of ideas^Q
4. Activity level increased and energy increased
5. Sleep (decreased need for sleep^Q) (e.g. patient feels rested after 2 hours of sleep)
6. Talkativenss (overtalkativeness)
7. Grandiose ideas and increased self esteem (e.g. patient believes himself to be the richest, most powerful, most goodlooking person on the earth, etc.)
8. **Distractibility**^{Q} (not able to concentrate on task in hand)
9. Painful consequences (involvement in activities with potentially painful consequences like foolish investments, sexual indiscretions)

Duration criterion - **7 days**^{Q}

Psychotic symptoms: Apart from the above mentioned symptoms, patient may also develop psychotic symptoms (delusions and hallucinations). These may be mood congruent (e.g. delusion of grandiosity) or mood incongruent (e.g. delusion of persecution). In the presence of psychotic symptoms, the diagnosis made is manic episode with psychotic symptoms.

Hypomania: The symptoms of hypomania are similar to mania however they are not severe enough to cause marked impairment in social and occupational functioning. Also, the duration criterion for hypomania is **4 days.**

Mixed episodes: Mixed episodes have both manic and depressive symptoms lasting for at least 7 days.

Etiology

- *Neurotransmitters:* Increased levels of dopamine has been implicated in pathophysiology of manic episode. The changes in depression have been already discussed.
- *Genetic factors:* The chromosomes **18q^Q** and 22q have the strongest evidence of linkage to bipolar disorder. Chromosome 21q has also been linked.

Treatment

The treatment in bipolar disorder depends on the phase. Patient requires treatment during acute illness (acute manic or mixed or depressive episodes) and also need prophylaxis to prevent further episodes (maintenance treatment). The following classes of drugs are usually used in bipolar disorder:

A. **Mood stabilizers:** Commonly used mood stabilizing drugs include lithium, valproate, carbamazepine oxcarbazepine and, lamotrigine. Many atypical antipsychotics also have mood stabilizing properties:
   - Lithium is considered the **prototypical mood stabilizer^Q**. However it takes around **1-2 weeks** to start acting. It is usually supplemented by other mood stabilizers, antipsychotics or benzodiazepines in early phase of treatment.
   - *Valproate*: Valproate has surpassed lithium in use for acute mania due to better tolerability.
   - *Lamotrigine*: It is mostly used in treatment of acute depressive episode of bipolar disorder (**bipolar depression^Q**).

B. *Antipsychotics*: Usually atypical antipsychotics are used due to better tolerance and side effect profile.

C. *Benzodiazepines*: High potency benzodiazepines such as lorazepam and clonazepam are frequently used in acute mania due to their calming effect.

D. *Antidepressants*: Antidepressants are **never used** alone in bipolar disorder. When used alone in bipolar depression they can cause switch (patient may go into mania), hence they are always used along with mood stabilizers.

Treatment Guidelines

A. Acute manic or mixed episode:
   - For severe mania or mixed episode, initiate lithium in combination with an antipsychotic or valproate in combination with an antipsychotic.
   - For less ill patients, monotherapy with lithium, valproate or an atypical antipsychotic such as olanzapine may be sufficient.
   - Short-term treatment with benzodiazepines is often used.
   - For mixed episodes, valproate is preferred over lithium.
   - If patient has psychotic symptoms, antipsychotics must be added to the treatment regimen.

B. Acute depression (bipolar depression):
   - Initiate lithium or lamotrigine.
   - In severely ill patients, initiate treatment with both lithium and an antidepressant.
   - Quetiapine alone and combination of olanzapine and fluoxetine are other treatment options.
   - Antidepressant monotherapy should never be given.
   - Electroconvulsive therapy for patients with high suicide risk.

C. Maintenance:
   - Usually given after two or more acute episodes in bipolar I illness or after a single manic episode if it was associated with significant risk.
   - Lithium and valproate have the best evidence.
   - Treatment should be continued for at least two years.

Lithium

Lithium is used for treatment of acute episodes (both mania and depression) as well as prophylaxis in bipolar disorder. **John FJ Cade^Q**, an Australian psychiatrist was the first to establish effectiveness of lithium in treatment of mania and as a prophylactic drug.

Lithium is a monovalent cation and gets **rapidly and completely absorbed^Q** after oral administration. The plasma half life is initially **1.3 days** and gets increased to **2.4 days** after continued administration for more than one year. Lithium doesn't bind to plasma proteins^Q is not metabolized in the body and gets excreted unchanged through the **kidney**.

Indications

A. *Acute manic episode*: Lithium is an effective treatment for acute mania however since its onset of action is delayed (1 to 3 weeks), an antipsychotic, benzodiazepine or valproate is usually added for initial period. Lithium is also effective for prophylaxis against future manic episodes.

B. *Bipolar depression*: Lithium is effective for treatment of bipolar depression and prophylaxis of same, however the antimanic efficacy of lithium is more than its antidepressive efficacy.

C. *Maintenance treatment:* Maintenance treatment with lithium decreases the frequency, severity and duration of manic and depressive episodes in patients with bipolar disorders.

D. Lithium is an effective **antisuicidal**^Q agent and decreases the risk of suicide by 80% in patients with bipolar disorder.

E. Lithium is also used in patients with schizoaffective disorders as well as an adjuvant to antidepressants in major depressive disorder.

F. Other indications in which lithium has been used but is not the first line treatment include obsessive compulsive disorder, aggression, **headache (cluster, migraine**^Q), gout, epilepsy, movement disorders, **neutropenia**^Q, ulcerative colitis.

Correlates of lithium responsiveness: Lithium response in patient with bipolar disorder tends to be better in the following clinical conditions:

a. **Euphoric (elated) mania**^Q (in euphoric mania, patients predominant mood state is euphoria) {In patients with dysphoric mania, where in the predominant mood state is irritability, valproate is a better choice over lithium}

b. Three or fewer episodes (patients who have had four or more manic/depressive episodes tend to respond poorly to lithium)

c. MDI sequence (it means that patient in whom sequence of mood episodes has been mania→ depression→ interval, respond better to lithium)

d. Absence of rapid cycling

e. Family history of bipolar disorder

f. Absence of comorbidities like substance use. Lithium has a narrow therapeutic index and therapeutic drug monitoring is required. The effective serum concentration for treatment of acute mania is **1.0-1.5 mEq/dL**^Q. The serum concentration required for maintenance treatment is **0.6-1.2 mEq/dL**^Q.

Side Effects

A. *Neurological side effects*: Lithium can cause **postural tremors** (usually treated with beta blockers **like propranolol**^Q), lack of spontaneity and memory disturbances, rarely it can cause raised intracranial tension and peripheral neuropathy.

B. *Endocrine*: **Hypothyroidism**, rarely hyperthyroidism, hyperparathyroidism.

C. Renal: Most common is polyuria at time progressing to diabetes insipidus which is treated with use of thiazide diuretics or potassium sparing diuretics (like amiloride, spironolactone or triamterene). Rarely nephrotic syndrome, renal tubular acidosis or interstitial fibrosis can be seen.

D. Others include dermatological side effects such as **acne, psoriasis, hair loss and rashes**^Q. Nausea, vomiting, diarrhea, weight gain and benign T wave changes can also occur.

E. *Teratogenic effects*: Lithium, if taken in pregnancy, can cause malformation in cardiovascular system of fetus, most commonly **Ebstein's anomaly**^Q of tricuspid valves. The teratogenic risk of lithium is lower than that associated with valproate and carbamazepine.

Lithium toxicity: The risk factors of lithium toxicity include renal impairment, **dehydration**^Q and low **sodium diet**^Q. Usually the sign of toxicity starts to appear at levels above **1.5 mEq/dL** and hence lithium has a **narrow therapeutic index**^Q. The early signs include **GI symptoms** like abdominal pain, vomiting and neurological symptoms like **coarse tremors, ataxia**^Q and **dysarthria**. The later signs and symptoms include impairment of consciousness, muscular fasciculations, increased **deep tendon reflexes**^Q and convulsions. There might be circulatory failure and death. The management involves stopping lithium, correcting dehydration, use of polyethylene glycol (and not activated charcoal) to remove unabsorbed lithium from GI tract. In severe cases, hemodialysis may be required.

Pregnancy and Use of Mood Stabilisers

The following points must be remembered:

1. Risk of relapse of bipolar disorder, is increased during pregnancy and even more during the postpartum period. If a patient is on a mood stabiliser, and it is stopped abruptly, the risk of relapse becomes very high.

2. Relapse during pregnancy has an adverse effect on the health of both mother and child.

3. No mood stabiliser is safe. A risk vs benefit assessment must be done and decision to continue (or not continue) the treatment should be taken.

4. *Lithium use in pregnancy*: Lithium use during pregnancy can cause ebstein's anomaly, however the risk of the same is very low (1:1000). Lithium use can also cause atrial and ventricular septal defects.

   If lithium is used during pregnancy, high resolution ultrasound and echocardiography should be done at 6 and 18 weeks of gestation. At the end of pregnancy, rapid changes in the total body water occur and may predispose the mother to lithium toxicity. This requires fluid balance monitoring.

5. **Valproate use in pregnancy**: **Valproate is the most teratogenic**^Q **amongst the mood stabilsers and should be avoided.** Use of valproate, can cause neural tube defects (i.e. spina bifida). Valproate must be given only

if all other treatment methods have failed, in such a case, folate supplements must be given to the patient. Use of folate, for atleast one month before conception, decreases the chances of development of neural tube defects.

Few studies have reported that in utero exposure of valproate may adversely impact cognitive development in children, and children of mothers who took valproate during pregnancy, have low IQ scores.

6. *Carbamazepine use in pregnancy*: Carbamazepine is a teratogenic drug and should be avoided. Use of carbamazepine, can cause neural tube defects (i.e. spina bifida), although risk is lesser in comparison to valproate. Use of folate, for atleast one month before conception, decreases the chances of development of neural tube defects. If carbamazepine is used, prophylactic Vitamin K should be given to mother and neonate after delivery, to prevent hemorrhagic disease.

7. Limited studies have suggested that lamotrigine is safer than valproate or carbamazepine, in pregnancy.

8. Antipsychotics are safer than mood stabilisers and less likely to cause any teratogenic effects, if possible, should be preferred over, mood stabilisers for prophylaxis.

9. If a patient develops acute manic episode in pregnancy, **antipsychotics are again preferred**[Q] overuse of any mood stabilisers

OTHER MOOD DISORDERS

A. *Recurrent depressive disorder*: If there are more than one depressive episodes, diagnosis of recurrent depressive disorder is made.

B. *Premenstrual dysphoric disorder*: It's a new diagnosis that has been added in DSM-5. It is characterized by symptoms that have onset about one week before menses, symptoms start to improve after onset of menses and become minimal or absent in the week post menses. The symptoms include irritable mood, emotional lability, depressed mood and anxiety symptoms. Somatic symptoms like lethargy, changes in appetite and sleep, weight gain, edema, breast tenderness are also present. Symptoms are significant and cause socio occupational dysfunction. Treatment is symptomatic and involves analgesics, **diuretics**[Q] (for fluid retention). SSRIs and benzodiazepines are also effective.

DSM-5 Update

In DSM-5, the diagnosis of dysthymia has been removed. A new diagnostic category of "persistent depressive disorder" has been made, which includes both chronic depression and previous dysthymic disorder.

C. *Dysthymia*: It is the presence of mild depressive symptoms (not enough to diagnose a major depressive episode) for a period of more than two years.

Chronic depression: If the depression continues for more than 2 years, it is known as chronic depression.

Double depression[Q]: Superimposed development of depressive episode in a patient already suffering from dysthymia is double depression.

D. *Cyclothymia*: It is a milder form of bipolar disorder, in which manic symptoms and depressive symptoms occur, but they are never severe enough to make a diagnosis of mania/hypomania or depression. The symptoms should last for at least 2 years.

Rapid cycling: If a patient of bipolar disorder has four or more than four episodes of mania/hypomania/depression in one calendar year.

SUICIDE

The psychiatric illnesses associated with highest risk of suicide are **depressive disorder**, schizophrenia, **alcohol dependence** and other substance dependence and personality disorders (especially borderline personality disorder and antisocial personality disorder). Low CSF level of **5-hydroxyindoleacetic acid (5 HIAA)**[Q], which is a **metabolite of serotonin**, is associated with higher suicide risk.

The following are the **risk factors**[Q] for suicide:

- **Previous suicide attempt**[Q] (most important risk factor)
- Signals of suicide intent (e.g. **writing a suicide note**[Q], transferring money into account of a loved one etc). Most people who commit suicide tend to clearly communicate their intention to their loved ones or doctors
- **Hopelessness**[Q]
- Delusions or hallucinations
- **Substance abuse**[Q]
- **Male sex**[Q]
- Age > 45 years (suicide rate increases with age and peaks at 45 years, suicide is rare before puberty. Suicide rate is however increasing in youth)
- Divorced, separated or single marital status
- Unemployed
- Chronic illness
- Family history of suicide
- **Poor social support**[Q]
- Sexual abuse.

According to NCRB (National Crime Record Bureau), in 2014, the suicide rate in India was 10.6 per lac of population. The most common method of committing suicide is **Hanging**[Q] followed by use of **poisons**[Q].

Important Terms

Parasuicide: The term parasuicide is used when a person indulges in self injurious behaviour (e.g. making superficial cuts on skin) however, doesn't have the intention to kill self.

Physician suicide: Doctors have a higher risk of suicide than general population. Amongst doctors, psychiatrists have the highest risk, followed by ophthalmologists and anaesthetist.

Copycat suicide [Q]: There have been reports where adolescents belonging to the same group have committed suicide one after another. It is believed that suicide by one member, influences the behaviour of others, this is called as copycat suicide. Some studies have found increased rate of adolescent suicides after release of a television program/movie that shows suicide by an adolescent, or after suicide by some popular figure like a pop star.

PSYCHIATRIC ASPECTS OF PREGNANCY

1. ***Postpartum blues (baby blues):*** Most women develop transient depressive symptoms like tearfulness, emotional lability (frequent mood changes), tearfulness, sadness and at times sleep disturbances. These symptoms may last for days to weeks and need no professional treatment except for support to the mother.

2. ***Postpartum depression:*** In some cases, the symptoms may be more severe and prolonged and a diagnosis of 'postpartum depression' is made. According to DSM-5, depressive episode can develop after child birth or may develop before the delivery, collectively these episodes are referred to as Depressive episode with peripartum onset (or peripartum depressive episodes)

Table 2: Differences between postpartum blues and postpartum depression.

	Postpartum blues	Postpartum depression
Incidence	30 to 75 percent of women who give birth	10 to 15 percent of women who give birth
Time of onset	3 to 5 days after childbirth	Within 3 months of childbirth
Tearfulness	Yes	Yes
Emotional lability	Yes	Yes
Anhedonia	No	Common
Sleep disturbances	Occasional	Common
Suicidal thoughts/ Thoughts of harming baby	No	Sometimes
History of mood disorder	No association	Usually present
Family history of mood disorder	No association	Usually present
Guilt	Rare	Common
Increased risk of development of future episodes of depression	No	Yes
Treatment	Support to mother	Pharmacotherapy plus psychotherapy

Contd...

Brexanolone

In 2019, US FDA, has approved brexanolone IV infusion (60 hours continuous i.v. infusion), which is the first ever drug approved specifically for treatment of Postpartum depression.

Brexanolone is chemically identical to endogenous allopregnanolone, which is a hormone that decreases after childbirth. Brexanolone acts as a positive allosteric modulator of GABA-A receptors (which become dysregulated in postpartum period).

3. ***Postpartum psychosis (puerperal psychosis):*** Postpartum psychosis is usually seen within 2 to 3 weeks of delivery. The following are the important characteristics of post part psychosis:
   a. Initially, patient presents with symptoms like insomnia, tearfulness and emotional lability followed by development of delusions and hallucinations.
   b. The content of delusion may involve thoughts that 'baby is dead' or that patient did not give birth or some other persecutory ideas. Hallucinations may have similar content. Postpartum psychosis is considered as a psychiatric emergency as patient may act on hallucinations and delusions, and may rarely commit suicide or infanticide.
   c. Postpartum psychosis is essentially an episode of bipolar disorder (sometimes depressive disorder), and childbirth (and accompanying hormonal changes) is considered as a stressor, that triggered this episode
   d. Two third of patients, develop another mood episode (manic, depressive or mixed episode), within one year of childbirth.
   e. About 50 to 60 percent of affected women had given birth to the first child, and in 50% of cases, delivery was associated with a non psychiatric perinatal complication.
   f. 50% of affected women have a family history of mood disorder.
   g. Subsequent pregnancy carries a high risk of another episode of postpartum psychosis, risk is around 50%.
   h. In most of the cases, recovery is complete from acute illness.
   i. Treatment involves use of antipsychotics, often in combination with lithium and possibly antidepressants.

Multiple Choice Questions

Depression

Epidemiology and Etiology

1. **Most commonly depression is seen in:** *(AI 1996, 1998)*
   A. Middle aged men
   B. Middle aged female
   C. Young girl
   D. Children

2. **Neurotransmitters involved in depression are:** *(AI 1995)*
   A. GABA and dopamine
   B. Serotonin and norepinephrine
   C. Serotonin and dopamine
   D. Norepinephrine and GABA

3. **Higher cortisol levels are seen in which of the following conditions?** *(NIMHANS 2015)*
   A. Depression
   B. Phobia
   C. Schizophrenia
   D. Parkinsonism

4. **Which of the following is not a part of cognitive triad of beck?** *(AIIMS Nov 2015)*
   A. Hopelessness
   B. Worthlessness
   C. Helplessness
   D. Guilt

5. **All of the following about "Aaron Becks cognitive theory of depression" is true, except:** *(DNB Dec 2010)*
   A. Negative thought of past
   B. Negative thought of future
   C. Negative thought of environment
   D. Negative about self

6. **True about major depressive disorder:** *(PGI Nov 2011)*
   A. Abnormally diminished activity in prefrontal cortex
   B. Lesion of corticospinal tract
   C. Monoaminergic system disturbances
   D. Genetic predisposition is present

7. **Depression is seen in:**
   A. Hyperthyroidism
   B. Hypoglycemia
   C. Adrenal disorder
   D. Pheochromocytoma

8. **Depression is a feature of which of the following condition?**
   A. Hypopituitarism
   B. Hyperthyroidism
   C. Hypothyroidism
   D. Hypoglycemia

9. **Depression is not caused by:** *(NIMHANS 2012)*
   A. Clonazepam
   B. Levodopa
   C. Metformin
   D. Corticosteroid

10. **All are true regarding depression except?** *(PGI NOV 2017)*
    A. More common in women
    B. Most common psychiatric disorder overall
    C. Most common age group is the middle age
    D. Is genetic in origin

11. **Which of the following psychiatric disorder has been projected to be 2nd leading cause of DALYs by 2020?**
    A. Dementia *(NIMHANS 2019, NIMHANS 2018)*
    B. Depression
    C. Schizophrenia
    D. Generalized Anxiety Disorder

Symptoms and Diagnosis

12. **Persistent feeling of guilt is seen in:** *(DNB NEET 2014-15)*
    A. Obsessive compulsive disorder
    B. Mania
    C. Depression
    D. Schizophrenia

13. **Which among the following is not a criterion to diagnose depression?** *(PGI May 2017)*
    A. Unexplained visceral pains
    B. Feeling of guilt
    C. Hypersomnia
    D. Insomnia
    E. Worthlessness

14. **Which of the following symptoms must be present for the diagnosis of major depressive disorder?**
    A. Loss of interest or pleasure *(MH 2010, 2007)*
    B. Recurrent suicidal tendencies
    C. Insomnia
    D. Indecisiveness

15. **Disruption or disorganization of biological rhythm is observed in:**
    A. Schizophrenia
    B. Anxiety
    C. Depression
    D. Mania

16. **"Nihilistic delusions" are seen in:** *(PGI 2000)*
    A. Endogenous depression
    B. Double depression
    C. Depression in involutional stage
    D. Cyclothymia
    E. Dysthymia

17. **True about psychotic feature in depression:** *(PGI Dec 2004)*
    A. Found in severe depression
    B. Found in moderate depression
    C. Mood incongruent psychotic feature
    D. Cyclothymia
    E. Dysthymia

18. **Intense nihilism, somatization and agitation in old age are the hallmark symptoms of:** *(AIIMS)*
    A. Involutional melancholia
    B. Atypical depression
    C. Somatized depression
    D. Depressive stupor

19. **True about major depressive disorder:** *(PGI 2003)*
    A. Commonly seen in female
    B. Recovery is complete after treatment
    C. Associated with hypothyroidism
    D. Family history of major depression

20. **Dysthymia is:** *(NIMHANS 2015, DNB NEET 2014-15)*
    A. Chronic mild depression
    B. Chronic severe depression
    C. Bipolar disorder
    D. Personality disorder

21. **Double depression is:** *(NIMHANS 2012)*
    A. Two episodes of depression
    B. Depression with dysthymia
    C. Depression for 2 years
    D. Dysthymia

22. **Most common type of postpuerperal psychosis is:** *(PGI 1999)*
    A. Depression
    B. Anxiety
    C. Mania
    D. Suicide

23. **Which of the following is not a feature of depression:** *(NIMHANS 2015)*
    A. Depressed mood
    B. Loss of appetite
    C. Hyperactivity
    D. Suicidal ideas

24. **Somatic symptoms of depression include all except:** *(NIMHANS 2013)*
    A. Feeling of guilt
    B. Reduced libido
    C. Insomnia
    D. Weight change

25. **All are true about atypical depression except:** *(AIIMS May, 2018)*
    A. Increased sleep and appetite are present
    B. TCAs work better than MAOIs and SSRIs
    C. Fatigue and heaviness of the lower limbs is present
    D. Variable mood reactivity to positive stimulus is a feature

26. **Intense depression and misery, without any cause is seen in:** *(NEET 2019)*
    A. Melancholic depression
    B. Reactive depression
    C. Schizophrenia
    D. Mania

Clinical Vignettes

Controversial Question

27. A 41-year-old woman presented with a history of aches and pains all over the body and generalized weakness for four years. She cannot sleep because of the illness and has lost her appetite as well. She has lack of interest in work and doesn't like to meet friends and relatives. She denies feelings of sadness. Her most likely diagnosis is: *(AIIMS Nov 2002)*
    A. Somatoform pain disorder
    B. Major depression
    C. Somatization disorder
    D. Dissociative disorder

28. A 60-year-old male is brought by his wife. He thinks that he had committed sins throughout his life. He is very much depressed and has considered com- mitting suicide but has not taken any such steps. He is also taking sessions with a spiritual guru. He does not get convinced when his wife tells him that he has led a pious life. How will you treat him? *(AIIMS)*
    A. Antipsychotic plus antidepressant
    B. Antidepressant with cognitive behavioral therapy
    C. Guidance and recounselling with guru plus antidepressant
    D. Antidepressant alone

29. A 60-year-old man whose wife died 3 months back now starts to believe that his intestines have rotten away and that he is responsible for the death of his wife and should be sent to prison. The most likely diagnosis is: *(NIMHANS 2012)*
    A. Delusional disorder
    B. Psychotic depression
    C. Grief psychosis
    D. Schizophrenia

30. An 18-year-old student complaints of lack of inter est in studies for last 6 months. He has frequent quarrels with his parents and has frequent headaches. The most appropriate clinical approach would be: *(AI 2005)*
    A. Leave him as normal adolescent problem
    B. Rule out depression
    C. Rule out migraine
    D. Rule out an oppositional defiant disorder

31. A 40-year-old female patient presents with history of depressed mood, loss of appetite, insomnia and lack of interest in surroundings for past one year. These symptoms followed soon after a business loss one year back. Which of the following statements is true regarding the management of this patient? *(AIIMS)*
    A. No treatment is necessary as it is due to business loss
    B. SSRI is the most efficacious of the available drugs
    C. Antidepressant treatment is based on the side effect profile of the drugs
    D. Combination therapy of two antidepressants should be given

32. A patient presents with depressed mood, loss of sleep, loss of hope, feeling of worthlessness and diminished concentration for last 1 month. Which of the following is the drug of choice in this patient? *(DNB NEET 2014-15)*
    A. SSRIs
    B. Atypical antidepressants
    C. Lithium
    D. Tricyclic antidepressants

33. A postnatal mother who delivered 2 days back presents with increased tearfulness and sleeplessness. No features of anhedonia, suicidal or lack of interest present. Most probable diagnosis: *(Jipmer 2017, PGI May 2015)*
    A. Mania
    B. Postpartum psychosis
    C. Postpartum blues
    D. Postpartum depression

34. A 28-year-old female was brought to psychiatry OPD. She appeared agitated and claimed that her husband has "stolen baby from her womb". Patient was also muttering to herself and has not slept for last 4 days. She had delivered a healthy female child three weeks back, however was not taking care of the baby. The symptoms started in seconds week postpartum. The likely diagnosis is: *(NEET 2016)*
    A. Postpartum blues
    B. Postpartum depression
    C. Postpartum psychosis
    D. Schizophrenia

35. A patient presents to the emergency department with self harm and indicates suicidal intent. Which of the following conditions does not warrant an immediate specialist assessment? *(AI 2010)*
    A. Formal thought disorder
    B. Acute alcohol intoxication
    C. Chronic severe physical illness
    D. Social isolation

36. Mr A, comes to the psychiatry OPD with complaints of irritability, guilt of not being able to perform well in office and decreased interest in recreational activities since he left college 3 years back. *(AIIMS Nov 2017)*
    A. Adjustment disorder
    B. Dysthymia
    C. Cyclothymia
    D. Major depressive episode

Controversial Question

37. A patient is depressed for past 3 years, does not go out of his house much and is cut off from the society. But with normal sleep and normal weight. Most probable diagnosis is? *(DNB December 2011)*
    A. Major depression
    B. Dysthymia
    C. Chronic fatigue syndrome
    D. No psychiatric illness

38. Neurotic depression in ICD-9 is stated as ____ in ICD-10? *(JIPMER 2016)*
    A. Dysthymia
    B. Somatoform disorder
    C. Adjustment disorder
    D. Delirium

39. True about Premenstrual Dysphoric Disorder (PMDD) is: *(PGI May 16)*
    A. It starts before menses, continues during menses and is relieved after menses
    B. Associated with major depressive disorder in females
    C. Severity increases with increasing levels of estradiol
    D. Has serious effect on normal relationship and lifestyle
    E. Treated conservatively with diet change and diuretics

40. Drug of choice for "Premenstrual Dysphoric Disorder" is:
    A. Benzodiazepines
    B. TCAs
    C. Progesterone
    D. SSRIs

Treatment

41. Which of the following drugs is correctly matched with its common side effect? *(NIMHANS 2017)*
    A. Clozapine: dryness of mouth
    B. Mirtazapine: akathisia
    C. Bupropion: premature ejaculation
    D. Sertraline: delayed ejaculation

42. SSRIs should be carefully used in the young for the management of depression due to increase in: *(DNB NEET 2014-15)*
    A. Nihilism ideation
    B. Guilt ideation
    C. Suicidal ideation
    D. Envious ideation

43. A 22 year old female was diagnosed with depression and was started on escitalopram. All are the side effects of escitalopram except? *(AIIMS May, 2018)*
    A. Nausea
    B. Vivid dreams
    C. Anorgasmia
    D. Sialorhera

44. The clinical effects of the antidepressant drugs is mainly based on: *(DNB NEET 2014-15)*
    A. Change in neurotransmitter receptor sensitivity
    B. Decreased levels of neurotransmitters
    C. Change in efficacy of neurotransmitters
    D. None of the above

45. Mechanism of action of bupropion is: *(DNB NEET 2014-15)*
    A. Increased levels of GABA
    B. Increased levels of norepinephrine in the synaptic cleft
    C. Increased levels of dopamine in the synaptic cleft
    D. Both B and C

46. Repetitive transcranial magnetic stimulation (rTMS) is approved by USFDA for the treatment of: *(AI 2012)*
    A. Resistant schizophrenia
    B. Obsessive compulsive disorder
    C. Acute psychosis
    D. Depression

47. A young female on antidepressants presents to the emergency with altered sensorium and hypotension. ECG reveals wide QRS complexes and right axis deviation. What is the next best step? *(AIIMS Nov 2015)*
    A. Sodium bicarbonate
    B. Hemodialysis
    C. Fomepizole
    D. Flumazenil

48. A patient who is a known case of a psychiatric illness is on anitpsychotics, antidepressants and antihypertensives. He suddenly developed tachycardia and chest tightness. On evaluation he had metabolic acidosis. ECG showed – widened QRS complex and prolonged QT interval. Which of the following drug is responsible for this? *(AIIMS May 2017)*
    A. Amlodipine
    B. Amitriptyline
    C. Enalapril
    D. Chlorthalidone

49. Rathi, 26-year-old female has been diagnosed to be suffering from depression. Now for the past 2 days she has suicidal tendency, thought and ideas. The best treatment is: *(AIIMS 2001)*
    A. Amitriptyline
    B. Selegiline
    C. Haloperidol + chlorpromazine
    D. ECT

50. A patient comes in stuporous condition. Patient's parents give history of patient being continually sad and suicidal attempts and not eating and sleeping for most of the time. The treatment is: *(AIIMS 2000)*
    A. ECT
    B. Antidepressant
    C. Antipsychotic
    D. Sedative

51. A patient on antidepressant therapy developed sudden hypertension on consuming cheese. The antidepressant is possibly: *(PGI 1999)*
    A. Amitriptyline
    B. Tranylcypromine
    C. Fluoxetine
    D. Sertraline

52. Which of the following are side effects of mirtazapine? *(PGI Nov 2016)*
    A. Weight gain
    B. Weight loss
    C. Sedation
    D. Blurred vision

53. Tricyclic antidepressant side effects include: *(PGI May 2018)*
    A. Tremors
    B. Hypertension
    C. Weight loss
    D. Diarrhoea
    E. Gynaeomastia

54. A patient on treatment for psychiatric disorder takes overdose of a drug, develops bradycardia, hypotension, decreased sweating and salivation. The likely drug is: *(NIMHANS 2016, AIIMS 1999)*
    A. Amitriptyline
    B. Lithium
    C. Selegiline
    D. Amphetamine

55. Tricyclic antidepressant are contraindicated in: *(DNB 1997, AI 1991)*
    A. Glaucoma
    B. Brain tumor
    C. Bronchial asthma
    D. Hypertension

56. Which of the following medicines are associated with side effect of sexual dysfunction? *(NEET 2016)*
    A. Fluoxetine
    B. Mirtazapine
    C. Bupropion
    D. None

57. Following drugs have abuse liability except: *(DNB 2003)*
    A. Buprenorphine
    B. Alprazolam
    C. Fluoxetine
    D. Dextropropoxyphene

58. Tianeptine acts by: *(AIIMS 1998)*
    A. MAO inhibitor
    B. Serotonin uptake inhibitor
    C. Serotonin uptake enhancer
    D. 5HT agonist

59. What is/are the side effects of SSRI? *(PGI)*
    A. Insomnia
    B. Sedation
    C. Nausea
    D. Seizure precipitation
    E. Weight gain

60. Not true regarding serotonin syndrome is: *(AIIMS)*
    A. It is predictable and not idiosyncratic
    B. SSRIs and MAOIs cause it
    C. IV dantrolene is the treatment of choice
    D. Hypertension, hyperthermia and hyperreflexia are the signs

61. Stimulation of which of the following nerve cause elevation of mood? *(AIIMS Nov 2009)*
    A. Olfactory nerve
    B. Optic nerve
    C. Trigeminal nerve
    D. Vagus nerve

62. Following are the somatic therapies used in depression, except: *(DNB NEET 2014-15)*
    A. Electroconvulsive therapy
    B. Deep brain stimulation
    C. Transcranial magnetic stimulation
    D. Ultrasound brain stem stimulation

63. The evidence-based psychological therapy of choice for depression is: *(AIIMS May 2014)*
    A. Group discussion therapy
    B. Counselling
    C. Cognitive behavioral therapy
    D. Psychological psychotherapy

64. Phototherapy is used to treat which of the following psychiatric condition: *(DNB NEET 2014-15)*
    A. Depression
    B. Mental retardation
    C. Schizophrenia
    D. Obsessive compulsive disorder

65. Which of the following indications of deep brain stimulation is not FDA approved? *(AIPG 2013)*
    A. OCD
    B. Major depression
    C. Parkinsonism
    D. Dystonia

66. Sudden discontinuation of which of the following drugs can cause agitation, anxiety and insomnia? *(AIIMS May, 2018)*
    A. Imipramine
    B. Velnafaxine
    C. Olanzapine
    D. Valproate

67. Which is selective serotonin and noradrenaline reuptake inhibitors: *(PGI, Nov 2017)*
    A. Duloxetine
    B. Venlafaxine
    C. Milnacipran
    D. Dapoxetine
    E. Paroxetine

Suicide

68. Increased suicidal tendency is associated with: *(DNB NEET 2014-15)*
    A. Increased noradrenaline
    B. Decreased serotonin
    C. Decreased dopamine
    D. Increased GABA

69. Which of the following regarding "suicide" is not correct? *(PGI May, 2018)*
    A. Young age and male sex is a risk factor
    B. Hopelessness is one of the strongest risk factor
    C. Parasuicide is defined as a failed attempt to kill self
    D. Risk is increased with substance use
    E. History of previous suicide attempt is the most important risk factor

70. A 25-year-old female, living as a paying guest, consumed multiple number of sleeping pills. Which of the following is not a risk factor of suicide? *(NIMHANS 2017)*
    A. Hopelessness
    B. Insomnia
    C. Social isolation
    D. Substance abuse

71. Suicidal tendencies are most common in: *(PGI 2000)*
    A. Involutional depression
    B. Reactive depression
    C. Psychotic depression
    D. Childhood depression

72. Emile Durkheim is linked with work on which of the following conditions in psychiatry? *(DNB NEET 2014-15)*
    A. Suicide
    B. Obsessive compulsive disorder
    C. Anxiety disorder
    D. Schizophrenia

73. Incidence of suicide in India is: *(PGI June 2005)*
    A. 8-10/100 population
    B. 8-10/1000 population
    C. 8-10/10000 population
    D. 8-10/100000 population

74. Which of the following is not a suicide predictor? *(NIMHANS 2019)*
    A. Adolescence
    B. Substance abuse
    C. Suicide note written
    D. Previous suicidal attempt

75. Suicide risk is seen in all except: *(NIMHANS 2016)*
    A. Social isolation
    B. Male sex
    C. Drug dependence
    D. Somatization

76. Copycat suicide is seen at age of: *(FMGE 2017)*
    A. Adolescence
    B. Child age
    C. Adult age
    D. Old age

Bipolar Disorder

Classification

77. **Chromosome associated with bipolar disorder:**
    (PGI Dec 2005)
    A. Chromosome 16   B. Chromosome 13
    C. Chromosome 18   D. Chromosome 11
    E. Chromosome 23

78. **Bipolar II disorder includes:**
    (DNB NEET 2014-15, AIIMS 2011)
    A. Cyclothymic disorder
    B. Dysthymia
    C. Single manic episode
    D. Major depression and hypomania

79. **All of the following are included in diagnosis of bipolar disorder except:** *(AI 2007)*
    A. Mania alone   B. Depression alone
    C. Mania and depression D. Mania and anxiety

80. **Which of the following is/are included in bipolar disorders:** *(PGI Nov 2010)*
    A. Hypomania   B. Cyclothymia
    C. Paranoid disorder   D. Hyperthymia
    E. Kleptomania

81. **The period of normalcy is seen between two psychosis. The diagnosis is:** *(AI 1999)*
    A. Schizophrenia   B. Manic depressive psychosis
    C. Alcoholism   D. Depression

82. **All of the following are true about bipolar disorder except:** *(NIMHANS 2012)*
    A. Prevalence is more amongst females than males
    B. Lifetime prevalence is around 1%
    C. Mean age of onset is 21 years
    D. Prevalence varies according to socioeconomic status

Symptoms and Diagnosis

83. **According to the ICD, for establishing a diagnosis of mania, the symptoms should persist for at least:**
    (NEET 2016, AIIMS May 2014, DNB 2010)
    A. 1 week   B. 2 weeks
    C. 3 weeks   D. 4 weeks

84. **The clinical features of mania include:** *(PGI 2006, 2002)*
    A. Anhedonia   B. Elated mood
    C. Avolition   D. Delusion of grandiosity
    E. Distractibility

85. **Mania is characterized by:** *(PGI 1999)*
    A. Paranoid delusions B. Loss of orientation
    C. High self esteem   D. Loss of insight

86. **Mania is unlikely to present with:** *(PGI May, 2018)*
    A. Delusion of Grandiosity
    B. Delusion of guilt
    C. Delusion of persecution
    D. Delusion of enormity
    E. Hypochondriac delusion

87. **Sleep pattern seen in mania is:** *(NEET 2016)*
    A. Hypersomnia   B. Insomnia
    C. Decreased need for sleep D. Somnambulism

88. **Which of the following is not a feature of mania?**
    (NIMHANS 2015)
    A. Disorientation   B. Delusion of grandeur
    C. Elation   D. Pressure of speech

Clinical Vignettes

89. **A 20-year-old man has presented with increased alcohol consumption and sexual indulgence, irritability, lack of sleep, and not feeling fatigued even on prolonged periods of activity. All these changes have been present for 3 weeks. The most likely diagnosis is:** *(AI 2003)*
    A. Alcohol dependence
    B. Schizophrenia
    C. Mania
    D. Impulsive control disorder

90. **A 67-year-old lady is brought in by her 6 children saying that she has gone senile. Six months after her husband's death she has become more religious, spiritual and gives lots of money in donation. She is occupied in too many activities and sleepless. She now believes that she has a goal to change the society. She does not like being brought to the hospital and is argumentative on being questioned on her doings. The diagnosis is:** *(AI 2002)*
    A. Depression   B. Schizophrenia
    C. Mania   D. Impulse control disorder

91. **A 42-year-old male with a past history of a manic episode presents with an illness of 1 month duration characterized by depressed mood, anhedonia and profound psychomotor retardation. The most appropriate management strategy is prescribing a combination of:**
    (AIIMS 2004)
    A. Antipsychotics and antidepressants
    B. Antidepressants and mood stabilizers
    C. Antipsychotics and mood stabilizers
    D. Antidepressants and benzodiazepines

92. **A 25-year-old female with bipolar disorder wants to get pregnant. Which drug should be avoided?**
    A. Valproate   *(NIMHANS 2019)*
    B. Carbamazepine
    C. Lithium
    D. Lamotrigine

93. **What of the following statements is not true?**
    (NIMHANS 2019)
    A. Postpartum psychoses is usually associated with full recovery
    B. Previous history of bipolar disorder, is a risk for postpartum psychoses
    C. Postpartum blues occurs after 2 weeks of delivery
    D. Puerperal psychosis is usually related to bipolar disorders

Treatment

Controversial Question

94. **Drug of choice in acute mania is:** *(DNB NEET 2015)*
    A. Lithium   B. Chlorpromazine
    C. Valproic acid   D. Risperidone

Mood Disorders

95. A patient was brought to the ER with non stop talking, singing, uncontrollable behavior and apparent loss of contact with reality. It is diagnosed as a case of acute mania. Which of the following drugs is most suitable for rapid control of his symptoms?
    A. Lithium
    B. Haloperidol
    C. Valproate
    D. Diazepam

96. Use of lithium in pregnancy can result in which of the following abnormalities in the baby? *(AIIMS Nov 2018)*
    A. Cardiovascular defect
    B. Urogenital defect
    C. Neural tube defect
    D. Craniofacial deformity

97. Treatment of mania includes: *(PGI Nov 2017)*
    A. Antidepressant drugs
    B. Antipsychotics
    C. ECT
    D. Mood stabilisers

98. Drug of choice for rapid cycling manic depressive psychosis (bipolar disorder) is: *(DNB 2004, AI 1999)*
    A. Lithium
    B. Carbamazepine
    C. Sodium valproate
    D. Haloperidol

99. Prophylactic maintenance serum levels of lithium is: *(NIMHANS 2013, DNB 1997)*
    A. 0.2–0.8 mEq/L
    B. 0.7–1.2 mEq/L
    C. 1.2–2.0 mEq/L
    D. 2.0–2.5 mEq/L

100. How many days before surgery should lithium be stopped? *(AIIMS 2013)*
    A. 1 day
    B. 2 days
    C. 3 days
    D. 5 days

101. All of following can be seen in severe lithium toxicity except: *(PGI May 2016)*
    A. Ataxia
    B. Seizures
    C. Hyporeflexia with normal relaxation
    D. Stupor
    E. Muscle fasciculations

102. True about Lithium toxicity: *(PGI 2012)*
    A. Causes ebstein anomaly
    B. Decreases neutrophil count
    C. Decreases eosinophil count
    D. Optimum concentration is 0.2–0.6 mEq/L
    E. Decreases sodium excretion

103. True about Lithium treatment in mania:
    A. Commonest side effect is tremor
    B. Toxic level is <1.5 mg/dL serum level
    C. Amiodarone is DOC for Li induced diabetes insipidus
    D. Lithium is 90% protein bound
    E. Tremor is treated with propranolol

104. A patient is brought to the casualty in the state of altered sensorium. He was on lithium treatment for affective disorder and has suffered through an attack of epileptic fits. On examination he has worsening tremors, increased DTR's and incontinence of urine. He has also undergone an episode of severe gastroenteritis 2 days ago. The serum lithium was found to be 1.95 mEq/L. The probable cause for his present state is: *(AIIMS 2001)*
    A. Lithium toxicity
    B. Dehydration
    C. Manic episode
    D. Depressive stupor

105. Which of the following are dermatologic side effects of lithium? *(PGI May 2017)*
    A. Acne
    B. Rash
    C. Psoriasis
    D. Pemphigus
    E. Blisters
    F. Angioneurotic edema

106. Best use of lithium is in: *(DNB NEET 2014-15)*
    A. Treatment of schizophrenia
    B. Treatment of recurrent depression
    C. Treatment of first depressive episode
    D. Prevention of recurrence in bipolar mood disorder

107. A male patient with bipolar disorder is controlled on medications. Symptoms of mania start to appear whenever he himself tapers down the drugs. What type of treatment can improve compliance in this patient?
    A. Psychoeducation *(AIIMS Nov 2015)*
    B. CBT
    C. Supportive psychotherapy
    D. Insight oriented psychotherapy

108. Which of the following is true for lithium: *(FMGE 2018)*
    A. Delayed absorption
    B. Narrow therapeutic index
    C. Protein bound
    D. Can be given safely in renal dysfunction

109. Lamotrigine is used in the treatment of: *(NIMHANS 2012)*
    A. Euphoric mania
    B. Hypomania
    C. Bipolar depression
    D. Dysphoric mania

110. Mood stabilizer which is not used for treatment of mania in paediatric age group is: *(JIPMER 2017)*
    A. Lithium
    B. Valproate
    C. Carbamazepine
    D. Oxcarbazepine

111. What is the half life of valproate? *(NIMHANS 2019)*
    A. 3 to 5 hours
    B. 11 to 17 hours
    C. More than 36 hours
    D. 24 to 36 hours

112. Which Australian psychiatrist demonstrated that Lithium can be used for treatment of manic depressive psychosis? *(NIMHANS 2018)*
    A. John Cade
    B. Alexander Ure
    C. Humphrey Davy
    D. Alfred

Controversial Question

113. A 30-year-old pregnant woman comes to your clinic with decreased sleep, increased appetite and hyperactivity for last 2 weeks. A diagnosis of mania is made. Further probing reveals four episodes of major depression in the past two years. What drug will you prescribe to this patient? *(AIIMS Nov 2015)*
    A. Haloperidol
    B. Lithium
    C. Promethazine
    D. Clonazepam

114. Which of the following mood stabilisers has anti-suicide property? *(AIIMS 2017)*
    A. Lithium
    B. Carbamezipine
    C. Valproate
    D. Lamotrigine

115. **Valproate is preferred over lithium in all of the following conditions except:** *(NIMHANS 2014)*
    A. Elated mania
    B. In renal compromise
    C. Dysphoric mania
    D. Mania with psychosis

116. **False statement regarding myocardial infarction and depression is:** *(NIMHANS 2013)*
    A. Depression is a risk factor for MI
    B. MI is a risk factor for depression
    C. SSRI's can be used post MI for treatmemt of depression
    D. Only Cognitive behavioral therapy is used after MI

Prospective Questions

117. **This image is representative of the following procedure used in treatment of Depression?**
    A. rTMS
    B. VNS
    C. ECT
    D. DBS

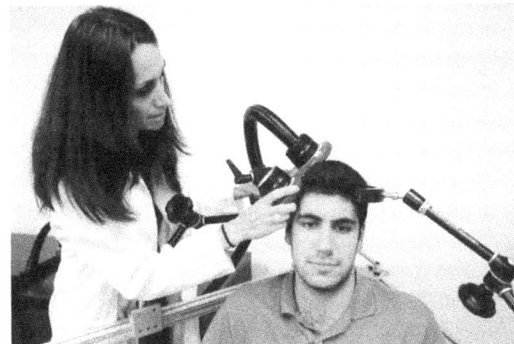

118. **The procedure described in the image is used for diagnosis of which of the following disorders?**

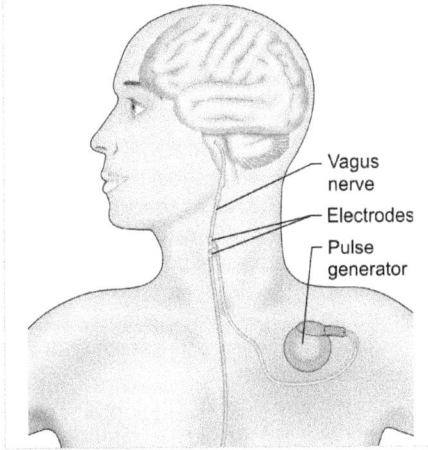

    A. Depression
    B. Mania
    C. Schizophrenia
    D. Obsessive compulsive disorder

119. **This image is representative of which of the following sign:**
    A. Veraguth fold seen in depression
    B. Omega sign seen in depression
    C. Veraguth fold seen in mania
    D. Veraguth fold seen in mania

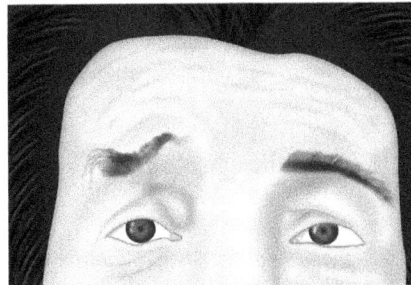

120. **This image is representative of which of the following signs:**
    A. Veraguth fold seen in depression
    B. Omega sign seen in depression
    C. Veraguth fold seen in mania
    D. Veraguth fold seen in mania

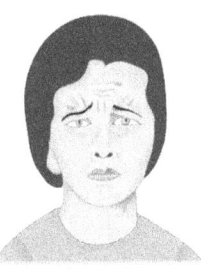

AIIMS New Pattern Question

121. **Reason assertion type**
    A. SSRIs are the first line treatment in patients with depression
    B. Amongst all the antidepressants, SSRIs have the fastest onset of action Statement (A) is the assertion and statement (B) is the reason
        A. Both Assertion and Reasons are independently true/correct statements and the Reason is the correct explanation for the Assertion
        B. Both Assertion and Reasons are independently true/correct statements, but the Reason is not the correct explanation for the Assertion
        C. Assertion is independently a true/correct statement, but the Reasons is independently a false/incorrect statement
        D. Assertion is independently a false/incorrect statement, but the Reasons is independently a true/correct statement
        E. Both Assertion and Reasons are independently false/incorrect statements

Answers With Explanations

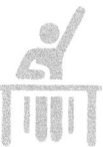

1. B. Middle aged female.
2. B. Serotonin and norepinephrine.
3. A. Depression.
4. D. Guilt.
5. A. Negative thought of past.
6. A, C and D.
7. A, C.
   Depression is the most common psychiatric illness associated with both hypothyroidism and hyperthyroidism. Also, in adrenal disorders like Cushing's syndrome and Addison's disease, depression is commonly associated.
8. A, B, C.
   In hypopituitarism, depression is commonly seen.
9. C. Few common medications which cause depression include antihypertensives (reserpine, methyldopa, beta blockers), steroids (corticosteroids, oral contraceptive pills), interferons, barbiturates and benzodiazepines (like clonazepam).
10. B. As a group, anxiety disorders are the commonest psychiatric disorder. Amongst the individual disorders, specific phobia is the most common psychiatric disorder.
11. B. Depression. According to Global Burden of Disease Study, Unipolar major depression would be the second leading cause of DALYs (disability adjusted life years) by 2020, with Ischemic heart diseases being the leading cause.

Symptoms and Diagnosis

12. C. Depression
13. A. Unexplained visceral pains.
14. A. According to DSM-IV and DSM-5, to diagnose depression at least one of the following two symptoms should be present (1) depressed mood (2) loss of interest or pleasure.
15. C. There are characteristic disturbances of sleep (early morning insomnia and reduced latency of REM sleep) in depression.
16. A, B, C.
    Psychotic symptoms are seen more commonly in both endogenous and melancholic depression (depression in involutional stage). It can also be seen in double depression, though less commonly (double depression is depression superimposed over dysthymia).
17. A, B, C.
    According to ICD-11, psychotics symptoms can be seen in both moderate and severe depression. The psychotic symptoms can be either mood congruent or mood incongruent.
18. A. Involutional melancholia.
19. A, C and D.
    The recovery is often incomplete in patients with depression.
20. A. Chronic mild depression.
21. B. Depression with dysthymia
22. A. The most common type of postpuerperal psychosis is depression.
23. C. Hyperactivity is not a common symptom of depression
24. A. Feeling of guilt. The somatic symptoms refers to the biological symptoms and includes amongst other things, sleep, appetite and sexual disturbances.
25. B. MAOIs and SSRIs are more effective than TCAs in the treatment of atypical depression.
26. A. Melancholic depression is characterised by a state of intensely depressed mood and feeling of misery.

Clinical Vignettes

27. B. In this case, patient has significant somatic symptoms such as aches and pain and generalized weakness. In a large number of patients, depression presents mostly with somatic complaints and patient may deny psychological symptoms such as sadness of mood. Further, in this patient there are sleep and appetite abnormalities along with loss of interest which clinches the diagnosis of depression.
28. A. This patient has depression with psychotic symptoms. The patient belief that he committed sins in his life, and the fact that despite his wife assurances he continues to hold the belief is suggestive of delusion. Hence, this patient should be treated with antidepressants and antipsychotics.
29. B. Psychotic depression. The symptoms in this question are suggestive of nihilistic delusions (intestine are rotting away) and pathological guilt (belief that patient is responsible for death). Both these symptoms are usually seen in patients with severe depression. The death of wife could have acted as the stressor that resulted in the development of severe depressive episode with psychotic symptoms (or psychotic depression). Please remember, whenever symptoms are severe enough to warrant an independent diagnosis, it's better to give an independent diagnosis, even if symptoms develop during the grief period.
30. B. In children and adolescents, depression frequently presents with irritability, lack of interest and changes in behavior such as withdrawn behavior or quarrelsome behavior. Its important to rule out depression first.
31. C. The diagnosis in this case is depression. The depression can be precipitated by various stressors, and irrespective of what precipitated it, it should always be treated. Further, all the available antidepressants have similar efficacy and the choice of antidepressants is usually dictated by the side effect profile of the drug. SSRIs are usually used as the first antidepressants because of their favorable side effect profile.
32. A. SSRIs.

33. C. Postpartum blues. These symptoms usually get resolved by 10th day postpartum.
34. C. Postpartum psychosis. Onset in postpartum period, and history of delusions (that husband has stolen baby from womb) and possibly hallucinations (as suggested by muttering to self) is suggestive of postpartum psychosis.
35. B. The suicidal intent in a person with formal thought disorder (most likely a patient with schizophrenia), chronic severe physical illness and social isolation, should be taken very seriously and immediate measures taken must include assessment by a specialist. If patient has expressed suicidal intent in an inebriated state, it must still be ensured that he doesn't harm himself however a specialist assessment can be deferred till he is sober.
36. B. Dysthymia. There are not enough symptoms to diagnose depression here, further the socio-occupational dysfunction history is not given (he appears to be going to office) which again goes against depression, and duration of symptoms is more than two years. The diagnosis of adjustment disorder is ruled out as there is no clear stressor (leaving college cannot be considered as one).
37. B. Dysthymia. This is a poorly framed question. "Cut off from the society" suggests decreased social interaction. Sleep and appetite is normal, and no other symptoms have been mentioned. Hence, we don't have enough symptoms to diagnose depression. Given the long duration of symptoms, dysthymia is the best answer.
38. A. Dysthymia. Neurotic depression of ICD-9 corresponds to dysthymia in ICD-10.
39. A, B, D, E.
    The symptoms are present in the week before menses, and start to improve within a few days of onset of menses and become absent or minimal in the week post menses. Hence, the symptoms increase when the levels of ovarian steroids are low (in the late luteal phase). Therefor option C here is wrong whereas option A is true.
    PMDD significantly affects the social and occupational functioning (Option D is correct)
    PMDD is usually treated symptomatically using analgesics. In some patients SSRIs, alprazolam and diuretics are use (Option E is correct).
    Depression is the most frequently reported previous disorder in individuals with PMDD (option B is correct).
40. D. SSRIs are considered as DOC for Premenstrual dysphoric disorder.

Treatment

41. D. Delayed ejaculation is a common side effect of SSRIs.
42. C. The use of SSRIs can increase suicidal ideations. This side effect is more common in children and adolescents and hence these medications should be used cautiously in that age group.
43. D. Sialorrhea is not a common side effect of SSRIs. It's a common side effect of clozapine.
44. A. The recent research has shown that its not the increase in neurotransmitters levels in synapse which causes antidepressant effect. Rather, secondary to increased neurotransmitter levels, the receptor sensitivity changes over a course of time and that is responsible for antidepressant effect.
45. D. Both B and C.
46. D. Depression.
47. A. This patient was most likely on tricyclic antidepressants and it appears to be a case of tricyclic antidepressant overdosage as the patient is experiencing arrhythmias, hypotension and has also developed altered sensorium. The mainstay of treatment in TCA induced cardiotoxicity is intravenous sodium bicarbonate. It is used if the QRS interval is prolonged (usually more than 100 milliseconds) and can reverse the toxic effects of TCAs. Because of large volume of distribution and high protein binding of TCAs, hemodialysis is not effective. Further flumazenil and fomepizole have no role.
48. B. Amitriptyline. The clinical presentation is consistent with tricyclic antidepressant toxicity.
49. D. In depression with suicide risk, ECT is the treatment of choice.
50. A. This patient most likely has depression with stupor. ECT is again the treatment of choice.
51. B. This is history of cheese reaction on MAO inhibitors.
52. A, C.
    Weight gain and sedation are common side effects of mirtazapine.
53. A, B, E.
    Tremors are one of the common neurological side effects of TCAs. Usually hypotension is a side effect, however hypertension can also be occasionally seen. TCAs (especially amoxapine) have also been found to be associated with hyperprolactinemia and may cause amennorhea, gynaecomastia, impotence, galactorrhea etc.
    TCAs often cause weight gain and anticholinergic side effects like constipation
54. A. The symptoms are suggestive of tricyclic antidepressants overdose (anticholinergic side effects).
55. A. Due to anticholinergic action, TCAs should be avoided in glaucoma.
56. A. Fluoxetine. SSRIs like fluoxetine are associated with sexual side effects.
57. C. SSRIs do not have any abuse liability. Both opioids (buprenorphine, dextropropoxyphene) and benzodiazepines (alprazolam) have abuse liability.
58. C. Serotonin uptake enhancer.
59. A, B, C, E.
    SSRIs can cause both sedation as well as insomnia. In long term they can cause weight gain. Nausea, diarrhoea, anxiety and sweating are some common side effects.
60. C. Dantrolene is not the treatment of choice, though it is at times used to control the hyperthermia.
61. D. Vagal nerve stimulation can be used for treatment of depression.
62. D. ECT, deep brain stimulation as well as transcranial magnetic stimulation can be used for treatment of depression.
63. C. Cognitive behavioral therapy.
64. A. Depression associated with a seasonal pattern can be treated with phototherapy.

65. B. Depression. FDA approved indications for deep brain stimulation are:
    a. Parkinson's disease and essential tremors
    b. Dystonia
    c. Obsessive compulsive disorder
66. B. Venlafaxine is most commonly associated with discontinuation syndrome.
67. A, B, C

Suicide

68. B. Decreased levels of 5 HIAA (which is a metabolite of serotonin) are related to increased risk of suicide.
69. A, C.
    Males have higher suicide risk than females. Please remember that females make more suicide attempts than males, however males complete suicide more commonly than females. This difference is mostly due to method used, males tend to use more lethal methods such as gun and hence are more likely to complete suicide. However young age is not a risk factor (age > 45 years is a risk factor).
70. B. Insomnia. Hopelessness, social isolation (poor social support) and substance abuse are risk factors for suicide
71. A, C.
    Endogenous depression, depression with psychotic symptoms (psychotic depression) and involutional depression (depression with melancholic features) are associated with higher suicide risk.
72. A. Emile Durkheim studied extensively the social factors associated with suicide.
73. D. The data for incidence of suicide is released by government every year. According to NCRB (National Crime Record Bureau), in 2014, the suicide rate in India was 10.6/lac of population.
74. A. Adolescent age is not considered a risk factor for suicide.
75. D. Somatization. The rest three are risk factors for suicide.
76. A. Copycat suicide is usually seen in adolescents.

Bipolar Disorder

Classification

77. C. Chromosome 18.
78. D. Major depression and hypomania.
79. B. Even a single episode of mania is sufficient to make a diagnosis of bipolar disorder.
80. A, B.
81. B. Manic depressive psychosis was the older name for bipolar disorder. In bipolar disorder, in between the episodes, patient is usually normal.
82. A. The prevalence if bipolar is almost equal in men and women with male to female ratio being 1.1:1

Symptoms and Diagnosis

83. A. 1 week.
84. B, D, E.
85. C, D.
    Insight is absent in mania and usually high self esteem is also a clinical feature.
86. B, D, E
    Delusion of grandiosity and delusion of persecution can be seen in manic patients. Delusion of persecution is often secondary to delusion of grandiosity (e.g. A patient said that 'I am the most intelligent person in the world and thats why government wants to kill me)
    Delusion of guilt and delusion of enormity, is usually seen in patients with severe depression.
    Hypochondriacal delusions (delusion of having a serious illness) is usually not seen in mania.
87. C. Decreased need for sleep
88. A. Disorientation. Please remember, presence of disorientation or disturbance of consciousness suggests an organic mental disorder like delirium.

Clinical Vignettes

89. C. Please remember that in manic stages, the substance intake also frequently increases.
90. C. Kindly don't get confused with the fact that the symptoms are following husband's death. Even negative life events can precipitate manic episode. This patient has increased religiosity, overspending (giving excessive donation), increased activity levels, decreased sleep, new interests and goals (of changing society) and lack of insight (doesn't want to come to hospital). All these symptoms are suggestive of mania.
91. B. The patient had a manic episode in past and currently he is in severe depression (as suggested by profound psychomotor retardation). The complete diagnosis would be bipolar disorder (currently severe depressive episode). Hence, this patient should receive both mood stabilizers and antidepressants.
92. A. Valproate is the most unsafe, amongst all the mood stabilsiers.
93. C. Postpartum blues usually have an onset within 3 to 5 days of delivery. All other options are correct statements

Treatment

94. D. Risperidone. Antipsychotics are considered as drug of choice if a patient develops acute mania as they have a faster onset of action. According to NICE guidelines, 'If a person develops mania or hypomania and is not taking an antipsychotic or mood stabiliser, offer haloperidol, olanzapine, quetiapine, or risperidone'.
95. B. Haloperidol. For rapid control of symptoms, antipsychotics are the preferred. For rapid control of agitation, and psychosis, usually parenteral antipsychotics are used. Benzodiazepines can also be used.
96. A. Lithium use in pregnancy can cause cardiovascular malformation in foetus, most commonly Ebsteins anomaly.
97. B, C, D.
    Mood stabilisers and antipsychotics are obviously used in treatment of mania. In cases of severe mania which is not responding to medications, ECTs can also be used. Antidepressants have no role in treatment of manic episode.
98. C. Sodium valproate.

99. B. 0.7–1.2 mEq/L.
100. B. Lithium should be stopped two days prior to surgery.
101. C. Hyporeflexia is not a feature of lithium toxicity. The neurological signs of lithium toxicity include blurred vision, muscle fasciculations, hyperactive deep tendon reflexes, convulsions, stupor and can finally result in death.

    # Important fact: Activated charcoal is not effective in lithium toxicity. To remove unabsorbed lithium, sodium polystyrene sulfonate or polyethylene glycol solution are used.

102. E > A.

    Dehydration as well as low sodium levels pre dispose to lithium toxicity. Ebstein anomaly is a teratogenic effect of lithium and as such is not a sign of lithium toxicity. Lithium causes neutrophilia and eosinophilia.

103. A, C, E
104. A. The gastroenteritis causes dehydration and may result in lithium toxicity (the body handles lithium similarly to sodium. In presence of dehydration, sodium absorption is increased and lithium absorption is also increased in kidneys). The lithium toxicity may present with tremors, increased reflexes and seizure.
105. A, B, C. The common dermatologic side effects of lithium include acne, hair loss, psoriasis and rash.
106. D. Prevention of recurrence in bipolar mood disorder
107. A. Psychoeducation is a form of psychological intervention in which patient as well as family members are educated about various aspects of disease and its treatment. It involves discussion about the symptoms, the need for medications as well as maintenance of a regular lifestyle. Psychoeducation decreases the chances of relapses in bipolar disorder.
108. B. Lithium has a narrow therapeutic index.
109. C. Lamotrigine is primarily used for management of bipolar depression.
110. D. Oxcarbazepine. Lithium, valproate and carbamazepine are all used in treatment of mania in paediatric age group. Oxcarbazepine has not been found to be useful for the same.
111. B. The plasma half life of valproate is 10-16 hours.
112. A. John Cade.
113. A. Haloperidol. If a patient develops acute manic episode in pregnancy, antipsychotics are preferred over use of any mood stabilisers, because of better safety profile.
114. A. Lithium. Lithium has been found to decrease both suicide attempts and completed suicides in a patient with bipolar disorder.
115. A. Elated mania. In elated or euphoric mania, lithium is preferred. In rest of the options, valproate is preferred. In renal compromise, lithium is avoided due to its renal side effects.
116. D. The first three options are correct. Depression and myocardial infarction are risk factors for each other. The treatment of depression after MI involves both medications and CBT.

Prospective Answers

117. A. rTMS. This image shows use of transcranial magnetic stimulation.
118. A. The image is illustrative of vagal nerve stimulation which is used for treatment of Depression.
119. A. The image shows a triangular skin fold on the nasal side of upper eyelid, referred as veraguth fold, seen in depression.
120. B. The image shows omega shaped skin folds on the forehead of the patient, referred to as omega sign, sen in depression.

AIIMS New Pattern Answer

121. C. Assertion is a correct statement. SSRIs are the first line treatment in depression. One of the SSRIs is usually the first drug that is used in the treatment of depression Reason is an incorrect statement. SSRIs do not have the fastest onset of action, all antidepressants take similar time for their onset of action

4
CHAPTER

Neurotic, Stress-related and Somatoform Disorders

According to the newer classifications (ICD-11 & DSM-5), the disorders have been reclassified under various diagnostic groups. For the sake of simplicity, they have been described together in this chapter.

4.1 ANXIETY DISORDERS

Anxiety

Anxiety is a common experience. It is an alerting signal and helps a person to take measures to deal with a threat. It must be differentiated from fear. Fear is the response one would have if he sees a snake. The fear is a response to a known, external and definite threat. Anxiety is the response one would have before exams. It is the response to an unknown, internal and vague threat.

Manifestations of Anxiety
- Feeling of nervousness
- Sweating, tachycardia, restlessness, tremors, mydriasis
- Diarrhea, urinary frequency
- **Cold clammy skin**^{Q}, hyperreflexia.

Anxiety Disorders

As a group, anxiety disorders are the **most common**^{Q} amongst all psychiatric disorders. Amongst individual psychiatric disorder, **phobias**^{Q} are the most common. They are a group of related disorders which include:
- Panic disorder
- Agoraphobia
- Specific phobia
- Social anxiety disorder
- Generalized anxiety disorder.

Panic Disorder

Panic attack is an acute attack of intense anxiety accompanied by "**feeling of impending doom**". The symptoms during panic attack usually involve sudden onset of **palpitations, chest pain, choking sensations**, dizziness and feeling of unreality (depersonalization or derealization). Along with these physical symptoms there is also a **fear of dying, losing control** or **going mad**.

In panic disorder, the patients have recurrent panic attacks which are not restricted to any particular situation or setting. The patient is usually free from anxiety symptoms in between the attack, however, anticipatory anxiety (fear that next panic attack can occur anytime) is common. The mean age of presentation is around 25 years and females are two to three times more commonly affected than men. Panic disorder presents with a number of comorbid conditions, most commonly **agoraphobia**.

The neurotransmitters which have been implicated in panic disorders include **norepinephrine, serotonin and GABA**^{Q}. Recently **cholecystokinin**^{Q} has also been found as a mediating neurotransmitter in panic disorder.

Differential Diagnosis

Due to predominance of somatic symptoms, panic disorder must be differentiated from common physical disorders such as **myocardial infarction**^{Q}, **angina, mitral valve prolapse, asthma, pulmonary embolism, pheochromocytoma, carcinoid syndrome, hypoglycemia, hyperthyroidism, anaemia, seizure disorder.**

Treatment

Usually a combination of pharmacotherapy and psychotherapy is used.

A. **Pharmacotherapy**: The drugs mostly used include **benzodiazepines**^{Q} **and SSRIs**. Frequently, both benzodiazepines and SSRIs are started concurrently, followed by slow tapering of benzodiazepines. Other medications which are used include venlafaxine, buspirone and clomipramine.

B. **Psychotherapy**: **Cognitive behavioral therapy**^{Q} is quite effective in management of panic disorder. Other less commonly used therapies include relaxation techniques and psychodynamic psychotherapy.

Agoraphobia

It is the fear of places from where **escape might be difficult**[Q]. This basic fear can manifest in various forms such as:
- Fear of being in open spaces[Q]
- Fear of crowded places[Q]
- Fear of enclosed places[Q]
- Fear of travelling alone[Q]
- Fear of using public transportations.

Agoraphobia and panic disorder usually coexist. Agoraphobia is the most disabling phobia and patient may become home bound.

Treatment

A. **Pharmacotherapy**: The pharmacotherapy usually includes benzodiazepines and SSRIs. Other medications which are used include venlafaxine, buspirone and clomipramine.
B. **Psychotherapy**: Cognitive behavioral therapy is frequently used. **Behavioral therapy (using techniques such as systematic desensitization, exposure and response prevention, flooding[Q])** is also effective. Less commonly used are **relaxation techniques** and **psychodynamic psychotherapy**.

Specific Phobias

A specific phobia is a strong, persistent and irrational fear of an object or a situation. The DSM-5 includes distinctive types of phobias:
1. Animal type (spiders, insects, dogs)

Table 1: Common phobias.

Acrophobia	Fear of heights
Ailurophobia[Q]	Fear of cats
Hydrophobia	Fear of water
Claustrophobia	Fear of closed spaces
Cynophobia[Q]	Fear of dogs
Mysophobia	Fear of dirt and germs
Pyrophobia	Fear of fire
Xenophobia	Fear of strangers
Zoophobia	Fear of animals
Thanatophobia	Fear of death
Nyctophobia[Q]	Fear of dark

2. Natural environment type (storms, water, height, etc.)
3. Blood-injection-injury type (needles, invasive medical procedures)
4. Situational type (cars, elevators, planes)
5. Others.

Treatment

A. **Pharmacotherapy**: The pharmacotherapy is at best used as an adjunct to psychotherapy and includes benzodiazepines, beta blockers, and SSRIs.
B. **Psychotherapy**: Behavior therapy is the most **effective treatment**[Q] for phobias. A variety of behavioral techniques, all of which involve exposure to phobic stimulus, have been used, which are described as follows:
- *Systematic desensitization*: In this method, the patient is exposed to a series of anxiety provoking stimuli, starting with the least anxiety provoking stimulus. After the exposure, relaxation techniques (usually progressive muscle relaxation) are used to induce relaxation. As the patient masters the technique of relaxation in the presence of an anxiety provoking stimuli, he moves up to the next stimulus.
- *Therapeutic graded exposure or in vivo exposure (or exposure and response prevention)*: It is similar to systematic desensitization except that no relaxation techniques are used. The patient learns to get habituated to anxiety.
- *Flooding (Implosion)*: Here, the patient is exposed to phobic stimulus in its most severe form. The patient experiences intense anxiety which gradually decreases.
- *Modeling* (**Participant modeling**[Q]): Here, therapist himself makes the contact with phobic stimulus and demonstrates this to the patient. Patient learns by imitation, primarily by observation. Apart from behavioral therapy, other less commonly used psychotherapeutic techniques include Psychodynamic psychotherapy (Insight oriented psychotherapy), hypnosis, supportive therapy and family therapy.

Social Anxiety Disorder (Social Phobia)

It involves the fear of social situations, including situations that involve contact with strangers. Patients with this disorder are afraid of **embarrassing themselves** in a social situation. The treatment is usually similar to specific phobias.

Generalized Anxiety Disorder

This disorder is characterized by excessive anxiety which is generalized and persistent and is not restricted to any particular situation (also called **"freely floating" anxiety**) and **excessive worries**. Patients are anxious about almost everything. This anxiety and worry is associated with the physical symptoms such as:
- Restlessness
- Being easily fatigued

- Poor concentration
- Irritability
- Muscle tension
- Insomnia

The treatment includes pharmacotherapy (SSRIs, benzodiazepines, buspirone and venlafaxine) and psychotherapy (cognitive behavioral therapy, insight oriented psychotherapy and supportive psychotherapy).

4.2 OBSESSIVE-COMPULSIVE AND RELATED DISORDERS

A. Obsessive-Compulsive Disorder (OCD)

The essential feature of this disorder includes recurrent obsessional thoughts and compulsive acts.

Obsessions are defined by the following properties:

- **Recurrent and intrusive** thoughts, images or impulses which cause marked anxiety or distress
- The person recognizes that the obsessional thoughts, images or impulses are a **product of their own mind**^{Q} (and not imposed by others such as is in thought insertion)
- The person recognizes that the thoughts, images or impulses are **irrational** and **senseless**^{Q} and experiences the obsessions and compulsions as **ego dystonic** (i.e. unwanted and unacceptable) **(in contrast a patient with a delusion, believes in the delusion and does not find it senseless or irrelevant)**
- The person attempts to suppress or resist such thoughts, images or impulses or tries to neutralize them, with some other thoughts or actions.

Compulsions are defined by following properties:

- Repetitive behaviors (such as handwashing, checking) or mental acts (such as counting, praying) that the person performs in response to an obsession.
- The repetitive behaviors and mental acts are done to reduce the distress and anxiety caused by obsessions.

The symptoms of obsessions and compulsions should be present for at least **two weeks** for the diagnosis of OCD. The lifetime prevalence of OCD is around 2-3%.

Depression is the most common comorbidity in OCD and both must be treated together.

Etiology

Serotonin dysregulation^Q is considered to be involved in the **etiopathogenesis** of OCD. Less evidence exists for dysregulation of noradrenergic system in OCD.

The neuroanatomical model of OCD emphasizes altered functioning in the circuit between orbitofrontal cortex (which is a part of prefrontal cortex), caudate (which is a part of striatum) and thalamus, the so called, **cortico-striatal-thalamic-cortical circuitry (CSTC)**. This circuit starts with prefrontal cortex and projects to striatum which further projects to thalamus and then back to prefrontal cortex. Dysfunction in this circuit is considered to be responsible for the symptoms of OCD. Studies have found **bilaterally small caudates**^{Q} in patients with obsessive compulsive disorder.

Symptoms

OCD has four major symptom patterns.

1. *Contamination*: **Most commonly** patients present with **obsession of contamination** followed by **washing behavior** and avoidance of situations which provoke obsessive thoughts. For example, a patient repeatedly gets thought that his hands are dirty, which causes anxiety, he understands that this thought is senseless and tries to stop this thought (obsessional thought), however, is forced to repeatedly wash his hands (compulsive behavior) which decreases this thought for some time. He further avoids using public toilet as these thoughts get increased in a dirty environment (avoidance).

   - Most common obsession is obsession of contamination.
   - Most common compulsion is compulsion of checking.

2. *Pathological doubt*: Second most common pattern is the **obsession of doubt** which is usually followed by **compulsion of checking**. For example, a patient would repeatedly doubt if he had locked the door properly (obsession) and would repeatedly check the lock (compulsion).

3. *Intrusive thoughts*: Here, patient gets **intrusive obsessional thoughts** without an observable compulsion, though mental compulsions are commonly present.

   The thoughts are usually with **sexual and aggressive content**^{Q}. For example, a patient repeatedly gets the thought about having sex with god, this thought causes intense anxiety and patient understand that this thought is senseless and tries to stop the thought but is not able to do so (obsessional thought), to decrease the anxiety patient starts to chant prayers in his mind which decreases the anxiety temporarily (mental compulsions).

4. *Symmetry*: The patient has a **need for symmetry** or **precision**. This can result in **compulsion of slowness**. For example, a patient would take hours while arranging pens on the table. He would ensure that all the pens are aligned exactly parallel to each other and are at exact same distance to each other.

Magical Thinking

This is a common symptom of OCD in which person believes that just because they thought about an event, it will occur in reality. In magical thinking, patient connects actions and events, that have no connection at all. E.g. A patient would repetitively have a thought "If I do not knock on the door four times, the house will catch fire".

PANDAS

In a small number of cases, OCD in children may be precipitated/worsened after infection with Group A β-hemolytic Streptococcus (GABHS). It has been hypothesised that an autoimmune response in basal ganglia may be triggered by the infection and can result in rapid development of OCD and tics. These cases of infection triggered OCD are referred to as Pediatric Autoimmune Neuropsychiatric Disorders Associated with Streptococcus Infections (PANDAS).

Course and Prognosis

Around 50% of patients with OCD have a sudden onset of symptoms. The course is usually chronic. Around 20–30% of patients have significant improvement in their symptoms, around 40–50% have moderate improvement and remaining 20–40% have no improvement or further deterioration.

Treatment

A **combination**^{Q} of pharmacotherapy and psychotherapy is the preferred approach.

- *Pharmacotherapy*: The standard approach is to start treatment with an **SSRI**^{Q}. Clomipramine is also considered the first line treatment, however, due to its adverse side effect profile, it is rarely used as a first drug. If treatment with SSRIs or clomipramine is unsuccessful, augmentation with antipsychotics (like **haloperidol**^{Q}, quetiapine, risperidone and olanzapine) is used. Other drugs which have been used include venlafaxine, lithium, valproate and **carbamazepine**^{Q}.
- *Psychotherapy*: Cognitive behavioral therapy relying primarily on behavioral technique of **exposure and response prevention**^{Q} (ERP) has the best evidence amongst all the psychotherapeutic techniques. Exposure and response prevention involves exposure of patient to a stimulus which is known to produce obsessional thoughts (**exposure**) followed by asking the patient to not indulge in the compulsive behavior (**response prevention**).

  Other types of behavioral therapy such as **desensitization, thought stopping, flooding,** and **aversive conditioning** have also been used.

  Psychodynamic psychotherapy, family therapy can also be used.

- *Other treatment modalities*: In extreme cases that are treatment resistant electroconvulsive therapy and psychosurgery can be considered. The psychosurgical techniques usually include **cingulotomy** and **capsulotomy** (also known as **subcaudate tractotomy**).

B. Hoarding Disorder

This disorder is characterised by acquiring and not being able to discard things that are considered to have little or no use. Patients keep on accumulating useless items and the house gets cluttered, to the point, that it becomes unsafe to live. The disorder is driven by fear of losing something important.

Earlier, hoarding disorder was considered as a subtype of OCD, but in both DSM-5 & ICD-11, it has been made a separate diagnostic entity.

Treatment involves use of Cognitive behavioral therapy and SSRIs. Exposure and response prevention, which is a standard treatment for OCD, is **not as effective**^{Q} in treatment of OCD.

C. Body Dysmorphic Disorder

It is characterized by the preoccupation with an **imagined defect**^{Q} in body appearance. In case a slight physical anomaly is present, patient's concern for the same is exaggerated. The location of the imagined defect is usually hair, nose and skin.

D. Olfactory Reference Syndrome

It is a new diagnostic entity added in ICD-11. It is characterised by preoccupation with the belief that one is emitting a foul body odour or breath that in reality is either unnoticeable or only slightly noticeable to others. The person who has the preoccupation feels self-conscious and may also believe that others are taking notice of the odour and talking about it. The patient may repeatedly check the odour or try to mask it or may start avoiding the social situations.

E. Body Focussed Repetitive Disorders

This diagnostic category involves repetitive actions that are directed at integument (e.g. hair pulling, skin picking etc), accompanied by unsuccessful attempts at stopping these actions. These include:

- *Trichotillomania*: It involves recurrent pulling of one's own hair leading to significant hair loss, accompanied by unsuccessful attempts to decrease or stop the behavior.
- Excoriation disorder: It involves recurrent picking of one's own skin leading to skin lesions, associated with unsuccessful attempts to decrease or stop the behavior.

4.3 TRAUMA AND STRESSOR-RELATED DISORDER

A. Post-traumatic Stress Disorder (PTSD)

This disorder follow significant traumatic events in which there is a serious injury or threat of serious injury to self or others and a feeling of helplessness and horror during the event. The traumatic events causing PTSD and ASD are sufficiently overwhelming to affect anyone (such as war, earthquake, floods, rape, serious accidents). The clinical symptoms are usually seen in the following three domains:

- *Intrusion symptoms*: These are characterized by **flashbacks**^{Q} (individual may feel as if trauma is reoccurring) and **nightmares** (dreams about the trauma).
- *Avoidance*: The patient avoids all those stimuli which can remind him of the trauma.
- *Arousal symptoms*: These include hypervigilance, exaggerated startle response, insomnia, poor concentration.

In addition, symptoms such as **emotional numbing**^{Q}, **emotional detachment**^{Q} and **anhedonia**^{Q} can also be present. The onset of symptoms may be delayed, if symptoms appear **6 months**^{Q} after the trauma, it is diagnosed as PTSD with **delayed onset**^{Q}.

For a diagnosis of post-traumatic stress disorder, the above mentioned symptoms should be present for more than one month, if the duration of symptoms is less than one month, a diagnosis of acute stress disorder is made. PTSD is mostly prevalent in young adults although children may also develop it. Females are more vulnerable than males. The area of brain involved in the pathogenesis of PTSD are **hippocampus** and **amygdala**^{Q}.

Treatment

Selective serotonin reuptake inhibitors **(SSRIs)**^{Q} are the first line pharmacological treatment in PTSD. Psychotherapeutic interventions include **cognitive behavioral therapy**^{Q} (treatment of choice), psychodynamic psychotherapy and eye movement desensitization and reprocessing (EMDR).

> **Complex PTSD**
>
> It is a new diagnostic category that has been added in ICD-11.
>
> Complex PTSD may develop following exposure to an event or series of events of extremely threatening nature (usually in cases where the event is repetitive, e.g. in cases of slavery, repeated childhood sexual or physical abuse, prolonged domestic violence). In complex PTSD, in addition to the symptoms of PTSD, the following are seen:
>
> *Contd...*

> *Contd...*
>
> ❖ Severe abnormalities of affect regulation (i.e. severe emotional regulation disturbances)
> ❖ Belief about oneself as being a defeated and worthless person and feelings of shame and guilt for the event
> ❖ Inability to feel close to others and sustain a relationship

B. Acute Stress Reaction (or Acute Stress Disorder)

Acute stress reaction (or corresponding DSM diagnosis of acute stress disorder) also develops after a traumatic event, like PTSD. However, it is usually short lasting and resolves rapidly within days. The symptoms include an initial state of "daze", depression, anxiety, anger, despair or withdrawal.

Treatment

The psychological treatment include Debriefing (which helps in promoting adaptation to traumatic event) and cognitive behavioral therapy. In pharmacotherapy, SSRIs are commonly used, TCAs also have some efficacy.

C. Adjustment Disorders

These disorders are characterized by emotional responses to stressful events like financial problems, medical illness, relationship problems or death of a loved one. The symptom complex that develops usually involve anxiety and depressive symptoms. The symptoms of adjustment disorders include depressed mood, anxiety, worry, a feeling of inability to cope and some degree of disturbance in individuals daily functioning. It is at times difficult to differentiate adjustment disorder from depression (depression can also follow a negative life event). If the symptoms are severe and a diagnosis of depression can be made, the diagnosis of depression will always get precedence over the diagnosis of adjustment disorder. Also, one needs to differentiate adjustment disorder from uncomplicated bereavement/grief reactions (in uncomplicated bereavement, the symptoms and dysfunctions which develop after death of a loved one are within expected limits, whereas in adjustment disorder the symptoms and dysfunction are beyond the expectable reaction to the stressor). Other differential diagnosis of adjustment disorder includes depression, PTSD and brief psychotic disorders. These diagnoses should be given precedence if their diagnostic criteria are met, irrespective of the presence of stressors.

Treatment

Psychotherapy is the treatment of choice. Supportive psychotherapy is commonly used. The medications are used as an adjuvant to psychotherapy and include antidepressants and antianxiety drugs.

4.4 DISSOCIATIVE DISORDERS (CONVERSION DISORDERS)

These disorders were previously classified as "Hysteria" however' that term is no longer used. Dissociative disorders are characterized by disturbances in one or more of mental functions such as memory, identity, perception, consciousness and motor behavior. These symptoms are produced by the "psyche" (mind) to deal with the unconscious conflicts that are producing anxiety. These symptoms are produced unconsciously and help the patient to get attention. The symptoms appear suddenly and are caused by psychological trauma (such as stressful events or disturbed relationship). Quite often, the genesis of dissociative disorders is explained in terms of primary, secondary and tertiary gains. All these gains function unconsciously.

- *Primary gain*: It refers to internal psychological motivation. For example, a person might be feeling guilty as he is not able to perform a task, however, if he suddenly develops paralysis, now his guilt will decrease, as it is understood that paralyzed patient can not work. So, this patients psyche is unconsciously producing symptoms of paralysis to reduce the unpleasant guilt feelings.
- *Secondary gain*: It refers to external psychological motivation. For example, this patient who developed sudden paralysis is now not expected to work outside or make money for the family and he is relieved of his duties.
- *Tertiary gain*: It refers to the gain that a third person derives because of patients symptoms. For example, the wife of this paralyzed patient starts to get lots of money from her parents as they feel sympathetic towards her.

Types

- *Dissociative amnesia*: Here, the main feature is loss of memory. The amnesia is usually for traumatic events of **personal significance**^{Q} (such as accidents or unexpected bereavements). For example, a rape survivor is not able to recall anything about her rape.

In DSM-5, dissociative fugue is not a separate diagnosis. Instead it has been made a specifier (special kind of) of dissociative amnesia. In ICD-11 too, the diagnosis of dissociative fugue has been removed.

- *Dissociative fugue*: It is characterized by a **sudden, unexpected travel**^{Q} away from home or work place, with inability to recall some or all of one's past. The **basic self-care is maintained**^{Q} during the travel and patients behavior during this time may appear completely normal to independent observers. Alongside when asked, the patient may be confused about his personal identity or may even assume a new identity (e.g. a doctor may claim that he is in fact a cab driver and give a different name when asked).
- *Trance disorder*: Trance disorder is characterized by 'trance states' in which the person experiences significant change in individual's state of consciousness or a loss of sense of 'personal identity'. The awareness of surroundings becomes very restricted and there may be restriction of movements, and speech, which may be experienced as being outside one's control. However, there is no experience of being replaced by an alternate identity.
- *Possession trance disorder*: There is a significant change in individual's state of consciousness and the individual's experiences that his personal identity has been replaced by an external 'possessing' identity, and that the individual's behaviours are experienced as being controlled by the possessing identity. For example, a middle aged women claimed that she has been possessed by a goddess and demanded that everybody should pray in front of her.
- *Dissociative neurological symptom disorder*: Here the patient presents with symptoms that suggest deficit in motor, sensory or cognitive functions, however, there is no evidence of any physical disorder. The symptoms are instead caused by psychological factors. The symptoms often **do not confirm**^{Q} with **anatomical** and **physiological principles** (e.g. sensory loss which does not confirm to any nerve lesion).

The DSM-5 uses the diagnosis of **conversion disorder**^{Q} (functional neurological symptom disorder) specifically for this category and classifies it along with the somatic symptom disorders.

La belle indifference^Q is a phrase used to describe the feeling of indifference which patients of conversion disorders have towards their symptoms. For example, if a person suddenly has a sensory loss, say loss of vision, he would be expected to get extremely concerned about it, however, the patient of conversion disorder looks completely unconcerned and this unconcern/indifference towards their symptoms is called **"la belle indifference"**^{Q}.

- *Depersonalization/derealization disorder*: In depersonalization patient has a **feeling of unreality of self**. He feels "as if" he has changed. The patients frequently report that they feel as if they have detached from their body and are watching themselves like in a movie. The depersonalization is often accompanied by derealization, which is a feeling of unreality of the external world, as if the world is unreal.

- *Dissociative identity disorder (multiple personality disorder)*: Here, two or more distinct personalities exist within an individual, with only one of them being evident at any particular time. The different personalities are known as **"alters"** and the personalities are unaware of eachothers existence.
- *Other dissociative disorders*: This category includes **Ganser^Q syndrome**. The characteristic symptom is **approximate answers^Q (Vorbeigehen)**. The approximate answer are the answers which are not correct, but bear an obvious relation to the question, indicating that the question was understood. For example, when asked the color of sky, patient may answer it red. Although, the answer is not correct but it is obvious that patient understood that the question was about color. Other symptoms include **clouding of consciousness^Q, auditory and visual hallucinations^Q** and other dissociative symptoms. Ganser syndrome is frequently seen in **prisoners**, however is **not confined only to them^Q** and can be seen in other populations also.

Treatment

Usually psychological modalities are used in the treatment of dissociative disorders. It is important that patient is not encouraged to assume a "sick-role" and it must be emphasized that the patient is normal. The secondary and tertiary gains should not be allowed otherwise the symptoms tend to become persistent. The treatment modalities include behavioral therapy, **abreaction^Q** (in abreaction, attempt is made to bring the unconscious memories and emotions, into conscious awareness using hypnosis, medications and other techniques) and psychoanalysis.

The use of drugs is limited. Benzodiazepines, thiopentone and amytal have been used for abreaction.

4.5 SOMATIC SYMPTOMS AND RELATED DISORDERS

The patients with somatic symptoms and related (earlier called as somatoform disorders) typically present with prominent physical symptoms that cause significant distress and impairment. Many a times, the symptoms cannot be explained by any known medical condition (**also called as MUS, medically unexplained symptoms^Q**). These patients persistently request for investigations despite repeated negative findings and reassurances by doctors.

There are various types of somatoform disorders:
- *Somatic symptoms disorder (earlier called as somatization disorder or Briquet's syndrome)*: The main feature is presence of one or more somatic symptoms and excessive thoughts (excessive thoughts about seriousness of symptoms), excessive feelings (excessive anxiety about symptoms) and excessive behaviors (too much time and energy spent on these symptoms) related to these somatic symptoms. In earlier classifications, the focus was on MUS 'medically unexplained symptoms' to make a diagnosis of somatoform disorder, however, later it was felt that just the absence of a medical explanation of a symptom, should not be the criterion to diagnose a psychiatric disorder.

In ICD-11, the corresponding diagnosis for somatic symptom disorder is **bodily distress disorder.**

The patient usually refuses to accept the advice or reassurance of the doctors that there is no physical cause of the symptoms. The onset and progression of symptoms usually bears a close relationship to unpleasant life events and psychological stressors.

Treatment usually involves psychotherapy. The patient should be made aware that the physical symptoms are expression of underlying emotions and should be helped to cope with the symptoms and underlying emotions.

ICD-11 continues to use the diagnosis of hypochondriasis. The DSM-5 uses the diagnosis of illness anxiety disorder, for the same illness.

- *Hypochondriasis*: This disorder is characterized by a **preoccupation** with the fear of having, or the idea that one has one or more **serious physical illnesses^Q**. The preoccupation persists despite **normal investigation^Q** results as well as doctors reassurances. It is important to differentiate hypochondriasis from somatic symptoms disorder. The emphasis in hypochondriasis is on the diagnosis whereas the emphasis in somatic symptom disorder is on the symptoms.

Also, hypochondriasis must be differentiated from delusional disorder (somatic type). In patients with hypochondriasis the belief is not as fixed as it is in delusional disorder. The patient with hypochondriasis may doubt his belief at least for short-term, after a normal investigation or medical reassurance. In contrast in delusional disorder, the belief is fixed and totally unshakeable.

> **Body Integrity Dysphoria: New Diagnosis in ICD-11**
>
> It is characterised by an intense and persistent desire to become physically disabled in a significant way (e.g. amputation of a limb or become blind). The patients report a sense of 'alienation' from a body part and a discomfort with the currently non-disabled body part.
>
> They have a preoccupation with becoming physically disabled and may pretend to be disabled (pretenders) or may request a surgical amputation.
>
> Not much is known about etiology and treatment.

Other Neurotic Disorders

Neurasthenia

This disorder is characterized by complaints of increased mental and physical fatigue after mild efforts. The patient is often concerned about lowered physical and mental efficiency. Associated symptoms include muscular aches and pain, sleep disturbances, irritability, dyspepsia, headache and inability to relax. The ICD-10 includes the diagnosis of fatigue syndromes under the category of neurasthenia.

Chronic Fatigue Syndrome (Myalgic Encephalomyelitis)

This syndrome is frequently diagnosed in western countries. The criterion (centre for disease control and prevention criterion) for diagnosis of chronic fatigue syndrome includes:
- Severe unexplained fatigue for over **6 months**^{Q} that is:
  - Of a new or definitive onset
  - Not due to continuing exertion
  - **Not resolved by rest**^{Q}
  - Causes functional impairment
- Four or more of the following new symptoms:
  - **Impaired memory**^{Q} and concentration
  - Sore throat
  - Tender lymph nodes
  - Muscle pain
  - Pain in several joints
  - New pattern of headaches
  - **Unrefreshing sleep**^{Q}
  - Postexertional malaise lasting for more than 24 hours.

There are no pathognomonic features and symptoms are often **nonspecific**^{Q}. **Epstein-Barr virus**^{Q} has been implicated as causative agent in some studies but mostly studies have been inconclusive and inconsistent. There are no reliable pattern of laboratory abnormalities though in some cases immunological abnormalities have been found. Comorbid psychiatric symptoms are common. Depression is the most common comorbidity. The diagnosis of chronic fatigue syndrome is not covered by either ICD-10 or DSM-5, however, the symptoms have some resemblance to neurasthenia. Treatment is mostly supportive and involves use of symptomatic treatment such as analgesics for pain. In many cases, psychotherapy shows good response with cognitive behavioral therapy^Q being particularly useful.

Pseudocyesis

This disorder is characterised by development of classical signs of pregnancy like abdominal enlargement (although umbilicus does not become everted), reduced menstrual flow or amenorrhea, subjective sense of fetal movements, breast engorgement and labour pains at the expected date of delivery, all in a nonpregnant woman. Some endocrine changes may also be present. The patient usually has a **false belief too, that she is pregnantQ**.

Culture Bound Syndrome

These are limited to a particular culture and are not seen worldwide. It is believed that local cultural beliefs and patterns of behavior have strong influence on the presentation of these syndromes. Few common culture bound syndromes are:
- **Dhat syndrome**^{Q}: It is prevalent in Indian subcontinent. The patient has a belief that he is passing semen in urine and this is resulting in physical and mental weakness.
- **Koro**^{Q}: The patient has a fear that his penis will retract into the abdomen and would result in death
- **Latah**: This is characterized by automatic obedience, echolalia and echopraxia.

Factitious Disorder (Munchausen Syndrome^Q)

Factitious disorder (also known as **hospital addiction**) is a disorder in which patients produces fake symptoms with the sole aim of obtaining medical attention (hence called **professional patients**^{Q}) and assume "**sick role**" (these patients want that they should be treated as if they are sick or ill). Unlike malingering, in which the motive is usually financial gains or avoidance of duty, the patients with factitious disorders have no recognizable motives apart from wish to get medical attention. These patients distort the history and make stories (**pseudologia fantastica**) to convince the doctors. The patients are often from the **medical and related fields**^{Q} and have basic **understanding** of symptoms/signs of various disorders. When a caregiver produces fake symptoms in those who are in their care (usually children) with the aim of gaining attention for them, it is called **Munchausen syndrome by proxy.**^{Q}

Malingering

Malingering is not a psychiatric disorder. Its discussed here just for purpose of maintaining continuity. Malingering involves intentional production of false physical or psychological symptoms, with a motivation of getting some external incentives such as financial incentives, avoiding military or some other tough duty, or avoiding legal cases. Malingering should be suspected if (a) there is a medicolegal case involved, including referrals by **courts of law**[Q], (b) there is marked **discrepancy** in complaints by patient and objective findings, and (c) lack of cooperation by patient during diagnostic evaluation and treatment.

Psychological Factors Affecting Other Medical Conditions

The concept of psychosomatic disorders (physical disorders caused by or aggravated by psychological factors) has been known for a long time. It is clear that stress can result in many somatic symptoms. Stress is described as any circumstance, that disturbs or is likely to disturb, the normal physiological or psychological functioning of an individual.

Hans Selye described a model of stress that is known as **general adaptation syndrome**[Q]. According to this model, body reacts to stress in three stages.

- *Stage 1, the alarm reaction*: This is the immediate response characterized by fight or flight response.
- *Stage 2, the stage of resistance*: This is also known as stage of adaptation. Here, the body adapts to the stress. For example, if the stress is starvation, body reduces the energy consumption and decreases physical activity.
- *Stage 3, the stage of exhaustion*: If the stress continues, the resistance of body gradually decreases and finally collapses.

Almost all the organ systems may be involved in psychosomatic disorders. The important ones include:

- *Gastrointestinal system*: A large number of GI disorders such as peptic ulcers, Crohn's disease, ulcerative colitis are affected by psychological causes. Irritable bowel syndrome, which is characterized by symptoms such as abdominal pain, cramps, alteration of bowel habits (diarrhea or constipation) is a well-known example of psychosomatic disorder.
- *Respiratory system*: Asthma, COPD and hyperventilation syndrome are known to have psychological component. Hyperventilation syndrome is characterized by rapid and deep breathing for several minutes and accompanying symptoms of suffocation, giddiness, paraesthesia and syncope due to falling PCO_2 levels in blood.
- *Cardiovascular system*: Cardiovascular disorders such as hypertension, coronary artery diseases, cardiac arrhythmias are known to be affected by psychological causes. Of particular interest is the association of so called **type A personality with coronary artery disease**[Q]. The type A personality is characterized by easily aroused anger, impatience, aggression, competitive striving and hostility. Type A pattern is associated with a nearly two fold risk of MI and CAD related mortality. In comparison type B-personality is characterized by calmness, relaxed attitude, low competitiveness and lesser chances of coronary artery diseases.
- *Musculoskeletal system*: Disorders like rheumatoid arthritis, systemic lupus erythematosus are known to have psychological components. Of particular note is fibromyalgia, a disease characterized by pain and stiffness of soft tissues such as muscle and ligaments. The patient often reports of local areas of tenderness, also known as "trigger points". There might be associated symptoms such as anxiety, fatigue and inability to sleep.
- Other disorders such as endocrinological disorders, skin disorders, headaches also have psychological contributions.

Treatment

Patients with all forms of somatic symptom and related disorder usually resist psychiatric treatment. The treatment is usually focused on helping the patient understand the effect of psychological factors in the genesis of symptoms while acknowledging that the symptoms are real and distressing to the patient. Psychotherapeutic techniques like group psychotherapy, insight oriented psychotherapy, behavior therapy, cognitive therapy and hypnosis may be useful. Relaxation techniques and stress management training may also be required.

4.6 DEATH AND DYING

When an individual is informed about his impending death, he usually goes through a series of responses. These stages of death and dying, were proposed by **Elisabeth Kübler-Ross**[Q].

Stage 1: Denial and shock—This is characterized by refusal to accept the diagnosis and a reaction of shock.

Stage 2: Anger—In this stage patients become irritable and angry at family members, friends, doctors and even God.

Stage 3: Bargaining—In this stage patient tries to bargain with family members and even God. For example, they may pledge to god that they will regularly go to temples if god cures them.

Stage 4: *Depression*—The patient now start showing symptoms of depression such as sadness of mood, withdrawal and suicidal thoughts

Stage 5: *Acceptance*—Finally patient accepts that death is inevitable and their feelings may change to neutral or even happiness.

Grief, Bereavement and Mourning

Although these terms have been used interchangeably, they have specific meanings. **Bereavement** means the **state** of being deprived of someone due to death. **Grief reaction** is the **psychological feeling** precipitated by the death of a loved one. **Mourning** is the **process** through which grief is resolved. Mourning involves societal practices like funerals, burial and memorial services.

In grief patient experiences intense sadness although positive emotions are also mixed with negative emotions. Patient may have **longing to join**[Q] the deceased person and may even experience **transient hallucinations**[Q].

Complicated Bereavement (Complicated Grief Reactions)

Complicated bereavement includes **prolonged grief reactions (chronic grief)** or extraordinarily intense grief reactions **(hypertrophic grief)** or delayed grief reactions **(delayed grief)**. **Traumatic Bereavement** refers to grief that is both chronic and hypertrophic.

Bereavement and Depression

Grief is a complex experience in which both positive emotions (happy memories of the deceased) and negative emotions (sadness) coexist and alternate. In depression, the negative emotions predominate and do not change. Also the symptoms in depression are severe and cause significant dysfunction. Finally, the symptom such as excessive guilt, suicidal thoughts, ideas of worthlessness and psychomotor retardation are not seen in grief and their presence is suggestive of depression.

Multiple Choice Questions

General

1. **All of the following are seen in anxiety *except*:**
   (Kerala 1996)
   A. Decreased sweating
   B. Hyperventilation
   C. Cold extremities
   D. Palpitations
   E. Pupillary dilatation

2. **General adaptation syndrome (GAS) is seen in:** *(AI 2012)*
   A. Panic attacks
   B. Depression
   C. Anxiety
   D. Stressful situations

3. **General adaptation syndrome relates to:** *(AI 2012)*
   A. How we achieve homeostasis
   B. How well we adapt to new situations
   C. Pattern of psychological response to stress
   D. Pattern of autonomic nervous system (ANS) and physiological response when we are aroused by a stressful situation

4. **Which of the following is the most common psychiatric disorder?** *(NEET 2016, DNB NEET 2014-15)*
   A. Anxiety disorders
   B. Schizophrenia
   C. Mood disorders
   D. Mania

Generalized Anxiety Disorders

5. **All are seen in generalized anxiety disorder *except*:**
   A. Muscle tension *(DNB June 2009)*
   B. Irritability
   C. Fear of impending doom
   D. Restlessness

6. **Drug of choice for generalized anxiety disorder is:**
   (DNB NEET 2014-15)
   A. Alprazolam
   B. Buspirone
   C. Venlafaxine
   D. Beta-blockers

7. **True about generalized anxiety disorder is/are:**
   A. Insomnia *(PGI Nov 2017)*
   B. Hypersomnia
   C. Episodes last for minutes to hours
   D. Free floating anxiety
   E. Benzodiazepine is treatment of choice
   F. Autonomic symptoms

Controversial Question

8. **A 25-year-old lady presented with sadness, palpitation, loss of appetite and insomnia. There is no complaint of hopelessness, suicidal thoughts and there is no past history of any precipitating event. She is remarkably well in other areas of life. She is doing her office job normally and her social life is also normal. What is the probable diagnosis in this case?** *(AI 2010)*
   A. Generalized anxiety disorder
   B. Mixed anxiety depression
   C. Adjustment disorder
   D. Mild depressive episode

Panic Disorder

9. **A 30-year-old lady presents with sudden onset breathlessness, anxiety, palpitation and feeling of impending doom. Physical examination does not reveal any abnormality. What is the probable diagnosis in this case?**
   (AIIMS Nov 2010)
   A. Panic attack
   B. Anxiety disorder
   C. Conversion disorder
   D. Acute psychosis

10. **Panic attack is associated with a disturbance in all of the following neurotransmitters *except*:** *(AIIMS Nov 2011)*
    A. Serotonin
    B. GABA
    C. Glutamate
    D. Dopamine, CCK, pentagastrin

11. **Differential diagnosis of panic disorder are:**
    (PGI June 2004)
    A. Pheochromocytoma
    B. Myocardial infarction
    C. Mitral valve prolapse
    D. Depression
    E. Carcinoid syndrome

12. **Which of the following is the most appropriate treatment for panic disorder?** *(AIIMS 2009)*
    A. Buspirone plus benzodiazepines
    B. Benzodiazepines plus supportive therapy
    C. Short-term benzodiazepine plus SSRI plus CBT
    D. Long-term benzodiazepine plus venlafaxine

Controversial Question

13. **A patient comes in emergency with feeling of impending doom, intense ghabrahat and palpitations. All of the following investigations should be done in emergency to find the cause of anxiety**
    (AIIMS May 2016)
    A. T3, T4, TSH
    B. Glucose levels
    C. Hemoglobin
    D. ECG

14. **Which of the following does not resemble panic attack?**
    A. Hypoglycemia *(NIMHANS 2019)*
    B. Generalised tonic clonic seizures
    C. Temporal lobe epilepsy
    D. Myocardial infarction

15. **Which of the following is not true regarding treatment of panic disorder?** *(NIMHANS 2019)*
    A. MAO-I are given in associated atypical depression
    B. Dose of SSRI is doubled to control initial symptoms of panic disorder
    C. Voluntary exposure is a part of psychotherapy
    D. Acute management of anxiety is with benzodiazepines

Phobic Anxiety Disorders

16. **Fear of dark is called as:** *(NEET 2019)*
    A. Nyctophobia
    B. Agoraphobia
    C. Claustrophobia
    D. Acrophobia

17. **True about social phobia is:** *(UP 2001)*
    A. Fear of closed spaces
    B. Irrational fear of situation
    C. Irrational fear of activities
    D. Irrational fear of specified objects

18. **A middle aged person reported to psychiatric OPD with the complaints of fear of leaving home, fear of travelling alone and fear of being in a crowd. He develops marked anxiety with palpitations and sweating if he is in these situations. He often avoids public transport to go to his place of work. The most likely diagnosis is:**
    A. Generalized anxiety disorder *(AIIMS May 2006)*
    B. Schizophrenia
    C. Personality disorder
    D. Agoraphobia

19. **Agoraphobia is often seen in patients with:**
    A. Generalised anxiety disorder *(NIMHANS 2018)*
    B. Social anxiety disorder
    C. Panic disorder
    D. OCD

20. **A 50-year-old male feels uncomfortable in using lift, being in crowded places and traveling alone. The most appropriate line of treatment is:**
    A. Counseling *(NIMHANS 2016, AIIMS Nov 2005)*
    B. Relaxation therapy
    C. Exposure and response prevention
    D. Covert sensitization

21. **Treatment of choice in phobic disorder is :**
    A. Psychotherapy
    B. Benzodiazepines
    C. Behavior therapy
    D. 5-HT reuptake inhibitor

22. **Agoraphobia is treated with:** *(PGI Dec 2007)*
    A. Systematic desensitization
    B. Psychodynamic therapy
    C. Exposure therapy
    D. Relaxation therapy
    E. Behavior therapy

Obsessive-Compulsive Disorder

Controversial Question

23. **Feeling of uncertainty and excessive sense of responsibility is seen in:** *(AIIMS May 2015)*
    A. Generalized anxiety disorder
    B. OCD
    C. Phobia
    D. Personality disorder

24. **A drug for Obsessive Compulsive Disorder, with maximum anticholinergic effect is:** *(NIMHANS 2019)*
    A. Fluvoxamine
    B. Sertraline
    C. Clomipramine
    D. Buspirone

25. **True statements about obsession:** *(PGI 2003)*
    A. It is a repetitive thought or image
    B. Patient believes that the images or thoughts are imposed by others
    C. Content of obsession are about sex or God
    D. Patient gets disturbed when unable to remove the ideas or thoughts

26. **Which of the following statements differentiates obsessional idea from delusion:** *(DNB NEET 2014-15, AIIMS Nov 2005)*
    A. Obsessional idea is not a conventional belief
    B. Obsessional idea is held in spite of evidence to the contrary
    C. Obsessional idea is regarded as senseless by patient
    D. Obsessional idea is held on inadequate ground

27. **Following are the major symptoms of obsessive compulsive disorder:** *(DNB NEET 2014-15)*
    A. Doubts of contamination
    B. Pathological doubts
    C. Intrusive thoughts
    D. All of the above

28. **True about obsessive compulsive disorders are all *except*:** *(DNB NEET 2014-15)*
    A. Obsessions are ego alien
    B. Patient tries to resist against obsessions and compulsions
    C. Obsessions are egosyntonic
    D. Insight is present

29. **Most common presentation of obsessive compulsive disorder in adults is:** *(AIIMS May 2018)*
    A. Pathological doubt
    B. Symmetry
    C. Sexual thoughts
    D. Aggression

30. **Brain areas involved with obsessive compulsive disorder include all *except*:** *(NIMHANS 2016)*
    A. Claustrum
    B. Orbitofrontal cortex
    C. Basal ganglia
    D. Head of caudate nucleus

31. **A 22-year-old male comes to your office with complains of frequenting checking of doors even when they are locked. He is distressed about this fact. He is subsequently diagnosed to have Obsessive Compulsive disorder. Consider the following statements:** *(AIIMS Nov 2016)*
    a. Repression and reaction formation are the defense mechanisms involved
    b. SSRIs are the drug of choice
    c. Risperidone may be used in SSRI resistant cases to augment the response
    d. Systematic desensitization is the psychotherapy of choice

    Which of the above are correct statements?
    A. a and b
    B. b and c
    C. b, c, and d
    D. a, b, c, and d

32. A 15-year-old boy feels that the dirt has hung onto him whenever he passes through the dirty street. This repetitive thought causes much distress and anxiety. He knows that there is actually no such thing after he has cleaned once but he is not satisfied and is compelled to think so. This has led to social withdrawal. He spends much of his time thinking about the dirt and contamination. This has affected his studies also. The most likely diagnosis is:
    A. Obsessive compulsive disorder *(AI 2003)*
    B. Conduct disorder
    C. Agoraphobia
    D. Adjustment disorder

33. An obsessive compulsive disorder patient is likely to develop: *(AIIMS 1993)*
    A. Hallucination
    B. Depression
    C. Delusion
    D. Schizophrenia

34. Drug of choice for OCD is: *(DNB June 2009)*
    A. Clomipramine
    B. Fluoxetine
    C. Carbamazepine
    D. Chlorpromazine

Controversial Questions

35. In obsessive-compulsive disorder, which is not given: *(DNB 2002, Jharkhand 2006)*
    A. Clomipramine
    B. Haloperidol
    C. Sertraline
    D. Carbamazepine

36. All drugs are used for treatment of OCD except: *(DNB 2009, PCI 1999; JIPMER 2002; MAHE 2003)*
    A. Carbamazepine
    B. Lithium
    C. Fluoxetine
    D. Diazepam

37. Drug used for long-term treatment of OCD includes: *(PGI May 2013)*
    A. Clomipramine
    B. Fluoxetine
    C. Fluvoxamine
    D. Citalopram
    E. Trifluperidol

38. Treatment of obsessive-compulsive disorder includes: *(PGI Dec 2008)*
    A. Exposure and response prevention
    B. Flooding
    C. Psychoanalytic therapy
    D. Supportive psychotherapy involving family members
    E. Systematic desensitization

39. Which of the following is least useful in treatment of OCD? *(NIMHANS 2014)*
    A. Clomipramine
    B. SSRIs
    C. Cognitive behavioral therapy
    D. Systematic desensitization

40. Treatment of choice for OCD is: *(DNB 2004, MP 2006)*
    A. Behavior therapy
    B. Drug therapy
    C. Psychosurgery
    D. Combination of behavior and drug therapy

41. A 35-year-old female has been diagnosed with obsessive compulsive disorder and she washes her hands many times a day. Which would be the best CBT technique for her treatment? *(AI 2012)*
    A. Thought stopping
    B. Response prevention
    C. Relaxation
    D. Exposure

42. Exposure and response prevention technique is/are used in: *(PGI May 2015)*
    A. Schizophrenia
    B. OCD
    C. Phobia
    D. Mania
    E. Depression

Controversial Question

43. A woman comes to psychiatrist with history of spending a lot of time in washing her hands. She is distressed about it but says that she is not able to stop washing. This has started to affect her social life as well. What is the best mode of treatment for her? *(AIIMS May 2015)*
    A. Cognitive behavioral therapy
    B. Exposure and response prevention
    C. Systematic desensitization
    D. Pharmacological agents

44. The following modes of therapy may be useful for treatment of Obsessive compulsive disorder except: *(NIMHANS 2015)*
    A. Fluoxetine
    B. Clomipramine
    C. Behaviour therapy
    D. Electroconvulsive therapy

45. In a child with OCD, MRI will reveal reduced volume (atrophy) of: *(JIPMER Nov 2018)*
    A. Putamen
    B. Globus pallidus
    C. Caudate nucleus
    D. Cerebellum

46. Which of the following types of OCD, responds poorly to exposure and response prevention (ERP), and has poor prognosis: *(NEET 2019)*
    A. Contamination
    B. Pathological doubts
    C. Hoarding disorder
    D. Magical thinking

47. The psychiatric disorder that has been found to be associated with PANDAS is: *(NIMHANS 2018)*
    A. OCD
    B. Depression
    C. Schizophrenia
    D. ADHD

Trauma and Stress-related Disorders

48. Most common disorder(s) after trauma is: *(PGI May 2015)*
    A. Major depression
    B. Mania
    C. Schizophrenia
    D. PTSD
    E. Acute stress reaction

49. An elderly female had her house destroyed in an earthquake. Following this, she presented to your office with complaints of anxiety, sadness, lack of sleep, anger, palpitations and despair. *(AIIMS Nov 2016)*
    Consider the following statements.
    a. The lady is suffering from acute stress reaction
    b. The defense mechanism involved is projection
    c. Drug of choice in this situation is Risperidone
    d. She needs referral to a psychiatrist for psychotherapy
    Which of the following statements are true?
    A. a and c
    B. b and d
    C. a, b, and c
    D. a and d

50. Which of the following is not a clinical feature of post-traumatic stress disorder (PTSD)? *(NIMHANS 2015, AI 2008)*
    A. Flashbacks
    B. Hyperarousal
    C. Hallucinations
    D. Emotional numbing

51. Post-traumatic stress disorder is associated with all *except*: *(PGI 2000)*
    A. Flashback
    B. Severe traumatic injury
    C. Re-experiencing of stressful event
    D. Anhedonia
    E. It does not develop after 6 months of stress

52. False statement about post-traumatic stress disorder: *(DNB NEET 2014-15)*
    A. Symptoms develop immediately after the event
    B. Symptoms include insomnia, poor concentration
    C. It is the response to an exceptionally stressful or catastrophic stimuli
    D. Anxiolytics are given only, if anxiety develops

53. All are true statements about PTSD, *except*: *(NIMHANS 2014)*
    A. Women are more likely to develop PTSD than men
    B. Children are less likely to experience PTSD after trauma than adults
    C. War veterans are commonly at risk for PTSD
    D. Most people having experienced a traumatizing event will develop PTSD

54. True for PTSD are all *except*: *(PGI 2001)*
    A. Patients have past history of psychiatric illness
    B. Women are more predisposed
    C. Occur in intellectuals
    D. Feeling of numbness
    E. Feeling of detachment

55. Post-traumatic stress disorder (PTSD) is differentiated from other disorders by presence of: *(AIIMS May 2012)*
    A. Nightmares about events
    B. Autonomic arousal and anxiety
    C. Recall of events and avoidance of similar experiences
    D. Depression

56. All are true for PTSD *except*: *(PGI 2002)*
    A. Hippocampus and amygdala are the brain areas involved in PTSD
    B. Anhedonia
    C. Depression and guilt
    D. Insomnia and poor concentration
    E. Anxiolytics are the treatment of choice

57. A patient with a history of road traffic accident, two months back, presents with complaints of dreams about the accident. He has visualisations of the same scene whenever he visits the place and is afraid to go back to the accident site. Identify the type of disorder that he might be suffering from? *(NEET 2018)*
    A. Adjustment disorder
    B. PTSD
    C. Anxiety disorder
    D. Major depression

58. Which of the following is the most effective treatment modality for post-traumatic stress disorder (PTSD)?
    A. Cognitive behavioral therapy *(AIIMS Nov 2014)*
    B. Eye movement desensitization and reprocessing
    C. Hypnosis
    D. Rational and emotive therapy

59. SSRIs are first line treatment for: *(PGI 2010)*
    A. OCD
    B. Panic disorder
    C. Social phobia
    D. Post-traumatic stress disorder
    E. Adjustment disorder

Grief and Adjustment Disorder

Controversial Question

60. A man coming from mountain whose wife died 6 months prior says that his wife appeared to him and asked him to join her. The diagnosis is: *(AIIMS 2000)*
    A. Normal grief
    B. Grief psychosis
    C. Bereavement reaction
    D. Supernatural phenomenon

61. Which of the following is not a part of Kubler-Ross's stages of impeding death? *(DNB Dec 2010)*
    A. Depression
    B. Bargain
    C. Aggression
    D. Anger

Controversial Question

62. An elderly house wife lost her husband who died suddenly of myocardial infarction couple of years ago. They had been staying alone for almost a decade with infrequent visits from her son and grandchildren. About a week after the death she heard his voice clearly talking to her as he would in a routine manner from the next room. She went to check but saw nothing. Subsequently she often heard his voice conversing with her and she would also discuss her daily matters with him. This however, provoked anxiety and sadness of mood when she would remain preoccupied with thoughts about him. She should be treated with: *(AIIMS May 2003)*
    A. Clomipramine
    B. Alprazolam
    C. Electroconvulsive therapy
    D. Haloperidol

63. Ms B a 27-year-old nurse had extracurricular interests in trekking and painting. She broke up relationship with her boyfriend. Two months later she lost interest in her hobbies and was convinced that she would not be able to work again. She thought life was not worth living and consumed 60 tablets of phenobarbitone to end her life. She is most likely suffering from: *(AI 2004)*
    A. Adjustment disorder
    B. Acute stress disorder
    C. Depressive disorder
    D. Post-traumatic stress disorder

64. Two months after knowing that his son was suffering from leukemia, a 45-year-old father presents with sleep deprivation, lethargy, headache, and low mood. He interacts reasonably well with others, but has absented himself from work. The most probable diagnosis is: *(AI 2008)*
    A. Depression
    B. Psychogenic headache
    C. Adjustment disorder
    D. Somatization disorder

65. A girl feels very depressed as her father died one month back. She feels moody and won't join with others and she thinks about joining her father. The most likely diagnosis is: *(NIMHANS 2015)*
    A. Post-traumatic stress disorder
    B. Grief
    C. Depression
    D. Bipolar disorder

66. A young girl comes to the OPD with symptoms of 'breaking down crying whenever she sees photos of her mother or items that her mother used to use. She developed these symptoms after death of her mother, which happened one month back. What is the diagnosis? *(NIMHANS 2018)*
    A. Normal grief
    B. Complicated grief
    C. Adjustment disorder
    D. Major depression

Somatic Symptom and Related Disorders & Factitious Disorders

67. All of the following are somatic symptoms and related disorder *except*: *(PGI Nov 2017)*
    A. Somatic symptom disorder
    B. Illness anxiety disorder
    C. Conversion disorder
    D. Somatic passivity
    E. Adjustment disorder

Controversial Question

68. Which of the following is not a specific somatoform disorder? *(AIIMS Nov 2011)*
    A. Somatization disorder
    B. Chronic fatigue syndrome
    C. Irritable bowel syndrome
    D. Fibromyalgia

69. A 45-year-old male presents with history of headache, and vague body pains, off and on diarrhea and constipation, impotence and tingling and paresthesia in glove stocking pattern. The most probable diagnosis is: *(AI 2K, JIPMER 2002, DNB 2004)*
    A. Hypochondriasis
    B. Somatization disorder
    C. Conversion disorder
    D. Factitious disorder

70. Which of the following is NOT a somatic symptom: *(NIMHANS 2013)*
    A. Anhedonia
    B. Constipation
    C. Impotence
    D. Numbness

71. A 41-year-old married female presented with headache for the last 6 months. She had several consultations. All her investigations were found to be within normal limits. She still insists that there is something wrong in her head and seeks another consultation. The most likely diagnosis is:
    A. Phobia *(NEET 2016, AI 2003)*
    B. Psychogenic headache
    C. Hypochondriasis
    D. Depression

72. Hypochondriasis is: *(AI 1994)*
    A. Normal preoccupation with abnormal body function
    B. Abnormal preoccupation with abnormal body function
    C. Normal preoccupation with normal body function
    D. Abnormal preoccupation with normal body function

73. A nondiabetic, nonhypertensive patient has some extra beats in pulse. Doctor informed that it is benign and no intervention is required. But patient is worried that it is a serious cardiac disorder and is still going for repeated investigations and going from doctor-to-doctor. This is a type of: *(FMGE 2017)*
    A. Conversion disorder
    B. Hypochondriasis
    C. Somatoform pain
    D. Depression

74. A 35-year-old male, with premorbid anxious traits and heavy smoker believes that he has been suffering from 'lung carcinoma' for a year. No significant clinical finding is detected on examination and relevant investigations. In the process, he has spent a huge amount of money, time and energy in getting himself unduly investigated. He is most likely suffering from: *(AIIMS Nov 2004)*
    A. Carcinoma lung
    B. Hypochondriacal disorder
    C. Delusional disorder
    D. Malingering

75. A young 20-year-old girl presents with complaints of pain in legs, intermittent vomiting, and headache since 2 months. Her physical examination was normal. What is the most possible diagnosis? *(AIIMS Nov 2009)*
    A. Generalized anxiety disorder
    B. Conversion disorder
    C. Somatoform pain disorder
    D. Somatization disorder

76. A 40-year-old male is admitted with complaints of abdominal pain and headache. General physical examination revealed six scars on the abdomen from previous surgeries. He seems to maintain a sick role and seeks attention from the nurses. He demands multiple diagnostic tests including a liver biopsy. The treating team failed to diagnose any major physical illness in the patient. His mental status examination did not reveal any major psychopathology. One of the treating staff recognized him to have appeared in several other hospitals with abdominal pain and some other vague complaints. He is most likely suffering from:
    A. Schizophrenia *(AIIMS Nov 2003)*
    B. Malingering
    C. Somatization disorder
    D. Factitious disorder

77. A 30-year-old lady presented to physician with complaints of hematuria. On evaluation RBCs were found in urine but no cause was found. On further enquiry it was found that she has gone to many doctors with the same complaints and would demand inpatient care. She would prick her finger and mix blood in urine sample. Her diagnosis is:
    A. Malingering *(Karnataka 2011)*
    B. Factitious illness
    C. Dissociative disorder
    D. Hypochondriasis

78. Munchausen's syndrome by proxy involves:
    A. Drug abuse *(MH 2011)*
    B. Toxin mediated neuropsychiatric disorder
    C. Illness caused by caregiver
    D. All of the above

79. Maintaining sick role by any means is a characteristic feature of: *(JIPMER 2002, Mahe 2004, Rohtak 2002, DNB 2003)*
    A. Hypochondriasis
    B. Somatization disorder
    C. Conversion disorder
    D. Factitious disorder

80. A person has been referred to you by the court. You find a discrepancy between the history and examination findings. Which of these conditions you should be aware of in this situation? *(AIIMS Nov 2016)*
    A. Malingering
    B. Factitious disorder
    C. Somatization syndrome
    D. Dissociative fugue

81. True about chronic fatigue syndrome is: *(PGI May 2016)*
    A. Symptoms are present for more than six months period
    B. Can be caused by EBV virus
    C. Shows characteristic symptoms
    D. Examination and investigations are usually normal
    E. Cognitive behavioral therapy is the management.

82. About chronic fatigue syndrome which one is not true? *(NIMHANS 2019)*
    A. Fatigue gets relieved by taking rest
    B. Patient complaints of non refreshing sleep
    C. Memory disturbances
    D. Benzodiazepines can be used in treatment

Dissociative Disorders (Conversion Disorders)

83. La belle indifference is seen in: *(DNB NEET 2014-15, AIIMS 1998)*
    A. Conversion disorder
    B. Schizophrenia
    C. Mania
    D. Depression

84. In conversion disorder, all of the following statements are true *except*: *(DNB NEET 2014-15)*
    A. Autonomic nervous system is involved
    B. There is primary and secondary gain
    C. La belle indifference is a feature
    D. Patient does not intentionally produce symptoms

85. All are true about conversion disorder *except*: *(DNB June 2011)*
    A. Presence of secondary gain
    B. Onset in late age
    C. Patient does not consciously produce symptom
    D. Relation with stress

86. Which of the following is a conversion disorder? *(DNB June 2009)*
    A. Hysterical fits
    B. Derealization
    C. Depersonalization
    D. Amnesia

87. In conversion disorders, all are found *except*: *(DNB NEET 2014-15)*
    A. Jealousy
    B. Paralysis
    C. Anesthesia
    D. Abnormal gait

88. Following are included in dissociative disorder: *(PGI June 2007, 2003)*
    A. Multiple personality disorder
    B. Fugue
    C. Hypochondriasis
    D. Somatization disorder
    E. Obsession
    F. Borderline personality

89. Which of the following can differentiate hysterical fits from epileptic fits? *(DPG 2009, Calcutta 2002)*
    A. Occur in sleep
    B. Injuries to person
    C. Incontinence
    D. Occur when people are watching

90. The most common form of dissociative hysteria is:
    A. Fugue *(MH 2000)*
    B. Amnesia
    C. Multiple personality
    D. Somnambulism

91. Psychogenic amnesia is characterized by: *(AIIMS 1997)*
    A. Anterograde amnesia
    B. Retrograde amnesia
    C. Both with confabulation
    D. Patchy impairment of personal memories

92. A person missing from home is found wandering purposefully. He is well-groomed and denies remembering how he reached at the new place. Most likely diagnosis is: *(AI 2001)*
    A. Dementia
    B. Dissociative amnesia
    C. Dissociative fugue
    D. Schizophrenia

93. An 18-year-old boy came to psychiatry OPD with a complaint of feeling as, if he is changed from inside. He reports feeling strange as, if he is different from his normal self. He was very tense and anxious yet could not point out the precise change in him. This phenomena is best called as:
    A. Delusional mood *(AI 2005)*
    B. Depersonalization
    C. Autochthonous delusion
    D. Overvalued idea

94. A young female presents with history of abdominal pain, headache, nausea and vomiting and sudden loss of movement of right upper limb. What is the most likely diagnosis? *(AIIMS May 2017)*
    A. Conversion disorder
    B. Migraine
    C. Right lower limb paralysis
    D. Acute intermittent porphyria (AIP)

95. All are true about Ganser's syndrome *except*: *(JIPMER/UP 2K, PGI 1999, DNB 1998)*
    A. Approximate answer
    B. Apparent clouding of consciousness
    C. Only found in prisoners
    D. Hallucinations

96. Ganser syndrome is a type of: *(DNB NEET 2014-15)*
    A. Dementia
    B. Malingering
    C. Dissociative disorder
    D. Personality disorder

97. **All is true about pseudocyesis *except*:**
    A. Abdominal enlargement *(DNB NEET 2014-15)*
    B. Patient is pregnant
    C. Labor pains at expected date of delivery
    D. Amenorrhea

98. **The difference between malingering and hysteria is:** *(AI 1994, DNB 2006)*
    A. Hypnosis
    B. Malingering has poor prognosis
    C. Hysteria is more common in females
    D. Conscious motive in malingering

99. **Differential diagnosis of premenstrual tension includes all of the following *except*:** *(AIIMS Nov 2002)*
    A. Psychiatric depressive disorder
    B. Panic disorder
    C. Generalized anxiety disorder
    D. Chronic fatigue syndrome

100. **A feeling of detachment from own body and a sense of unreality is called as:** *(NIMHANS 2018)*
    A. Depersonalisation
    B. Derealisation
    C. Dissociation
    D. Trance

Miscellaneous

101. **An 18-year-old boy presented with a belief that his penis is retracting in the abdomen and he will die when it complete retracts. What is this disorder called as?** *(NEET 2016)*
     A. Dhat syndrome
     B. Koro
     C. Latah
     D. Munchausen syndrome

102. **All of the following are correctly matched *except*:** *(NIMHANS 2015)*
     A. Continuous irrelevant intrusive thoughts about having HIV infection and handwashing-Hypochondriasis
     B. Sudden loss of limb movements Conversion disorder
     C. Avoidance and safety behavior-OCD
     D. Negative symptoms- Schizophrenia

103. **Which of the following is NOT an anxiolytic drug?** *(NIMHANS 2013)*
     A. Melatonin
     B. Haloperidol
     C. Alprazolam
     D. Sertraline

104. **Thyrotoxicosis is most commonly associated with:** *(NIMHANS 2012)*
     A. Anxiety   B. Mania
     C. Delirium   D. Paranoid state

105. **Which of the following is incorrectly matched?** *(NIMHANS 2019)*
     A. Generalised anxiety disorder-excessive worries
     B. Generalised anxiety disorder-avoidance
     C. Phobia-Fear of situations
     D. Panic attack-Fear of symptoms

106. **MUS stands for:** *(NIMHANS 2019)*
     A. Medically unexplained syndrome
     B. Medically unexplained symptoms
     C. Medically undifferentiated symptoms
     D. Mentally unstable symptoms

AIIMS New Pattern Question

107. **The correct statements about Obsessive compulsive disorder includes:**
     a. Obsessions are disorders of 'possession' of thought
     b. The most common type of compulsion is washing
     c. Systematic desensitization is the psychotherapy of choice
     d. OCD in children can be precipitated by streptococcal infections

     A. If a, c are correct
     B. If a, d are correct
     C. If b, d are correct
     D. If all four (a, b, c, and d) are correct

Answers With Explanations

General

1. A. Decreased sweating.
2. D. Stressful situations.
3. D. Pattern of autonomic nervous system (ANS) and physiological response when we are aroused by a stressful situation.
4. A. As a group anxiety disorders are the most common psychiatric disorders, followed by mood disorders. When individual disorders are compared, the most common psychiatric disorder is "specific phobia" followed by "depression". Many a times, the question asked in exam does not have the option of either phobia or anxiety disorder, in that case the answer becomes depression.

Generalized Anxiety Disorders

5. C. Fear of impending doom is typically seen in panic attacks.
6. A. Benzodiazepines are the drugs of choice for generalized anxiety disorder. However, it must be remembered that benzodiazepines can cause dependence. The other drugs which can be used include SSRIs, buspirone and venlafaxine.
7. A, D, E, F. According to Kaplan and Sadock's 'Synopsis of Psychiatry, benzodiazepines are the drugs of choice for generalized anxiety disorder.
8. B. In this patient the best answer would be "mixed anxiety depression". This patient has some depressive symptoms (sadness, loss of appetite and insomnia), however, the question explicitly mentions that there is no hopelessness, no suicidal thoughts and that her job and social life is normal. The question goes on to add that "she is doing remarkable well in other areas of life". Please remember that even in a patient with mild depression, it is expected that there would be at least some disturbance in professional and social life. Further her symptoms are not enough to make a diagnosis of depression. In view of the above, the diagnosis of mild depression cannot be made. This patient does not have any history of precipitating event hence the diagnosis of adjustment disorder can be easily ruled out. Few guides are giving the answer as generalized anxiety disorder which does not make any sense as the only anxiety symptom mentioned here is palpitation. The core feature of generalized anxiety disorder, i.e. "generalized and persistent anxiety" is not there. Hence, we are left with mixed anxiety depression. The diagnosis of mixed anxiety depression is made when there are "symptoms of both anxiety and depression, but neither set of symptoms is severe enough to make an independent anxiety or depressive disorder diagnosis". This description suits best to the clinical scenario provided here.

Panic Disorder

9. A. Panic attack.
10. C. Serotonin, norepinephrine and GABA are the major neurotransmitters involved. Cholecystokinin and pentagastrin (which acts on CCK receptors) are known to cause panic attacks.
11. A, B, C, E.
12. C. Short-term benzodiazepine plus SSRI plus CBT.
13. C. Hemoglobin. This is an interesting question, First of all, in all likelihood, "except" at the end of question got omitted due to typographical error. Hence, our answer is keeping that in mind. This patient's presentation is suggestive of panic attack. Before diagnosing panic attack, we must rule out organic (medical) causes of anxiety. Myocardial infarction, angina, arrhythmias, hypoglycemia, hyperthyroidism (thyroid storm), anaemia are all differentials of panic attacks. So all four tests given in this question should be done. The sequence in which these tests should be done depends on which diagnosis we want to rule out first which in turn depends on how life threatening that diagnosis is. So, first investigation in this case should be ECG, as we want to rule out life threatening cardiac conditions first. We should also do random blood sugar and thyroid function tests too. Hemoglobin levels need not be done in emergency as anaemia is least likely to present as a life threatening condition and can be tested for later on.

    One of the view point on this question is that since thyroid function tests are not available in emergency and reports come after a day, hence thyroid function test should be the answer. This is an erroneous view. First of all while answering a MCQ, you presume ideal situation, that is you have all the facilities possible. Secondly, what we seen in our routine practice should not be used as an argument while solving questions, and finally, emergency thyroid profile tests can actually be done, so it is not that they are not available.
14. B. Patients with GTCS have tonic clonic movements which are not seen in panic attack. Temporal lobe epilepsy can present with psychic symptoms (such as anxiety symptoms) and hence can be a differential diagnosis for panic attack.
15. B. SSRIs should not be started at high dosages as they may actually increase anxiety, when treatment is initiated. That is why mostly SSRIs are usually started in combination with benzodiazepines. Exposure therapy is used in treatment of panic disorder. MAOI and SSSRIs are used for treatment of atypical depression

Phobic Anxiety Disorders

16. A. Nyctophobia
17. B. Social phobia is defined as irrational fear of social situations. Though it can be said that it also includes

Neurotic, Stress-related and Somatoform Disorders

certain activities, however, please remember that it is the context (situation) that is central to social phobia and not the activity. For example, many patients with social phobia have difficulty eating in a restaurant. However, they have no problem doing the same activity (i.e. eating) when alone. It's the situation (i.e. the restaurant) that produces anxiety.

18. D. Agoraphobia.
19. C. Panic disorder and agoraphobia are usually comorbid conditions.
20. C. The diagnosis here is agoraphobia as this gentleman is uncomfortable with closed places (lift), crowded places and also travelling alone. The best treatment option here is exposure and response prevention.
21. C. Behavior therapy.
22. A, B, C, D, and E.

Obsessive-Compulsive Disorder

23. B. The cognitive theory of OCD says that the typical abnormalities in OCD include, "excessive or inflated sense of responsibility", "feeling of uncertainty" and "overestimation of threat". Few books are giving the answer as "generalized anxiety disorder" which is incorrect.
24. C. Clomipramine (which is a Tricyclic antidepressant) has significant anticholinergic activity
25. A, C, and D. Obsessions are repetitive thoughts, images or impulses. Often the content of thoughts is about sex or god and patient tries to stop these anxiety provoking thoughts unsuccessfully. Please remember, that a patient with obsession identifies the repetitive thought as his "own thought" and not something that is imposed by others. Also remember, if the patient indeed believes that the thought has been imposed by others, it would then be diagnosed as "thought insertion" and not an obsession.
26. C. Obsessions are considered senseless by the patient whereas patient has full belief in the delusions. For example, a patient who gets obsessive thoughts that "his hands are unclean" understands that his thought is not true and gets bothered by this repetitive thought whereas a patient with "delusion of infidelity" actually believes that his wife is cheating on him and continues to believe so irrespective of what others say.
27. D. All of the above.
28. C. Obsessions are egodystonic and not egosyntonic.
29. A. Pathological doubt

    The most common presentation of OCD involves obsession of contamination and compulsions of checking, however, that is not in the options. The second most common presentation involves pathological doubts.
30. A. Orbitofrontal cortex, caudate (which is a part of basal ganglia) and thalamus are involved in OCD.
31. B. b and c are correct statements. The defense mechanisms involved in OCD are undoing, reaction formation, isolation of affect and inhibition (defense mechanisms are discussed in chapter of Psychoanalysis). SSRIs are the first line agent and antipsychotics like risperidone can be used as an adjuvants. Exposure and response prevention is the psychotherapy of choice.
32. A. Obsessive compulsive disorder.
33. B. Most of the patients with OCD, develop secondary depression.
34. B. Both SSRIs and clomipramine are considered first line treatment, however due to better side effect profile, SSRIs are preferred.
35. D. Many guides are giving the answer as haloperidol but that is not the right answer here. The American Psychiatric Association guidelines clearly state that, if patients do not respond to SSRIs and clomipramine, one of the treatment strategy is augmentation with antipsychotics. The best evidence is for haloperidol, risperidone, quetiapine and olanzapine. In comparison, carbamazepine is rarely used in OCD and has very weak evidence in comparison to haloperidol. Hence, the best answer here would be carbamazepine.
36. D. Again, we have to choose between carbamazepine and diazepam. Now, diazepam is a benzodiazepine and can improve anxiety temporarily however it doesn't act at core symptoms of OCD. Whereas, carbamazepine, though has minimal evidence, but it has been found to act on core symptoms of OCD.
37. A, B, C, D. SSRIs and clomipramine are first line agents. Trifluperidol does not have any evidence in management of OCD.
38. A, B, C, D and E.
39. D. SSRIs, Clomipramine and CBT are all first line treatment. Systematic desensitization is least effective of all.
40. D. A combination of pharmacotherapy and psychotherapy has the best evidence in the management of OCD.
41. B. The technique is actually exposure and response prevention. In OCD, the primary aim is to stop the compulsions; hence response prevention is the better answer here.
42. B, and C.
43. B. According to American Psychiatric Association Guidelines "The first line treatments for OCD are cognitive behavioral therapy that relies on behavioral technique of exposure and response prevention and serotonin reuptake inhibitors". Now, this question is just mentioning pharmacological agents without specifying anything about which agent. Also few studies have found, that exposure and response prevention has more lasting effect than pharmacological agents. Said that, the choice of treatment between ERP and pharmacological agents depends on patients characteristics, which have not been provided, hence it is tough to choose. However in this case, exposure and response prevention appears to be the best answer.
44. D. Electroconvulsive therapy has no major role in treatment of OCD.
45. C. Studies have found **bilaterally small caudates** in patients with obsessive compulsive disorder.
46. C Hoarding disorder. According to Textbook of Anxiety Disorders, Stein, Hollander & Rothbaum (American Psychiatric Publishing), "Consistent evidence is emerging to suggest that patients who present with primarily hoarding symptoms respond less well to ERP than do patients with other presentation of OCD"
47. A. OCD

Trauma and Stress-related Disorders

48. A, D, E.
49. D. A and D are correct statements. The onset of symptoms after a traumatic event (loss of house in earthquake) followed by onset of symptoms such as despair, anxiety, sadness, etc. is consistent with the diagnosis of acute stress reaction. The treatment should be offered, and hence referral to psychiatrist should be done. Risperidone is not normally used and projection is not involved as a defence mechanism.
50. C. Hallucinations.
51. E. PTSD may have a delayed onset, i.e. after 6 months of trauma.
52. A. Symptoms develop immediately after the event.
53. D. Last statement is not correct. Most people who experience trauma do not develop any disorder.
54. C. The patients who have a past history of psychiatric illness are more predisposed and so are women. There is no such correlation with intellect.
55. C. Recall of events and avoidance is quite typical of PTSD. Nightmares, autonomic arousal and depressive symptoms can be seen in other disorders also.
56. E. The treatment of choice is cognitive behavioral therapy. All other statements are correct.
57. B. Posttraumatic stress disorder.
58. A. Cognitive behavioral therapy.
59. A, B, C, D, E.

Grief and Adjustment Disorder

60. A. The answer here is debatable. First of all, lets review some facts. There is no clear-cut duration in which grief should get resolved. The most accepted duration for grief is 6–12 months. However, every single textbook says that grief usually continues beyond that period. Second, brief hallucinations can be a part of normal grief, however continuous hallucinations are not seen. In this case, the history is that the man reported that wife asked him to join her. The question has not mentioned if it was an auditory perception (i.e. he heard voice of wife) or visual perception (i.e. he saw his wife), what was the state of consciousness (whether he was awake or sleeping). In view of above its difficult to even call this phenomenon as a hallucination. Even if we accept it as a hallucination, it appears to be a single episode. There is no history of any other associated symptoms. Hence, the better answer here would be normal grief. Also, please remember that grief and bereavement are often used interchangeably, however strictly speaking, bereavement is a state of loss, whereas grief is the emotional and behavioral response to loss. The question is talking about the behavioral and emotional response here. All in all, its a poorly framed and incomplete question.
61. C. Aggression.
62. D. In this case, death happened "couple of years ago". The first time she had auditory hallucinations was after a week of his death and since then it has been happening. Now, in grief "brief hallucinations" can occur, however, here the hallucinations are often and patient is even discussing the daily matters with the "voice". This clearly shows presence of psychotic symptoms which should be diagnosed separately. Please remember patient can develop all kind of psychiatric disorders like depression, anxiety, PTSD in association with grief and if the symptoms are severe enough, they should receive separate diagnosis. This patient has psychotic symptoms (i.e. hallucinations) and should be treated with an antipsychotic, haloperidol. The treatment depends on symptoms, in case of occasional anxiety, alprazolam could have been used. In case of significant depressive symptoms antidepressant could have been used, but since the psychotic symptoms are prominent, we must use an antipsychotic.
63. C. This question has been answered wrongly by most of the guides. Please remember few basic things about adjustment disorder and depression. Adjustment disorder is always seen after a stressful event, which is usually a negative life event. The symptoms of adjustment disorder are quite similar to depression and include depressed mood, anxiety, worry, a feeling of inability to cope and some degree of disturbance in individuals daily functioning. Now, a negative life event can also precipitate the depressive episode. So, the presence of a stressor cannot be used to differentiate between adjustment disorder and depression. If a patient has the symptoms severe enough to qualify the diagnosis of depression, depression would always be diagnosed ahead of adjustment disorder, irrespective of whether there was a stressor or not. In this case patient has severe symptoms such as loss of interest, ideas of hopelessness (patient is convinced that she would not be able to work again) and most importantly suicide attempt, all of which are highly suggestive of depression. Hence, the diagnosis would be depressive disorder.
64. C. Here, the diagnosis is adjustment disorder. The symptoms are not severe enough to qualify for the diagnosis of depression and there is a clear history of a stressor (diagnosis of leukemia in son).
65. B. Grief. Feeling depressed, mood changes and longing after death of a loved one are all suggestive of grief.
66. A. Normal grief

Somatic Symptom and Realated Disorders & Factitious Disorders

67. A, B, C.
    According to DSM-5, the category, somatic symptom and related disorder consists of the following: 1) Somatic symptom disorder (the DSM IV diagnosis of somatization disorder, somatoform pain disorder, undifferentiated somatoform disorder have all been clubbed under this diagnosis in DSM-5); 2) Illness anxiety disorder and 3) conversion disorder.
68. A. The classification of somatoform disorders mentioned in the preceding answer is frequently not used by nonpsychiatrist practitioners. These practitioners use other diagnoses, which are frequently referred to as functional somatic syndromes. These include chronic fatigue syndrome, fibromyalgia and irritable

bowel syndrome. Somatization disorder is not a part of functional somatic syndromes.

69. B. This patient has pain symptoms, gastrointestinal symptoms, sexual symptoms and pseudoneurological symptoms.
70. A. Anhedonia. The somatic symptoms as defined in somatization disorder give special importance to GI symptoms (constipation here), sexual symptoms (impotence here), numbness (neurological symptoms).
71. C. The patient had multiple normal investigations but continues to believe that there is something wrong in her head and continues to seek multiple consultations. The most likely diagnosis is hypochondriasis.
72. D. Abnormal preoccupation with normal body function.
73. B. Hypochondriasis. Preoccupation with as serious illness (serious cardiac disorder) on the basis of misinterpretation of a benign symptom, and continuation of preoccupation despite reassurance by doctor is suggestive of hypochondriasis.
74. B. Hypochondriacal disorder.
75. D. The best answer here is somatization disorder. The patient has pain symptoms and gastrointestinal symptoms. Going by strict definition of DSM-IV, there should be 4 pain symptoms, 2 GI symptoms, 1 sexual symptom and 1 pseudoneurological symptoms. However the ICD-10, simply says that there should be "multiple and variable physical symptoms for which no adequate explanation has been found". The other plausible option is somatoform pain disorder, however it is characterized by only pain symptoms whereas in this patient intermittent vomiting is also present.
76. D. The history of multiple scars from previous surgeries, seeking attention from nurses, maintenance of sick role, demands for multiple diagnostic tests and identification by a staff all suggest a factitious disorder.
77. B. Factitious illness.
78. C. Illness caused by caregiver.
79. D. Sick role means that the patient wants others to accept him as "sick" and treat him accordingly by giving attention and care. Patients with factitious disorders frequently fake symptoms to get the "sick role".
80. A. Malingering. Referral by court and discrepancies, both are suggestive of malingering.
81. A, B, E.
The duration should be more than six months. Although yet not proved, EBV has been implicated. Given that the language of option is "EBV **can**", it becomes a correct statement. Symptoms are quite nonspecific and definitely not "characteristic". Mostly investigations are normal and cognitive behavioural therapy is effective.
82. A. The fatigue present in chronic fatigue syndrome does not improve with rest.

Dissociative Disorders (Conversion Disorders)

83. A. La belle indifference is a phrase used to describe the feeling of indifference which patients of conversion disorders have towards their symptoms.
84. A. Sensory and motor system are involved and not the autonomic nervous system.
85. B. The onset of conversion disorder is usually seen in late childhood to early adulthood and is rare after 35 years of age.
86. A. The term "hysterical fits" is no longer used in modern terminology. The current classificatory system will use the diagnosis of conversion disorder with seizure. The DSM diagnosis of conversion disorder can present with either motor symptoms, sensory symptoms or convulsions. Please remember that in ICD-10, conversion disorder is another name for dissociative disorders. So, if we follow ICD-10, all four options are true. But usually, in examinations the term conversion disorder refers to the DSM diagnosis and not the ICD.
87. A. Jealousy is not a neurological sign, the rest three are.
88. A, B.
89. D. Hysterical fits or dissociative convulsions/seizures or conversion disorders with convulsions/seizures do not occur in sleep, are not associated with any injuries, are not associated with any incontinence and there is no post seizure amnesia or confusion. They usually occur when others are watching.
90. B. Dissociative amnesia is the most common type of dissociative disorder.
91. D. In psychogenic amnesia (or dissociative amnesia), usually memory is lost for events which have some personal significance, whereas memories for neutral events (e.g. national events) is intact. Hence, the memory loss is patchy and mostly for personal memories.
92. C. Dissociative fugue.
93. B. Depersonalization.
94. D. Acute intermittent porphyria. The history of a young female presenting with abdominal symptoms and sudden neurological symptoms should raise the suspicion for AIP. AIP is an important differential diagnosis of conversion disorders. Conversion disorders are usually precipitated by a psychological stressor and present with altered voluntary motor or sensory symptoms. History of abdominal pain and other GI symptoms is not usually seen and their presence is more consistent with the diagnosis of AIP.
95. C. Though Ganser syndrome is usually seen in prisoners but it is not exclusive to them.
96. C. Dissociative disorder.
97. B. Patient is not pregnant is pseudocyesis. Though she falsely believes that and there are also associated changes suggestive of pregnancy.
98. D. The symptoms is malingering are produced consciously for some conscious motive (e.g. monetary gain). In hysteria (dissociative disorders), the symptoms are produces unconsciously and the motive is also unconscious (e.g. attention or love from others).
99. D. Premenstrual tension or Premenstrual syndrome is characterized by depressive and anxiety symptoms one week before the onset of menses, and their resolution after the onset of menses or within few days of onset of menses. These symptoms are not present during the other period of menstrual cycles. If the depressive and anxiety symptoms are present throughout the

cycle the differential diagnose is depression, anxiety disorders such as generalized anxiety disorder, panic disorder. Chronic fatigue syndrome is not a differential here.

100. A. Depersonalization

Miscellaneous

101. B. Koro
102. A. Continuous irrelevant thoughts about having HIV and handwashing is consistent with OCD and not hypochondriasis.
103. A. Melatonin. SSRIs and benzodiazepines are the main stay of treatment. Antipsychotics like haloperidol can be used as adjunct. Melatonin has no clearly defined indication in anxiety disorder.
104. A. Anxiety
105. B. Avoidance is not a core feature of generalized anxiety disorder. In panic attack, patient tends to misinterpret benign physical signs such as tachycardia, as suggestive of something serious (e.g. MI) and is afraid of them.
106. B. Medically unexplained symptoms.

AIIMS New Pattern Answer

107. B. (a and d are correct statements)
    a. Correct. Obsessions are disorders of possession of thought
    b. Incorrect. The most common type of compulsion is 'compulsive checking'
    c. Incorrect. Exposure and response prevention is the psychotherapy of choice in OCD
    d. Correct. In a small number of cases, OCD in children may be precipitated/worsened after infection with Group A β-hemolytic streptococcus (GABHS)

5. Substance-related and Addictive Disorders

SUBSTANCE USE DISORDERS

The substance related disorders encompass 10 separate classes of drugs which includes alcohol, caffeine, cannabis, hallucinogens, inhalants, opioids, sedatives and hypnotics, stimulants, tobacco and other substances.

Terminology

A. ***Dependence***: It is defined as a pattern in which the use of a substance or a class of substances takes on a much higher priority for a given individual than other behaviors that once had a greater value. It encompasses **behavioral dependence (substance seeking behaviors), physical dependence (physiological effects of multiple episodes of substance use)** and **psychological dependence (continuous or intermittent craving)**.

According to ICD-11, the presence of the following in past 1 year is required for diagnosis of dependence on a substance:
- Strong desire or sense of compulsion to take a substance **(craving)**
- Difficulty in controlling substance taking behavior in terms of its onset, termination or levels of use
- **Withdrawal symptoms** (typical physiological symptoms that develop when substance use is reduced or stopped)
- **Tolerance** (increased doses of substance is required to achieve the effects originally produced by lower doses)
- Progressive neglect of alternative pleasures or interests because of substance use
- Persistence with substance use despite clear evidence of harmful consequences.

B. ***Harmful use***: It is a state where substance use is causing harm but still criterion of dependence are not met.

According to ICD-11, the harmful use is defined as a pattern of substance use which is causing damage to person's **physical health** (e.g. hepatitis due to alcohol use) or **mental health** (e.g. episode of depression secondary to heavy alcohol consumption) or has resulted in behaviour leading to harm to the health of others.

C. ***Single episode of harmful use***: A single episode of substance use that has caused damage to a person's physical or mental health or has resulted in behaviour leading to harm to the health of others.

 DSM-5 Update

DSM-5, doesn't use the categories of "dependence" and "harmful use" and instead uses a single diagnostic category of "substance use disorders".

D. ***Intoxication***: A transient condition that develops following administration of a substance, in which various mental functions such as consciousness, thinking, perception or behavior are altered.

E. ***Withdrawal***: Specific symptoms that occur after stopping or reducing the amount of substance that has been used regularly over a prolonged period.

Etiology

The development of substance use disorders is best explained by a **biopsychosocial model**. It means that there is an interaction of biological factors, psychological factors and social factors which results in development of substance use disorders (dependence, harmful use or abuse). The drugs act on particular receptors and brain pathways and these receptors and pathways have been found to play a central role in development of substance use disorders. Of particular importance are the dopaminergic neurons in the ventral tegmental area which project to cortical and limbic regions, especially the nucleus accumbens. This pathway is involved in the sensation of reward (or pleasure) and is believed to be the major mediator of effects of substances. This pathway is also known as **"brain reward pathway"**.

 DSM-5 Update

Pathological gambling has been included along with substance related disorders under the diagnostic entity of "gambling disorder". ICD-11 has included gambling disorder & gaming disorders, as addictive behaviour disorders, and they have been classified along with substance related disorders.

The major neurotransmitters involved in development of substance used disorders include opioids, catecholamines (particularly dopamine) and γ-aminobutyric acid (GABA).

The evidence from studies of twin, adoptees and siblings has also suggested the role of genetic factors in development of substance abuse.

Apart from biological factors, learning and conditioning is also known to contribute to development of the substance use disorder. The use of substance can result in an intense sense of euphoria, it also frequently alleviates the negative emotions (such as sadness, anxiety). This results in reinforcement of substance taking behavior. Other factors like peer pressure, social acceptance, easy availability and the personality type of the individual also contribute to the development of substance use disorders.

ALCOHOL

Ethyl alcohol is the active ingredient of alcoholic drinks. The concentration of ethyl alcohol (ethanol) varies across the preparations. The standard drink or a unit of alcohol corresponds to 10 mL of absolute alcohol or 7.8 gram of absolute alcohol (specific gravity of alcohol = 0.78).

Table 1: Absolute alcohol concentration in various preparations.

Preparation	Concentration of alcohol by volume (% ABV)
Spirits (whiskey, rum, gin, vodka, brandy, etc.)	40
Arrack	33
Fortified wines	14–20
Wines	5–13
Beer (strong)	8–11
Beer (standard)	3–4

One standard drink = 1 peg (30 mL) of spirits = 1 glass (125 mL) of wine = 1 glass (60 mL) of fortified wine = 1/2 packet of arrack = 1/2 bottle of standard beer = 1/4 bottle of strong beer.

Arrack is the country made liquor. Fortified wines are prepared by adding brandy to wine.

Absorption: About 20% of alcohol is absorbed from stomach and remainder from **small intestine (80 percent from duodenum and jejunum)**^{Q}. However, when alcohol is consumed with food, due to slowing down of gastric emptying, stomach becomes the main site for absorption. Peak blood alcohol concentration is reached in 30–90 minutes, depending on whether the alcohol was ingested on an empty stomach (absorption is faster) or with food (absorption is slower).

Mellanby effect^Q: Studies have shown that intoxicating effects of alcohol are greater at a given blood alcohol level when BAC (blood alcohol concentration) is increasing than for the same BAC when the blood alcohol level is falling.

Reverse tolerance: This refers to the phenomenon where the intoxicating effects of alcohol are seen progressively with **lower dosages**^{Q}. A patient may report that he gets intoxicated with much smaller amounts of alcohol now in comparison to the past. It is believed to be secondary to decreasing levels of alcohol metabolizing enzymes secondary to progressive liver dysfunction. A similar concept of **"sensitization"** is seen in cocaine, amphetamines, opioids and cannabis wherein augmented stimulant response is observed with repeated, intermittent exposure to a specific drug. It is believed to be due to changes in the brain reward pathways.

Metabolism: About 90% of absorbed alcohol is metabolized through oxidation in the liver, the remaining 10% is excreted unchanged by the kidneys and the lungs. The alcohol in alveolar air is in equilibrium with alcohol in blood passing through pulmonary capillaries, hence determining the alcohol levels in breath by breath analyzer gives a good estimate of blood alcohol levels.

The rate of oxidation by the liver is constant and is around 7–10 gram an hour (which equals to amount of alcohol in one standard drink). Alcohol is converted by activity of enzyme alcohol dehydrogenase into acetaldehyde, which is further oxidized by aldehyde dehydrogenase into acetate. Acetate is converted to carbon dioxide and water.

Acute Intoxication

Alcohol is a depressant of the central nervous system. The excitement that follows alcohol use is due to decrease in conscious self control. The symptoms and signs of alcohol intoxication depend on the blood alcohol concentration. Following symptoms develop:

Blood levels	Symptoms
20-30 mg/dL:	Slowness of motor performance and decreased thinking ability. **30 mg/dL**^{Q} is the legal limit for driving in India
30-80 mg/dL:	Worsening of motor performance and further decrease in thinking ability
80-200 mg/dL:	Incoordination, judgment errors, mood lability
200-300 mg/dL:	Nystagmus, slurring of speech, **alcoholic blackouts**^{Q}
>300 mg/dL:	Impaired vital signs and possible death.

Alcoholic blackout: It refers to **anterograde amnesia**^{Q} seen during intoxication. The person is unable to recall the events that happened when his blood alcohol levels were between 200-300 mg/dL.

Alcohol Withdrawal

It refers to the symptoms which develop after cessation of alcohol intake. In most patients the following sequence is seen, though all symptoms do not necessarily occur in all patients.

After 6-8 hours: The classic and most common sign of alcohol withdrawal is **tremulousness (coarse tremors)**^{Q}. Other symptoms include gastrointestinal symptoms (like nausea and vomiting), sympathetic autonomic hyperactivity including arousal, anxiety, sweating, hypertension, mydriasis and tachycardia.

After 12-24 hours: **Alcoholic hallucinosis**^{Q}. It refers to hallucinations in the absence of any disturbances of consciousness. Usually auditory hallucinations are present.

After 24-48 hours: Alcohol withdrawal seizures. The seizures are usually generalized and tonic-clonic. Usually patients have more than one seizures in a span of 3-6 hours, hence often the term **cluster seizures** is used for alcohol withdrawal seizures.

After 48-72 hours: Delirium tremens. Alcohol withdrawal delirium is a medical emergency and if untreated the mortality rate is around 20%. The symptoms and signs include disturbances of consciousness, disorientation to time, place and person, hallucinations (most commonly visual, but also auditory and tactile hallucinations) coarse tremors and autonomic hyperactivity.

Alcohol Induced Disorders

The use of alcohol may be associated with development of various mental disorders. Usually alcohol induced disorders, resolve within one month of cessation of alcohol intake. If the symptoms of mental disorder persist beyond that, the possibility of an independent mental disorder should be entertained. The following disorders have been described:

1. Alcohol induced psychotic disorders.
2. Alcohol induced bipolar disorders.
3. Alcohol induced depressive disorders.
4. Alcohol induced anxiety disorders, alcohol induced sleep disorder.
5. Alcohol induced sexual dysfunction.
6. Alcohol induced neurocognitive disorders.

Alcohol induced neurocognitive disorders: Long-term alcohol use can cause amnestic disorders characterized by disturbances in short-term memory. The classic names for alcohol induced amnestic disorders are **Wernicke's encephalopathy** and **Korsakoff's syndrome**.

A. *Wernicke's encephalopathy*: It is the acute neurological complication characterized by the following symptoms (pneumonic GOA):

G: Global **confusion**^{Q}

O: **Ophthalmoplegia,**^{Q} usually 6th nerve palsy (second most common is 3rd nerve palsy) causing, horizontal nystagmus and gaze palsy)

A: **Ataxia**^{Q}

Although Wernicke's encephalopathy can be **completely reversed** with treatment, often **residual ataxia**^{Q} and horizontal nystagmus remain despite treatment. Ophthalmoplegia responds rapidly to thiamine treatment and may get reversed within hours. Wernicke's encephalopathy may clear spontaneously in days to weeks or progress to Korsakoff's syndrome.

B. *Korsakoff's syndrome*: It is the **chronic** neurological complication of long-term alcohol use. It is characterized by impaired recent memory, **anterograde amnesia**^{Q} (inability to form new memory), **retrograde amnesia**^{Q} (inability to recall old memories) and **confabulations**^{Q} (making of false stories to fill memory gaps, which is unintentional). The anterograde amnesia is much more prominent than the retrograde amnesia.

The pathophysiology for both Wernicke's syndrome and Korsakoff's syndrome is **thiamine deficiency**^{Q}.

The neuropathological lesions are usually symmetrical and involve **mammillary bodies**^{Q}. Other sites of lesion include thalamus, hypothalamus, midbrain, pons, medulla, fornix and cerebellum.

The treatment of Wernicke's encephalopathy is high dose of parenteral thiamine. Treatment of Korsakoff syndrome is oral thiamine for 3-12 months. Only around 20% of patients with Korsakoff syndrome recover.

C. *Marchiafava bignami disease*: It is a rare neurological complication of long-term alcohol use. It is characterized by epilepsy, ataxia, dysarthria, hallucinations and intellectual deterioration. The pathophysiology is demyelination of **corpus callosum**, optic tracts and cerebellar peduncles.

Evaluation

A. *Screening test*: One of the most commonly used screening test is **CAGE questionnaire**^{Q}, which includes the following four questions:

- Have you ever felt that you should **C**ut down on your drinking?
- Have people **A**nnoyed you by criticizing your drinking?
- Have you ever felt bad or **G**uilty about your drinking?
- Have you ever had a drink first thing in the morning to steady your nerves or to get rid of hangover (**E**ye opener)?

A positive response on **two or more** than two of the above questions, is suggestive of alcohol use disorder. Another commonly used screening test is **AUDIT**[Q] (**alcohol use disorders identification test**). Others tests such as **SADQ (severity of alcohol dependence questionnaire)** are used to determine the severity of dependence.

B. *Diagnostic markers*: Apart from the screening tests, the blood test may also help in the identification of heavy drinkers who are susceptible to development of alcohol use disorders.
   - *Blood alcohol concentration*: It can be used to judge tolerance to alcohol. For example, if a person has high blood alcohol concentration without showing any signs of intoxication, it indicates the presence of tolerance and high chances of presence of alcohol use disorders.
     Blood alcohol concentration is usually measured using breath analyzers. It can also be estimated by using **Widmark formula**, if the amount of alcohol consumed and body weight is known.
   - *Carbohydrate deficit transferrin (CDT)*: The **most sensitive** and **specific** laboratory test for the identification of heavy drinking is elevated blood levels of carbohydrate deficit transferrin.
   - *Gamma-glutamyl transferase (GGT)*: Elevated levels of GGT are again suggestive of heavy drinking. However, GGT has a poor sensitivity and specificity (50-60%). The levels of both CDT and GGT return towards normal within days to weeks of stopping drinking.
   - *Alanine aminotransferase (ALT) and Aspartate aminotransferase (AST)*: These liver enzymes are even less sensitive than GGT, however have higher specificity. Out of two **ALT has higher specificity**[Q] as it mostly found in liver. A ratio of AST: ALT is a good marker for heavy alcohol consumption.
   - *Mean corpuscular volume*: MCV is frequently elevated in individuals who indulge in heavy drinking.
   - Other test include elevated levels of alkaline phosphatase, which indicate liver injury secondary to heavy drinking.

Treatment

The treatment of alcohol dependence is done in the following phases.
A. *Detoxification*: It is the first phase of treatment which involves management of withdrawal symptoms. The usual duration of detoxification is 7-14 days. **Benzodiazepines**[Q] are the drugs of choice (particularly **chlordiazepoxide**[Q]) for all the withdrawal symptoms ranging from common ones like tremors and nausea to severe withdrawal symptoms like alcohol withdrawal seizures and delirium tremens. In addition vitamins (particularly thiamine) must be given as patients usually are deficient in vitamins. **Carbamazepine** can also be used in place of benzodiazepines however other anticonvulsants do not have any role. The antipsychotics can be used in patients with delirium tremens and alcoholic hallucinosis.

B. *Maintenance of abstinence*: After the completion of detoxification, the next phase involves long-term treatment to maintain the abstinence. It involves both pharmacological and nonpharmacological treatment.
   - *Pharmacological treatment*: The drugs used are of two types:
     a. *Deterrent agents*: The most commonly used deterrent agent is **disulfiram**[Q]. It is an irreversible inhibitor of aldehyde dehydrogenase, the enzyme which metabolites acetaldehyde. Acetaldehyde is the first breakdown product of alcohol. If a patient who is on disulfiram, consumes alcohol, it results in accumulation of toxic levels of acetaldehyde and causes a number of unpleasant signs and symptoms, termed as **disulfiram ethanol reaction (DER)**.
        Other deterrent agents include citrated calcium carbimide and metronidazole.
     b. *Anticraving agents*: These agent reduce craving, which is an important reason for relapse. The anticraving agents include **naltrexone**[Q], **acamprosate**[Q], topiramate, serotonergic agents like fluoxetine and baclofen.
   - *Nonpharmacological treatment*: These are psychosocial treatment methods and include:
     a. *Cognitive behavioral therapies*: A large number of therapies have been found to have efficacy in maintaining abstinence. These include **motivational enhancement therapy**, relapse prevention model and cognitive therapy.
     b. *Alcoholic anonymous*: It is a self help group, which follows 12 steps to quit alcohol use. The members include patients who have recovered from alcoholism, current alcohol users and also volunteers.
     c. Family therapy.
     d. Group therapy.

OPIOIDS

The term **opiates** is used to describe the psychoactive alkaloids (like morphine and codeine) which are present in opium (derived from papaver somniferum, the poppy plant). The term **opioids** is a broader term which also includes synthetic compounds like heroin and methadone, which share the action and effects of opiates.

Heroin (diacetyl morphine) is the **most commonly**[Q] abused opioid. Since, it is more lipid soluble than morphine, it crosses blood brain barrier faster and has a more rapid onset of action. Heroin was initially used as a treatment for morphine addiction, however, it was realized that dependence forming potential of heroin is higher than morphine. The street names of heroin includes **"smack"** and "brown sugar" amongst others. The street forms are often impure and have adulterants like starch (fructose and sucrose), quinine, chalk powder, paracetamol and talcum powder, etc.

Opioids can be taken orally, snorted intranasally (also called chasing the dragon), and injected intravenously or subcutaneously. The intravenous users tend to gradually shift from peripheral veins to larger veins (a phenomenon called **mainlining**[Q]). The user may progress to subcutaneous administration, once he is not able to find any patent vein. The subcutaneous route is known as **"skin popping"**.

Intoxication

Opioids when taken (especially intravenously) produce a feeling of intense euphoria. The other symptoms include a feeling of warmth, heaviness of extremities and facial flushing. This initial euphoria is followed by a period of sedation (known as "nodding off").

Opioids overdose can be lethal due to **respiratory depression**[Q]. The symptoms of overdose include coma, slow respiration, hypothermia, **hypotension**[Q], bradycardia, pin point pupils, cyanosis.

Withdrawal Symptoms

The sudden stopping of opioids after prolonged use or intake of opioid antagonists like naltrexone can produce withdrawal symptoms. The short-term use of opioids decreases the activity of noradrenergic neurons and the long-term use results in compensatory hyperactivity. When opioids are suddenly stopped, there are symptoms of rebound noradrenergic hyperactivity. This hypothesis also explains the mechanism of action of clonidine (alpha-2 adrenergic receptor agonist, which decreases norepinephrine release) in management of opioid withdrawal.

The withdrawal symptoms usually appear around **6-8 hours**[Q] after the last dose, peak during the second or third day and subside during the next 7-10 days. The withdrawal from opioids produces a **flu-like syndrome**[Q] with the following symptoms.

1. **Lacrimation**[Q], **rhinorrhea**[Q], sweating, **diarrhea**[Q]
2. **Yawning** and **piloerection**[Q]
3. Pupillary dilation[Q]
4. Muscle cramps and generalized bodyache
5. **Insomnia**[Q], anxiety, hypertension and tachycardia
6. Nausea, vomiting and anorexia.

Treatment

A. ***Detoxification***: In this stage, the main focus is on the management of withdrawal symptoms. The medications used are usually long acting opioids like **methadone**[Q] or **buprenorphine**. Both medications, in view of their agonist action at opioid receptors, suppress the withdrawal symptoms. Other opioids like dextro-propoxyphene can also be used. Usually detoxification medicines are required for 2-3 weeks. Another method is use of **clonidine**[Q] for detoxification. However, clonidine provides considerably less reduction in symptoms in comparison to buprenorphine or methadone. Clonidine is thus mostly used as an adjunct to methadone or buprenorphine during detoxification.

   Accelerated detoxification: In this method, initially low doses of naltrexone is given to patient. Naltrexone being an opioid antagonist, produces severe withdrawal symptoms. After that, clonidine is used to control the symptoms. This method reduces the detoxification period to 4-5 days.

B. ***Maintenance treatment***: It follows the detoxification and the aim is to prevent the relapse. There are two different pharmacological approaches for maintenance phase.

   - ***Opioid substitution therapy***: In this method, the illicit, parenterally administered and short acting opioids (like heroin) are replaced by medically safe, orally taken and long acting opioids. The long acting opioids such as **methadone**, buprenorphine are mostly used. Levo alpha acetylmethadol was also used in past, however it has since been stopped as it is known to cause torsades de pointes.

     These orally used opioids are given at government approved centres. Though the patient continues to remain dependent, however he is protected from medical consequence of parenteral opioids (like HBV, HIV infection) and does not need to indulge in criminal activities to fund the illicit opioid use.

   - ***Opioid antagonist treatment***: **Naltrexone**[Q] can be given to the patient after detoxification is complete. The rationale is that naltrexone will block the opioid receptors and any opioid use would fail to produce the euphoric response and hence would not be repeated.

- Nonpharmacological approaches like cognitive behavioral therapy, narcotic anonymous (12 step self help groups), family therapy and group therapy are also useful.
C. **Overdose treatment**: The opioids are lethal in overdose. The drug of choice for treatment of opioid over-dose is i.v. **naloxone**^{Q} (short acting opioid antagonist).

CANNABIS

Cannabis is derived from the hemp plant, *cannabis sativa*. The plant has several varieties named after the regions where it is found (e.g. cannabis sativa indica in India, cannabis sativa americana in USA). Cannabis is the **most commonly used illegal drug**^{Q} in the world and in India. The street names include joints, marijuana, grass, pot, weed, etc.

The active ingredient, which is responsible for the psychoactive effects of cannabis is δ-**9 tetrahydrocannabinol (THC)**^{Q}. The various preparations of cannabis are tabulated below.

Table 2: THC concentration in various cannabis preparations.

Cannabis preparation	THC content (%)
Bhang (derived from dried leaves)	1
Ganja (derived from inflorescence)	1–2
Hashish/Charas (derived from resinous exudates)	8–14
Hash oil (lipid soluble plant extract)	15-40

The cannabis can be ingested orally or is more commonly smoked. It is unsuitable for intravenous use because of poor solubility in water and risk of anaphylaxis due to undissolved particulate matter.

Intoxication

It is characterized by euphoria, subjective sense of slowing of time, sense of floating in air, **reddening of conjunctiva**^{Q} (due to dilatation of conjunctival blood vessels), **increased appetite** and dryness of mouth. Other symptoms include depersonalization, derealization, **synesthesia**^{Q} (cross over of sensory perceptions. For example, patient may report that he is "seeing" music and "hearing" lights).

Sometimes, after consumption of cannabis, the person might feel restless, fearful, extremely anxious (similar to panic attack) and may feel that he is about to go crazy. This unpleasant experience is known as **"bad trip"**^{Q}.

Withdrawal Symptoms

It was earlier believed that cannabis does not cause physical dependence and produces no withdrawal symptoms, however recent studies have shown that there are mild withdrawal symptoms within 1-2 weeks of cessation and includes **irritability**^{Q}, anxiety, decreased appetite, depressed mood and sleep difficulties (including insomnia and strange dreams). Physical complaints such as abdominal pain, tremors, headache, sweating, fever or chills can also be present.

Cannabis Related Disorders

1. *Cannabis induced psychotic disorder*: It is also sometimes referred to as "hemp insanity". The patient has psychotic symptoms such as delusions and hallucinations.
2. *Cannabis induced anxiety disorders*.
3. *Flashback phenomenon*^{Q}: It is characterized by a recurrence of cannabis use experience in the absence of current cannabis use.
4. *Running amok*^{Q}: It is described as development of rage following cannabis use, in which person may hurt or even kill others in an indiscriminate fashion.
5. *Amotivational syndrome*^{Q}: It is characterized by an unwillingness to persist in any task, whether at school or at work. The patient appears uninterested, lethargic and apathetic.

Treatment

As withdrawal symptoms are mild, no medications are usually used. If required, benzodiazepines can be used for short-term.

Long-term treatment usually involves the psychotherapeutic approach and patient may be offered cognitive behavioral therapy, family therapy or group therapies.

HALLUCINOGENS

This class includes a variety of drugs like LSD (Lysergic acid diethylamide), mescaline, psilocybin, methylenedioxyamphetamine (MDMA, also called ecstasy), phencyclidine (**angel dust**^{Q}) and ketamine.

Intoxication

The characteristic symptoms of LSD (and other hallucinogens) intoxication are depersonalization, derealization, **synesthesia**^{Q} (also called as reflex hallucinations wherein patient may report cross over of sensory perceptions), illusions and hallucinations, autonomic hyperactivity features such as pupillary dilatation, tachycardia, sweating, palpitations, tremors, etc.

Similar to cannabis, at times, patient may become restless, fearful and may develop panic reaction (**bad trip**[Q]). Usually patient can be calmed down by reassurance. However in cases with extreme agitation, benzodiazepines or antipsychotics may be required.

Phencyclidine (PCP) and Ketamine are closely related compounds and are termed as "dissociative anesthetics", because they produce a condition where patient appears dissociated or cutoff from the environment though he is awake. Both of them act by blocking NMDA receptors[Q]. The symptoms in PCP and Ketamine intoxication are closely similar to schizophrenia[Q]. Phencyclidine intoxication also produces few characteristic symptoms such as vertical or horizontal nystagmus[Q], ataxia, dysarthria and extreme agitation and assaultiveness.

Withdrawal Symptoms

Hallucinogens do not cause any physical dependence, hence tolerance and withdrawal symptoms are not seen. The use of hallucinogens like LSD can be associated with **flashback phenomenon**[Q] which refers to recurrence of LSD use experience in the absence of current LSD use.

Treatment

Mostly psychotherapeutic techniques are used to prevent relapse.

STIMULANTS

Cocaine

Cocaine is derived from the plant **erythroxylum coca**. **Sigmund Freud**[Q] had studied its pharmacological effects and is also believed to be addicted to cocaine for a long time. Coca cola used to contain cocaine till 1903 after which it ceased to be an ingredient.

Cocaine was initially used as a **local anesthetic**[Q] and still is used in **eye, nose and throat surgery**[Q]. The local anesthetic effect is mediated by blockade of fast, sodium channels.

Cocaine acts primarily by **blocking dopamine receptors**[Q] (D1 and D2) and **increasing dopamine concentration** in synaptic cleft. It is also an inhibitor of uptake of norepinephrine and hence has significant sympathomimetic effect. It causes marked vasoconstriction of peripheral arteries, which results in **hypertension**[Q], further, vasoconstriction of the epicardial coronary arteries, can lead to **ischemic myocardial injury**[Q]. Cocaine use can also cause seizures. Cocaine (most common) and amphetamines (second most common) are the substances associated with **seizures**[Q].

Cocaine is usually inhaled (known as snorting). Due to its vasoconstrictive properties nasal inhalation of cocaine causes nasal congestion and can even result in **nasal septal perforation**[Q]. Long-term use can also cause **jet black pigmentation of tongue**[Q].

Other methods of intake are smoking (known as **freebasing**[Q]) and subcutaneous or intravenous injections. Freebasing involves mixing street cocaine (which usually has procaine or sugar as adulterants) with freebase (chemically extracted pure cocaine). A particular potent way is consumption of cocaine and heroin (called speedball) together.

Crack, is a freebase form of cocaine which is smoked. It is extremely potent and even a single use can cause intense craving.

Intoxication: The intoxication is characterized by euphoria, pupillary dilatation, tachycardia, hypertension and sweating. Acute intoxication with moderate to high dose of cocaine may be associated with **paranoid ideations**, **auditory hallucinations**[Q] and visual illusions. The patients also occasionally report of tactile hallucinations (feeling of insects crawling under the skin), also known as **cocaine bugs**. (also known as **formication** and **magnan phenomenon**[Q]).

Withdrawal symptoms: Cocaine causes **strong psychological dependence**[Q] however physiological dependence (tolerance and withdrawal symptoms) is **mild**[Q] in comparison. The withdrawal symptoms includes feeling low, exhaustion, lethargy, fatigue, insatiable hunger. The most severe withdrawal symptom is depression, which can be associated with suicidal ideation.

Cocaine induced psychotic disorder: It is most commonly seen with intravenous use and crack users. The hallmark is **paranoid delusions (delusion of persecution)** and **auditory hallucinations**[Q]. Visual and tactile hallucinations (cocaine bugs) can also be present. The disorder is quite similar to **paranoid schizophrenia**[Q] in its presentation.

Treatment: The withdrawal symptoms are usually mild and no specific pharmacological agents reduces the intensity of withdrawal. Treatment mostly relies on psychotherapeutic interventions like cognitive behavioral therapy, group therapy, and support groups such as narcotic anonymous.

Amphetamines

The major amphetamines include dextroamphetamine, methamphetamine. Methylphenidate is also an amphetamine like compound. Amphetamines are used to increase performance and induce a euphoric feeling. Long-term use can result in amphetamine induced psychotic disorder, whose hallmark is presence of **paranoid delusions (delusion of persecution**[Q]**)** and auditory **hallucinations**[Q].

TOBACCO

It is the most commonly used substance in India (caffeine not considered) and is used in a variety of ways which includes smoking, chewing, applying, sucking and gargling. Beedi smoking is the most common form followed by cigarette smoking. The active ingredient of tobacco, which causes addiction is nicotine. The constituents responsible for cardiovascular disorders are **nicotine** and carbon monoxide.

Nicotine has a stimulant action and improves the attention, learning, reaction time and problem solving ability.

The withdrawal symptoms can develop within two hours of smoking the last cigarette and peak in 24-48 hours. These symptoms include:
- **Craving for nicotine**^{Q}
- **Irritability**^{Q}
- **Anxiety**^{Q}
- **Poor concentration**^{Q}
- **Bradycardia**^{Q}
- **Drowsiness and paradoxical trouble sleeping**^{Q}
- **Increased appetite and weight gain**^{Q}.

Treatment

Pharmacotherapy

1. *Nicotine replacement therapy*: It is used to relieve the withdrawal symptoms by substituting nicotine in tobacco with nicotine in safer forms as they do not contain other harmful constituents present in tobacco. The various preparations include nicotine gums, nicotine lozenges, nicotine patches, nicotine inhalers and nicotine spray.
2. Medications which can be used include varenicline, **bupropion,** and clonidine and nortriptyline (second line).

Varenicline^Q: Varenicline is a new first line treatment for smoking cessation. It acts as a **partial agonist at $\alpha4\beta2$ nicotinic acetylcholine receptors**^{Q}, which is responsible for its clinical effectiveness. When a person smokes cigarette, the nicotine that gets absorbed binds to $\alpha4\beta2$ nicotinic acetylcholine receptors which results in release of dopamine in nucleus accumbens that is responsible for the 'high' as well as reinforcement of smoking behaviour. When a person stops smoking, the nicotinic acetylcholine receptors are unstimulated and dopaminergic activity also falls, which results in the craving and withdrawal symtoms.

Varenicline acts as a partial agonist and when it binds to $\alpha4\beta2$ nicotinic acetylcholine receptors, it results in much lesser dopamine release and hence lesser reinforcement and lesser potential for dependence, at the same time since receptors are occupied, it also controls craving and withdrawal symptoms. Further, it competitively inhibits the nicotine from binding to $\alpha4\beta2$ nicotinic acetylcholine receptors, and hence even if a person smokes, the reinforcement of smoking behaviour is prevented.

Before starting varenicline, patient sets a quit date (the day on which he will stop smoking) Varenicline is started a week before the quit date. Varenicline is started at dosages of **0.5 mg/day**^{Q} for first three days; from fourth day, the dose is increased to 0.5 mg twice a day and finally from 8th day, it is increased to 1 mg, twice a day. The treatment is continued for 3 months. For those, who have successfully stopped smoking at the end of 12 weeks, an additional course of 12 weeks treatment with varenicline is recommended to further increase the likelihood of long-term abstinence.

The most common adverse effects include nausea, headache and insomnia. In some patients, neuropsychiatric side effects such as depression, anxiety and **suicidal ideations**^{Q} have been reported and should be monitored for.

Apart from medications behavioral therapy is also considered beneficial.

OTHER DRUGS

1. *Inhalants or volatile solvents*: These include gasoline (petrol), glues, thinners, industrial solvents. These solvents are soaked in a cloth and than are sniffed (vapors are inhaled). It is more commonly seen in children and adolescents. Long-term use may cause irreversible damage to livers and kidneys, peripheral neuropathy and brain damage.
2. *Benzodiazepines and other sedative hypnotics*: Benzodiazepines can produce physical and psychological dependence. The withdrawal symptoms usually include anxiety, irritability, insomnia and in some cases seizures. The treatment usually involves slow tapering and then stopping of benzodiazepines along with supportive measures.
3. *Caffeine*: Caffeine is the most widely used psychoactive substance worldwide. Caffeine use is associated with feeling of improved efficiency, increased energy levels and concentration. Excessive use can produce anxiety, restlessness, irritability. Caffeine can also produce physiological dependence and withdrawal symptoms include anxiety, irritability, mid depressive symptoms, nausea and vomiting.

Multiple Choice Questions

Substance Use Disorders

1. Which of the following is not an important factor in development of substance dependence?
   (AIIMS Nov 2009)
   A. Personality
   B. Family history
   C. Peer pressure
   D. Intelligence

2. Not included in definition of substance abuse syndrome:
   (PGI May 2011)
   A. Withdrawal symptom
   B. Use despite knowing that it can cause physical/mental harm
   C. Tolerance to drug
   D. Recurrent substance abuse
   E. Use despite substance related legal problems

3. All of the following are criteria for substance dependence except:
   (AI 2012)
   A. Repeated unsuccessful attempts to quit the substance
   B. Recurrent substance related legal problems/use of illegal substances
   C. Characteristic withdrawal symptoms; substance taken to relieve withdrawal
   D. Substance taken in larger amount and for longer than intended

4. Diagnosis of alcohol dependence includes all of the following except:
   (NIMHANS 2014)
   A. Impaired occupational and social functioning
   B. Need for daily drinking to function adequately
   C. Lack of tolerance for alcohol
   D. Inability to cut down on alcohol intake

5. Symptomatic treatment is not required in withdrawal of:
   (AI 1998)
   A. Cannabis
   B. Morphine
   C. Alcohol
   D. Cocaine

6. Drugs which cause both physical and psychological dependence are:
   (DNB NEET 2014-15)
   A. Opioids
   B. Alcohol
   C. Nicotine
   D. All of the above

Alcohol

7. Irresistible urge to drink alcohol is known as:
   (DNB June 2011)
   A. Kleptomania
   B. Pyromania
   C. Dipsomania
   D. Trichotillomania

8. All of the following statements are true about blackouts except:
   (AIIMS May 2014)
   A. The person appears confused to the onlookers
   B. Remote memory is relatively intact during the blackout
   C. It is a discrete episode of anterograde amnesia
   D. It is associated with alcohol intoxication

Controversial Question

9. A patient taking 120 mL alcohol every day since last 12 years is brought to the hospital by his wife and is diagnosed to have alcohol dependence syndrome. Which of the following drug should be avoided in the management?
   (AIIMS Nov 2014)
   A. Phenytoin
   B. Disulfiram
   C. Naltrexone
   D. Acamprosate

10. All of the following are true about alcohol dependence syndrome except:
    (DNB NEET 2014-15)
    A. No tolerance
    B. Withdrawal symptoms
    C. CAGE questionnaire
    D. Physical dependence

11. First symptom to appear in alcohol withdrawal is:
    (AIIMS May 2015)
    A. Visual hallucinations
    B. Sleep disturbance
    C. Tremors
    D. Delirium

12. Alcohol is maximally absorbed in:
    (NIMHANS 2019)
    A. Stomach
    B. Proximal small intestine
    C. Distal small intestine
    D. Large intestine

13. Which of the following is characteristic of alcohol withdrawal?
    (AIIMS 1991)
    A. Hallucination
    B. Illusion
    C. Delusion
    D. Drowsiness

14. Widmark formula is used for:
    (AIIMS 1993)
    A. Opium
    B. Cannabis
    C. Alcohol
    D. Amphetamine

15. AUDIT Test is used for which of the following?
    (JIPMER 2016, NEET 2016)
    A. Alcohol use disorder
    B. Opioid use disorder
    C. Sexual abuse
    D. Cannabis abuse

16. Male started drinking alcohol at age of 20 years, presently taking 3 quarters daily over 30 years, complains that now he gets the kick in 1 quarter. Probable diagnosis is:
    (AIIMS Nov 2012)
    A. Withdrawal
    B. Mellanby phenomenon
    C. Reverse tolerance
    D. Cross tolerance

17. Psychiatric complications of alcohol dependence are:
    (PGI 2001)
    A. Anxiety
    B. Suicide
    C. Depression
    D. Schizophrenia
    E. Mania

18. True about delirium tremens:
    (PGI Nov 2016)
    A. Visual hallucinations
    B. Auditory hallucinations
    C. Delusional perception
    D. Seen in alcohol withdrawal
    E. On EEG, slow waves are present

19. **True about delirium tremens:** *(PGI June 2005)*
    A. Clouding of consciousness
    B. Coarse tremors
    C. Chronic delirious behavior
    D. Hallucination
    E. Autonomic dysfunction

Controversial Question

20. **Thiamine dose in patients with delirium tremens is about:** *(NIMANS 2016)*
    A. 100-200 mg per oral/parenteral daily
    B. 250 mg per oral/parenteral daily for first 3-5 days
    C. 400 mg per oral/parenteral daily
    D. 500 mg per oral/parenteral daily

21. **Wernicke's encephalopathy involves which part of central nervous system?** *(PGI 2000)*
    A. Mammillary body
    B. Thalamus
    C. Frontal lobe
    D. Arcuate fasciculus

22. **A 45-year male with a history of alcohol dependence presents with confusion, nystagmus and ataxia. Examination reveals 6th cranial nerve weakness. He is most likely to be suffering from:** *(AI 2005)*
    A. Korsakoff's psychosis
    B. Wernicke encephalopathy
    C. De Clerambault syndrome
    D. Delirium tremens

23. **Disulfiram is a type of:** *(FMGE 2017)*
    A. Aversion therapy
    B. Anticraving therapy
    C. Detoxification
    D. Opioid management therapy

24. **Which of the following is included in the classical triad of Wernicke's encephalopathy?** *(DNB NEET 2014-15)*
    A. Peripheral neuropathy   B. Autonomic dysfunction
    C. Ataxia   D. Abdominal pain

25. **Not affected in Wernicke's disease:** *(DNB NEET 2014-15)*
    A. Hypothalamus   B. Thalamus
    C. Hippocampus   D. Mammillary bodies

26. **An alcoholic patient comes to your office, he can not tell his name. There is gross incoordination in walking, and his eyes are deviated to one side. What is the probable diagnosis?** *(Bihar 2006)*
    A. Wernicke's encephalopathy
    B. Korsakoff's psychosis
    C. Alcoholic hallucinosis
    D. Delirium tremens

27. **Feature(s) of Korsakoff's psychosis:** *(PGI Nov 2014)*
    A. Confabulation   B. Retrograde amnesia
    C. Ophthalmoplegia   D. Delirium

28. **Korsakoff's syndrome true is/are:** *(DNB NEET 2014-15)*
    A. Can be seen in chronic alcoholics
    B. Absence of intellectual decline
    C. Chronic amnestic syndrome
    D. All of the above

29. **All are relatively normal in Korsakoff's psychosis except:** *(MAHE 2003, KA 2003; J & K 2000)*
    A. Implicit memory   B. Intelligence
    C. Language   D. Learning

30. **True statement about Korsakoff's psychosis is:** *(Rohtak 2000; JIPMER 1999); (UP 1999; PGI 1997)*
    A. Severe anterograde + mild retrograde memory defect
    B. Mild anterograde + severe retrograde memory defect
    C. Only anterograde memory defect
    D. Only retrograde memory defect

31. **Wernicke's Korsakoff's syndrome is characterised by all except:** *(NIMHANS 2016)*
    A. Loss of remote memory
    B. Confabulations
    C. Ataxia
    D. Nystagmus and paralysis of certain ocular muscles

32. **A patient was brought with symptom of tremulousness, arousal, sweating, irritability and tachycardia. History of daily alcohol intake is present. The diagnosis is:** *(NEET 2016)*
    A. Alcohol withdrawal
    B. Delirium tremens
    C. Wernicke's encephalopathy
    D. Korsakoff's psychosis

33. **A 35-year-old male comes with h/o 10-years of alcoholism and past history of ataxia with bilateral rectus palsy. He was admitted and treated. What changes can be expected to be seen in such condition?** *(PGI June 2008)*
    A. Progression to Korsakoff's psychosis
    B. Residual ataxia in 50% of patients
    C. Extraocular palsy disappears in hours
    D. Immediate relief from symptoms

34. **Earliest symptoms showing improvement from the classical triad of Wernicke's encephalopathy to thiamine therapy is:**
    A. Ataxia
    B. Ophthalmoplegia
    C. Confusion
    D. All improve simultaneously

35. **A 30-year-old male with history of alcohol abuse for 15 years is brought to the hospital emergency with 'complaints' of fearfulness, misrecognition, talking to self, aggressive behavior, tremulousness and seeing snakes and reptiles that are not visible to others around him. There is history of last drinking alcohol 2 days prior to the onset of the present complaints. He is most likely suffering from:** *(AIIMS Nov 2003)*
    A. Delirium tremens   B. Alcoholic hallucinosis
    C. Schizophrenia   D. Seizure disorder

36. **A 55-year-aged chronic alcoholic male, presented with irrelevant talks, tremor and sweating. He had his last drink 3 days back. What will the probable diagnosis?** *(NEET 2018)*
    A. Delirium tremens
    B. Korsakoff's psychosis
    C. Post-acute withdrawal syndrome
    D. Discontinuation syndrome

37. Which of the following is most specific for alcohol use disorder? *(NIMHANS 2013)*
    A. AST
    B. ALT
    C. GGT
    D. ALP

38. A 40-year-old man presents to casualty with history of regular and heavy use of alcohol for 10 years and morning drinking for 1 year. The last alcohol intake was 3 days back. There is no history of head injury or seizures. On examination, there is no icterus, sign of hepatic encephalopathy or focal neurological sign. The patient had coarse tremors, visual hallucinations and had disorientation to time. Which of the following is the best medicine to be prescribed for such a patient? *(AI 2004)*
    A. Diazepam
    B. Haloperidol
    C. Imipramine
    D. Naltrexone

39. A chronic alcoholic patient stopped alcohol intake for 2 days due to religious reasons, developed symptoms of withdrawal on first day. On second day he had GTCS followed by another episode of GTCS after few hours. Drug which should be given to control the symptoms? *(AIIMS May 2013)*
    A. Sodium valproate
    B. Phenytoin
    C. Diazepam
    D. Clonidine

40. In alcohol withdrawal drug of choice is: *(NEET 2016; DNB NEET 2014-15; PGI June 2007)*
    A. Diazepam
    B. Acamprosate
    C. Naltrexone
    D. Disulfiram

41. Drugs used for treatment of delirium tremens is/are: *(DNB NEET 2014-15, MCI Screening)*
    A. Diazepam
    B. Quetiapine
    C. Chlordiazepoxide
    D. Both A and C

42. Naltrexone is used for treatment of which of the following substances? *(PGI May 2017)*
    A. Cocaine
    B. Cannabis
    C. Alcohol
    D. Bulimia
    E. Anorexia nervosa

43. In patients of substance-abuse, drugs used are: *(PGI 2002)*
    A. Naltrexone
    B. Naloxone
    C. Clonidine
    D. Lithium
    E. Disulfiram

44. All are anticraving agent for alcohol except: *(NEET 2016, AIIMS May 2009)*
    A. Lorazepam
    B. Naltrexone
    C. Topiramate
    D. Acamprosate

45. Which of the following is not used in delirium? *(PGI Dec 2005)*
    A. Haloperidol
    B. Lithium
    C. Diazepam
    D. Olanzapine
    E. Risperidone

46. Alcohol dependence is associated with all of the following except: *(JIPMER 2016)*
    A. Anxiety disorder
    B. Dementia
    C. Sexual dysfunction
    D. Alcohol amotivational syndrome

47. False about alcoholic anonymous is: *(NEET 2016)*
    A. It is a self-help group
    B. It follows 12 steps to quit alcohol
    C. It includes recovered patients and volunteers
    D. It provides incentives for quitting alcohol

48. How much do genes contribute (heritability) to the development of alcohol use disorders? *(NIMHANS 2019)*
    A. 10%
    B. 45%
    C. 60%
    D. 90%

Opioid

49. Which of the following is not an opioid peptide? *(AIIMS May 2005)*
    A. Endorphins
    B. Epinephrine
    C. Leu-enkephalins
    D. Met-enkephalins

50. All are seen in morphine poisoning except: *(AI 1997)*
    A. Cyanosis
    B. Pinpoint pupil
    C. Hypertension
    D. Respiratory depression

51. Opioids can cause which of the following? *(DNB NEET 2014-15)*
    A. Physical dependence
    B. Psychological dependence
    C. Both A and B
    D. None of the above

52. Usual sign of morphine withdrawal are all except: *(PGI May 2013, 1999, 1993)*
    A. Dryness of secretion
    B. Constipation
    C. Miosis
    D. Lacrimation, diarrhea, rhinorrhea
    E. Generally occur after 6-8 hours of last use

53. Withdrawal of which of the following causes yawning and piloerection? *(DNB NEET 2014-15)*
    A. Morphine
    B. Cannabis
    C. Smoking
    D. Alcohol

54. A boy is having diarrhea, rhinorrhea, sweating and lacrimation. What is the most probable diagnosis?
    A. Cocaine withdrawal *(AIIMS Nov 2010)*
    B. Heroin withdrawal
    C. Alcohol withdrawal
    D. LSD withdrawal

55. Treatment of opioid dependence includes: *(PGI May 2011)*
    A. Naloxone
    B. Naltrexone
    C. Acamprosate
    D. Buprenorphine
    E. Topiramate

56. Which drug is most commonly used worldwide in maintenance treatment for opioid dependence? *(AI 2011)*
    A. Naltrexone
    B. Methadone
    C. Imipramine
    D. Disulfiram

57. Which of the following is an alternative to methadone for maintenance treatment of opiate dependence?
    A. Diazepam *(AIIMS May 2005)*
    B. Chlordiazepoxide
    C. Buprenorphine
    D. Dextropropoxyphene

58. Naltrexone is used in opioid addiction because:
    (AIIMS May 2010, 2007, 2006, AI 2007)
    A. To treat withdrawal symptoms
    B. To treat overdose of opioids and prevent respiratory depression
    C. Prevent relapse
    D. Has addiction potential; used for detoxification of opioid

59. Which of the following is drug of choice for opioid overdose? *(NIMHANS 2019)*
    A. Naloxone   B. Clonidine
    C. Buprenorphine   D. Flumazenil

Cannabis

60. After use of some drug, a person develops episodes of rage in which he runs about and indiscriminately injures a person who is encountered in way. He is probably addict of: *(AIIMS 1997)*
    A. Alcohol   B. Cannabis
    C. Opium   D. Cocaine

61. A 40-year-old patient who has been consuming cannabis regularly for last 20 years comes to you in withdrawal. What is the most frequently seen withdrawal symptom? *(NIMHANS 2017)*
    A. Yawning   B. Seizures
    C. Irritability   D. Tremors

62. Which of the following substances is associated with flashback phenomenon? *(KA 1999)*
    A. Cannabis   B. LSD
    C. Psilocybin   D. All of the above

63. Amotivational syndrome is seen in:
    (DNB NEET 2014-15, MH 2010, TN 1999)
    A. Cannabis   B. Cocaine
    C. Amphetamine   D. Heroin

64. Which of the following substance intoxication causes conjunctival congestion, increased appetite, dry mouth, tachycardia and synesthesia? *(MH 2009)*
    A. Cannabis   B. Caffeine
    C. Cocaine   D. Codeine

65. Bad trip is seen with which of the following drugs?
    (DNB NEET 2014-15)
    A. Cocaine   B. Cannabis
    C. LSD   D. Heroin

Others

66. Correct statement about cocaine abuse: *(PGI May 2011)*
    A. Block uptake of dopamine in CNS
    B. Strong physical dependence
    C. Increased BP
    D. Severe tolerance
    E. Cause impairment of nerve conduction

67. All of the following are true about cocaine addiction except: *(NIMHANS 2014)*
    A. Myocardial infarction
    B. Seizures
    C. Comorbid addiction to alcohol
    D. Amantadine is the drug of choice

68. Magnan's phenomenon is associated with which of the following drug use? *(PGI Nov 2017)*
    A. Cocaine   B. Cannabis
    C. Alcohol   D. Tobacco

69. Jet black pigmentation of tongue with tactile hallucination is a feature of which substance use? *(FMGE 2018)*
    A. Cocaine   B. Cannabis
    C. Heroin   D. LSD

70. Paranoid psychosis observed with cocaine abuse can be explained by: *(AI 2011, 2012)*
    A. Tolerance   B. Intoxication
    C. Reverse tolerance D. Withdrawal

71. Formication and delusion of persecution, both are together seen in: *(AIIMS May 2011, 2009)*
    A. LSD psychosis
    B. Amphetamine psychosis
    C. Cocaine psychosis
    D. Cannabis psychosis

72. Which of the following is a stimulant? *(NEET 2016)*
    A. Cocaine   B. Alcohol
    C. Nicotine   D. Cannabis

73. A 16-year-old boy suffering from drug abuse presents with crossover of sensory perceptions, such that, sounds can be seen and colors can be heard. Which of the following is the most likely agents responsible for drug abuse? *(AI 2012)*
    A. Cocaine   B. LSD
    C. Marijuana   D. PCP (phencyclidine)

74. Psychosis resulting due to chronic amphetamine intake most commonly resembles: *(Odisha 1999)*
    A. Delirium   B. Mania
    C. Paranoid schizophrenia   D. Dissociative disorder

75. Used for averting tobacco dependence is:
    (DNB 2017, DPG 2008)
    A. Buspirone   B. Methadone
    C. Bupropion   D. Buprenorphine

76. Most common substance of abuse in India is:
    (NEET 2016, DNB NEET 2014-15, AIIMS May 2010, May 2007, AI 2007)
    A. Tobacco   B. Cannabis
    C. Alcohol   D. Opium

77. Which of the following statement is false about varenicline? *(NIMHANS 2017)*
    A. Acts as nicotinic cholinergic partial agonist
    B. Can lead to suicidal ideation
    C. Started at dosages of 0.5 mg per day
    D. Treatment is given initially for 6 weeks

78. Nicotine withdrawal symptoms include: *(PGI May 2017)*
    A. Irritability   B. Anorexia
    C. Loss of concentration   D. Weight gain
    E. Hypersomnia

79. Which is not a feature of caffeine withdrawal?
    (DNB Dec 2011)
    A. Headache   B. Hallucination
    C. Depression   D. Weight gain

80. **Which of the following is a date rape drug?** *(NEET 2016)*
    A. Cocaine
    B. Heroin
    C. Flunitrazepam
    D. Methamphetamine

81. **Which of the following is a rave drug?** *(NEET 2016)*
    A. Cocaine
    B. Methamphetamine
    C. Heroin
    D. Cannabis

82. **Angel dust is the street name for:** *(NIMHANS 2018, 2014)*
    A. Phencyclidine
    B. LSD
    C. Heroin
    D. Ketamine

83. **Which of the following drug effects closely mimics "schizophrenia"?** *(NIMHANS 2013)*
    A. Barbiturates
    B. Cocaine
    C. Phencyclidine
    D. Levodopa

84. **Match the following substances of use with their common names:** *(AIIMS Nov 2017)*
    a. LSD   1. White lady
    b. Abrus precatorius 2. Purple haze
    c. Cocaine   3. Hunan hand
    d. Capsaicin   4. Ratti
    A. a-2, b-1, c-4, d-3
    B. a-2, b-4, c-1, d-3
    C. a-4, b-1, c-3, d-2
    D. a-1, b-2, c-3, d-4

85. **Anticraving agent which acts as NMDA antagonist is:** *(NIMHANS 2018)*
    A. Naltrexone
    B. Acamprosate
    C. Baclofen
    D. Topiramate

86. **The drug used in treatment of smoking cessation and tobacco addiction:** *(NEET 2019)*
    A. Varenicline
    B. Acamprosate
    C. Naltrexone
    D. Baclofen

AIIMS New Pattern Question

87. **Match the substances mentioned in column A with their characteristic presentation in column B**

    Column A
    1. Alcohol relapse prevention
    2. Opioid overdosage
    3. Nicotine dependence treatment
    4. Opioid relapse prevention

    Column B
    a. Naloxone
    b. Naltrexone
    c. Methadone
    d. Clonidine
    e. Varenicline
    f. Diazepam

    A. 1-a, 2-b, 3-e, 4-c
    B. 1-b, 2-a, 3-e, 4-d
    C. 1-f, 2-b, 3-e, 4-c
    D. 1-b, 2-a, 3-e, 4-c

Answers With Explanations

Substance Use Disorders

1. **D.** The personality, **family history** and peer pressure all play a role in development of dependence. There is no correlation between intelligence and substance use.

2. **A, C.**
   The DSM-IV, diagnosis of substance abuse includes the following four criterion: (1) Recurrent use resulting in failure to fulfill major obligations at work, school or home, (2) recurrent use in situations in which it is physically hazardous (such as while driving), (3) substance use causing legal problems and (4) substance use causing social or interpersonal problems (e.g. fights with spouse). Withdrawal and tolerance are a criterion for "substance dependence" but not "substance abuse". Please remember in DSM-5, both these diagnosis of "substance dependence" and "substance abuse" have been removed and replaced by "substance use disorders".

3. **B.** Neither presence of legal problems related to substance use nor use of illegal substances, is a criterion for substance dependence.

4. **C.** Option C is clearly wrong as tolerance is a feature of dependence.

5. **A.** Since cannabis causes very mild withdrawal symptoms hence, no symptomatic treatment is required. LSD and other hallucinogens also do not cause any withdrawal symptoms or tolerance.

6. **D.** All of the above.

Alcohol

7. **C.** Dipsomania is compulsive drinking or an irresistible urge to drink alcohol.

8. **A.** In alcoholic blackouts, which is an anterograde amnesia, the person later does not remember, however, at that time he appears to be totally in control and his behavior appears purposeful to others. He does not look confused to the onlookers.

9. **B.** Since this patient, has been taking alcohol every day, at the time of presentation, disulfiram should be avoided as it may precipitate a severe disulfiram like reaction. Disulfiram should not be used until person has abstained from alcohol for atleast 12 hours. Also, please remember that phenytoin does not have any role in the management of alcohol dependence. However, this question is specifically asking for the drug that should be avoided and hence, disulfiram is the best answer.

10. **A.** Alcohol does produce tolerance.

11. **C.** Tremors usually appear 6-8 hours after last alcohol intake. Tremors are the most common withdrawal symptom of alcohol (excluding the hangover).

12. **B.** 80% of alcohol is absorbed from duodenum and jejunum.

13. **A.** Alcoholic hallucinosis is a characteristic withdrawal symptom of alcohol. Delusion of infidelity (morbid jealousy) is also seen in chronic alcoholism but it is not related to withdrawal state.

14. **C.**

15. **A.** AUDIT is used for screening of alcohol use disorders.

16. **C.** Reverse tolerance refers to the phenomenon where the intoxicating effects of alcohol are seen progressively with lower dosages.

17. **A, B, C, E.**
    See the list of alcohol induced disorders in the text.

18. **A, B, D.**
    In delirium tremens, EEG shows low voltage fast activity and not show waves.

19. **A, B, D, E.**
    Delirium tremens is usually not a chronic condition.

20. **B.** According to Maudsley prescribing guidelines (12th edition, 2015), in patients who are undergoing inpatient detoxification, parenteral thiamine 250 mg/day should be given for 5 days followed by oral thiamine. As delirium tremens is complicated alcohol withdrawal that is always treated inpatient, the same dosage should be used. Thiamine is used to prevent development of Wernicke's encephalopathy.

21. **A, B.**
    Kindly *see* text for explanation.

22. **B.** Wernicke encephalopathy

23. **A.** Disulfiram is an aversive agent. It helps in creating aversion for use of alcohol.

24. **C.** Ataxia

25. **C.** Kindly *see* text for explanation.

26. **A.** Here, there is history of ataxia (incoordination) and ophthalmoplegia. The inability to tell name might be because of confusional state. The likely diagnosis is Wernicke's encephalopathy.

27. **A, B.** Confabulation and retrograde amnesia

28. **D.** Korsakoff's syndrome is due to thiamine deficiency. Apart from alcoholism, malnutrition can also cause it. Also it presents with amnesia and confabulations.

29. **D.** In Korsakoff's psychosis, there is prominent anterograde amnesia. Whenever there is anterograde amnesia (i.e. new memories cannot be made), learning would be severely affected.

30. **A.** Severe anterograde + Mild retrograde memory defect

31. **A,** Remote memory is usually preserved.

32. **A.** These are symptoms of simple alcohol withdrawal.

33. **A, B, C.**
    The diagnosis in this patient is Wernicke's encephalopathy. The patients when treated adequately have

the following course: (1) Ophthalmoplegia starts to resolve within hours, though horizontal nystagmus often persists, (2) Ataxia begins to improve within first week however around 50% of patient will be left with some residual abnormalities, (3) Global confusion begins to recover within 2-3 weeks and would usually clear completely in 1-2 months. Despite treatment, patient can progress to Korsakoff's syndrome.

34. B. Ophthalmoplegia responds rapidly to thiamine, within hours of administration.
35. A. The onset of symptoms is after 2 days of last intake. There is history of chronic alcohol use. There is history of disorientation (misrecognition), visual hallucination (seeing snakes and reptiles), hyperactivity. All these put together is suggestive of delirium tremens.
36. A. Delirium tremens. The presence of 'irrelevant talks' is suggestive of disturbance of consciousness in this patient, which is consistent with diagnosis of Delirium Tremens. Post-acute withdrawal symptoms or the protracted withdrawal symptoms of alcohol are those symptoms that persists for a long period (months to years) after the cessation of substance intake, and after the acute withdrawal symptoms have subsided (usually within two weeks). They usually include symptoms such as irritability, mood swings, fatigue, lack of motivation etc.
37. B. Out of the given options, ALT has the highest specificity for alcohol induced liver damage.
38. A. The diagnosis is delirium tremens and the drug of choice is benzodiazepines like diazepam.
39. C. The diagnosis is alcohol withdrawal seizures and the drug of choice is benzodiazepines like diazepam.
40. A. Benzodiazepines are the drug of choice in alcohol withdrawal. If the question asks you to choose a specific benzodiazepine, the best choice would be chlordiazepoxide.
41. D. The best answer here is both diazepam and chlordiazepoxide as the benzodiazepines are the drugs of choice. However, please remember antipsychotics can also be used if patient is having excessive hallucinations or is excessively agitated and these symptoms are not responding to benzodiazepines alone.
42. C. Alcohol. Naltrexone is used for treatment of alcohol use disorders and opioid use disorders.
43. A, B, C, E.
    Naltrexone is used in alcohol as well as opioid dependence. Naloxone is used in opioid overdose. Clonidine can be used in opioid withdrawal and disulfiram in alcohol dependence.
44. A. *See* text for explanation.
45. B. As explained above, benzodiazepines and antipsychotics can be used in delirium.
46. D. Alcohol amotivational syndrome
47. D. No incentives are given in alcoholic anonymous.
48. B. The heritability of alcohol use disorder has been estimated to be 0.49. In other words, alcohol use disorder is 49% heritable. The option closest to this figure is 45%. Out of psychiatric disorders, autism spectrum disorders have the highest heritability approaching around 90%.

Opioid

49. B. Epinephrine is not an opioid peptide. The endogenous opioid peptides include endorphins, Met and Leu enkephalins and Dynorphins.
50. C. Hypotension is a feature and not hypertension.
51. C. Both A and B
52. A, B, C.
53. A. Morphine.
54. B. Heroin withdrawal.
55. B, D.
56. B. Methadone is used as methadone maintenance treatment, in long-term treatment of opioid dependence.
57. C. Methadone, buprenorphine, levo alpha acetylmethadol can be used for maintenance treatment of opiate dependence.
58. C. The only indication for naltrexone in opioid dependence is relapse prevention in highly motivated patients. For opioid overdose naloxone is used and not naltrexone.
59. A. Intravenous naloxone is the drug of choice for opioid overdosage.

Cannabis

60. B. The description is suggestive of run amok which is seen with cannabis use.
61. C. Irritability.
62. D. Cannabis and hallucinogens can cause flash back phenomenon.
63. A. Cannabis.
64. A. Cannabis.
65. B, C

Others

66. A, C and E.
    Cocaine causes strong psychological dependence, however, physiological dependence (tolerance and withdrawal symptoms) is mild in comparison. Cocaine blocks dopamine and norepinephrine uptake and hence causes hypertension. It blocks nerve conduction and is also used as an anesthetic agent.
67. D. No pharmacological agent has any reliable role in cocaine dependence. These patients frequently use other substances too.
68. A. Cocaine
69. A. Cocaine.
70. B. The delusion of persecution and auditory hallucinations can be seen in cocaine intoxication.
71. C. Cocaine psychosis
72. A. Cocaine and amphetamines are classified as stimulants.
73. B, C.
    The sign here is synesthesia (sounds can be seen and colors can be heard) which is in with LSD and cannabis intoxication.
74. C. The symptoms of amphetamine induced psychotic disorder include delusion of persecution and auditory hallucinations and it resembles paranoid schizophrenia.
75. C. Bupropion.

76. A. Tobacco. According to National Mental Health Survey (2016), tobacco is the most commonly used drug in India. Earlier, there was some controversy about this question, as DSM-IV used to give a strict definition for the diagnosis of 'abuse', and 'tobacco abuse' was not a a valid diagnosis in DSM-IV. However, DSM-5 has removed the diagnostic category of 'abuse' and now we can safely answer this question as tobacco
77. D. Initial treatment is given for 12 weeks and not 6 weeks.
78. A, C, D
79. B. *See* text for explanation.
80. C. Flunitrazepam, gamma hydroxybutyric acid (GHB) and ketamine are the three most commonly used date rape drugs. These drugs lower the alertness and make the victim more vulnerable to sexual assault, hence known as 'date rape drugs'
81. B. Methamphetamine. Rave drugs are party drugs which are used for recreational purposes. These include LSD, amphetamines, Gamma hydroxy butyric acid and ketamine.
82. A. Phencyclidine
83. C. Though both levodopa and cocaine can cause psychotic symptoms, phencyclidine resembles schizophrenia most closely
84. B. Purple haze is commonly used as a street name for a potent form of cannabis. It is also used as a street name for LSD. The common name for abrus precatorius plant is 'gunjaa' or 'ratti'. White lady is the street name for both cocaine as well as heroin due to white powder like appearance. Hunan hand syndrome, is a form of painful contact dermatitis, which is usually seen in people with continuous and prolonged exposure to chili peppers. The main ingredient in chili peppers is capsaicin.
85. B. Acamprosate
86. A. Varenicline

AIIMS New Pattern Answer

87. D. The drug of choice for relapse prevention (maintenance of abstinence) of alcohol is Naltrexone. In patients who have compromise liver functions, acamprosate is used. The drug of choice for opioid overdosage is intravenous naloxone (opioid antagonist).

    The drugs used for treatment of nicotine dependence include varenicline and bupropion.

    The preferred treatment for opioid dependence is opioid substitution therapy (methadone, buprenorphine). If one specific opioid is asked to be chosen, the best answer is methadone. Though, naltrexone can also be used in the maintenance treatment of opioids its not as effective as opioid substitution therapy.

    Clonidine can be used in the detoxification of opioids Diazepam and other benzodiazepines are used for detoxification of benzodiazepines.

CHAPTER 6

Neurocognitive Disorders (Organic Mental Disorders)

Neurocognitive disorders (**organic mental disorders**) are caused by either a **demonstrable cerebral disease, brain injury** or other insults leading to **cerebral dysfunction**. Following are the common symptoms seen in organic mental disorders:

A. *Cognitive impairment*: The term "cognition" is used to describe all the mental processes that are utilized to gain knowledge. These processes include memory, language, orientation, judgment, performing actions (praxis) and problem solving. At times the term "cognition" is used to describe the thoughts. In organic mental disorders one or more of cognitive functions are impaired. Frequently patient presents with **disorientation (to time, place and person)**, **impaired attention** and concentration, disturbances in memory (especially recent memory resulting in anterograde amnesia), etc. As organic mental disorders commonly have disturbances of cognition, they are also known as **cognitive disorders**.

B. *Disturbances of consciousness*: The consciousness has different levels ranging from alertness to coma. Usually the term "alertness" is used when one is aware of the internal and external stimuli and can respond to them. The patients with organic mental disorders usually have disturbances of consciousness which can be of varying severity. The term "somnolence or lethargy" is used when patient tends to drift off to sleep when not actively stimulated. The next level is "obtundation" in which patient is difficult to arouse and when aroused appears confused. The next level is "stupor or semicoma" in which patient is mute and immobile. When stimulated persistently and vigorously he may groan or mumble. Finally, in "coma", patient is totally unarousable and remain with their eyes closed. Various other terms such as "**confusional** state", "**clouding of consciousness**" and "**altered sensorium**" are used to describe the disturbances of consciousness in delirium.

C. *Hallucinations*: These patients most commonly have **visual hallucinations**^{Q} although auditory, olfactory, gustatory and tactile hallucinations can also be present.

D. *Delusions*: The delusions are usually **transient**^{Q}. Complex delusions are **rare**^{Q}.

The organic mental disorders are classified in the following groups:
A. Delirium
B. Dementia
C. Amnestic disorders

Disturbances of Consciousness

The disturbances of consciousness have been described by using different and confusing terms. According to strub and black, there are five basic levels of consciousness:
1. **Alertness**: Patient is awake, and aware of internal and external stimuli, and can respond to them.
2. **Lethargy (or somnolence)**: Patient is not fully alert, and if not actively stimulated, drifts into sleep. Even when aroused, patients are not able to give close attention
3. **Obtundation**: Patient is difficult to arouse, and when aroused, patient appears confused. Constant stimulation is needed to get even minimal cooperation from the patient
4. **Stupor (or semicoma)**: In stupor, patient doesn't show any spontaneous response and remains akinetic (lack of movement) and mute. They may respond only to persistent and vigorous stimulation, by groaning or mumbling.
5. **Coma**: Coma is a state of complete unawareness. The patient cannot be aroused with any kind of external stimulation, and doesn't respond to internal stimuli either. The patient remains with the eyes closed.

Apart from these standard states, few other abnormalities have been described in literature:
1. **Torpor**: Torpor is described as a lowering of consciousness, short of stupor.
2. **Twilight state**: It is the dream like state (also called as **oneroid state**^{Q}), in which awareness is restricted, and the patient may feels as if they were in a dream. Twilight state corresponds to 'obtundation' stage of strub & black classification.

DELIRIUM

It is the **most common**^{Q} organic mental disorder. It is characterized by an **acute onset**^{Q} of symptoms and a **fluctuating course**^{Q}. It is most commonly seen in elderly population. The patients who have been hospitalized for medical and surgical disorders frequently develop delirium. The patients with **hip fractures**^{Q}, **open heart surgeries**^{Q}, **severe burns**^{Q}, **pneumonia**^{Q}, **postoperative patients**^{Q} and critically ill patients have high prevalence of delirium. The history of a medical disorder followed by sudden development of disturbances of consciousness, cognition and psychiatric symptoms such as hallucinations and delusions is strongly suggestive of delirium. The other causes includes use of multiple medications (especially those with anticholinergic actions). Withdrawal of psychoactive substances (such as alcohol and sedatives/hypnotics) is another common cause. Delirium can develop in older patients wearing eye patches after cataract surgery (due to sensory deprivation), also known as **black-patch delirium**^{Q}.

Symptoms

The clinical features of delirium are:
- **Disturbances of consciousness**^{Q} (ranging from somnolence to coma)
- Impairment of attention
- **Disorientation** to time, place and person
- Memory disturbances (impairment of immediate and recent memory with **relatively intact remote memory**^{Q})
- Perceptual disturbances like illusions and hallucinations (**most commonly visual**^{Q}) and transient delusions
- Hyperactivity or hypoactivity, agitation
- Autonomic disturbances
- Disturbances of sleep wake cycle (insomnia or reversal of sleep wake cycle)
- *Sundowning*: It refers to diurnal variation of symptoms with worsening of symptoms in the evening (i.e. with downing of sun)
- *Floccillations (or carphologia)*: Aimless picking behaviour, where patient appears to be picking at his clothes/bed
- *Occupational delirium*: Patient behaves as if he is still on his job, despite being in hospital (e.g. a tailor may ask for clothes and scissors, while lying on the bed of the hospital).

The neurotransmitter involved in delirium is **acetylcholine** and the neuroanatomical area involved is the **reticular formation** (kindly remember reticular ascending system is responsible for arousal in a person).

Diagnosis

The diagnosis of delirium is made **clinically**^{Q}, on the basis of above mentioned symptoms. The sudden onset and fluctuations in symptoms are important pointers towards the diagnosis. Bedside examinations such as **mini mental status examination (MMSE)**^{Q} and mental status examination (MSE) are used to provide a measure of cognitive impairment. Diagnostic tools such as **confusion assessment method**^{Q} have been developed to identify the patients with delirium.

Generalized slowing^Q on EEG is a common finding in patients with delirium, however delirium caused by **alcohol** or **sedative hypnotic** withdrawal has **low voltage fast activity** on EEG.

Delirium versus dementia: The **acute presentation**^{Q} and **fluctuations of symptoms**^{Q} is suggestive of delirium. Dementia develops slowly and usually the symptoms are stable over time. Further, a patient with delirium presents with **disturbances of consciousness**^{Q} whereas a patient with dementia does not have any consciousness disturbances. In some cases, a patient of dementia may develop superimposed delirium, a condition called as "beclouded dementia".

Delirium versus schizophrenia: A patient of delirium may have pronounced hallucinations and delusion and may resemble schizophrenia. However, in delirium the hallucinations are not constant and delusions are transient and not systematized (not organized) whereas in schizophrenia the hallucination are more constant and delusions are also better organized. Further, the patient of delirium has disturbances of attention and disturbed consciousness which is not seen in patient with schizophrenia.

 MMSE^Q

Mini mental status examination (MMSE) is a tool that is used to assess **cognitive functioning**^{Q} of an individual. MMSE assesses the following five cognitive functions and gives them different weightage:

1. **Orientation (10 points)**^{Q}: Patient is asked, What is the (year) (season) (date) (day) (month) and Where are we (state) (country) (town) (hospital) (floor). Patient gets one point for all the correct responses
2. **Registration (3 points)**: Examiner names three objects, e.g. Home, Tree and Car. And patient is asked to repeat them. For every correct repetition he gets a point
3. **Attention and Concentration (5 points)**: Patient is asked to serially subtract 7 from 100 for 5 times and gets 1 point for every correct subtarction. Alternatively, patient can be asked to spell WORLD backwards (D-L-R-O-W)
4. **Recall (3 points)**: Patient is asked to recall the three objects that were named while testing registration
5. **Language (9 points)**:
   a. Patient is shown two objects (e. g watch and pencil) and asked to name them (2 points)
   b. Patient is asked to repeat the phrase "No ifs, ands or buts" (1 point)

Contd...

Contd...

c. Patient is asked to follow a 3 stage command "Take a paper in your hand, fold it in half and put it on the floor" (3 points)
d. Patient is asked to follow a written command (1 point) (paper is given which says "Close your eyes", patient is supposed to close his eyes after reading it)
e. Patient is asked to write a sentence (1 point)
f. Patient is shown a design and is asked to copy it (1 point)

The maximum score for MMSE is **30**[Q]. A score less than **24**[Q] is indicative of cognitive impairment

Treatment

A. Treat the underlying cause.
B. **Antipsychotics** can be used for management of delusions, hallucinations and agitation seen in delirium.
C. **Benzodiazepines** are used for insomnia and are the drugs of choice in alcohol withdrawal delirium (delirium tremens).

DEMENTIA

Dementia is defined as a progressive impairment of cognitive functions in the **absence of any disturbances of consciousness**[Q]. The prevalence of dementia increases with age, with prevalence of around 5% in the population older than 65 years and prevalence of 20–40% in the population older than 85 years. The underlying cause of dementia can be permanent or reversible.

 DSM-5 Update

The DSM-4 diagnosis of dementia and amnestic disorder are subsumed under the newly named entity major neurocognitive disorders (NCD).

 DSM-5 Update

In DSM-5, a new diagnostic category of mild neurocognitive disorders (NCD) has been added, for the patients who present with milder cognitive impairment (which is not severe enough of diagnosis of dementia or major neurocognitive disorder).

Symptoms

The following are the symptoms of dementia:

A. *Cognitive impairment*: The cognitive impairment is characterized by 4 A's: amnesia, aphasia, apraxia and agnosia.
 - **Amnesia** refers to the memory impairment. Initially there is loss of recent memory, which is followed by loss of immediate memory and lastly the remote memory is lost. Another way of describing memory impairment is in terms of episodic (memory for events), semantic memory (memory for facts such as rules, words and language) and visuospatial deficits. In episodic memory, there is a gradient of loss with more recent events being lost before remote events. Semantic memory is preserved in the early course of disease and is gradually lost as the disease progresses. Visuospatial skills deficits manifests with symptoms of disorientation in strange environments and later, wandering and getting lost in even familiar environments.
 - Aphasia refers to the disturbances of **language function**. The initial disturbance is usually "word finding difficulties" which gradually progresses to more severe abnormalities.
 - Apraxia is inability to perform learned motor functions. For example, patient may start having difficulties in functions like buttoning the shirt or combing the hair.
 - Agnosia is inability to interpret a sensory stimulus. One of the common disturbance is "prosopagnosia"[Q] which is inability to identify the face. At times patient may be unable to identify his own face, a condition known as "autoprosopagnosia".
 - Apart from the 4 A's, disturbances in executive functioning (i.e. planning, organizing, sequencing and abstracting) is another important cognitive impairment.

B. *Behavioral and psychological symptoms*: These may include:
 - *Personality changes*: There might be a significant change in the personality. Patient may become introvert and seem to be unconcerned about others or patients may become hostile. The personality changes are mostly seen in patients with frontal and temporal lobe involvement.
 - *Hallucinations and delusions*: Delusion mostly seen is delusion of persecution and delusion of theft.
 - Depression, manic and anxiety symptoms.
 - Apathy, agitation, aggression, wandering and circadian rhythm disturbances.
 - *Catastrophic reaction*: The subjective awareness of intellectual deficits while in a stressful situation may result in an emotional outburst in a patient of dementia. This is known as **"catastrophic reaction"**[Q].

C. *Focal neurological signs and symptoms*: These are usually seen in vascular dementia (multi-infarct dementia) and correspond to the site of vascular insults. These include exaggerated tendon reflexes, extensor plantar response, gait abnormalities, etc.

Types

The dementia can be divided into reversible and irreversible dementias. It is extremely important to do detailed work up of a patient of dementia as around 15% of cases are reversible. The **reversible causes of dementia**^{Q} are:

A. Neurosurgical conditions (subdural hematoma, normal pressure hydrocephalus, intracranial tumors, intracranial abscess).
B. Infectious causes (meningitis, encephalitis, neurosyphilis, lyme disease).
C. Metabolic causes (vitamin B12 or folate deficiency, niacin deficiency, hypo and hyperthyroidism, hypo and hyperparathyroidism).
D. Others (drugs and toxins, alcohol abuse, autoimmune encephalitis).

Dementia can also be classified into cortical and subcortical types depending on the area of brain which is affected first by the dementing process.

Cortical dementias: These disorders are characterized by early involvement of cortical structures and hence early appearance of cortical dysfunction. These disorders have early and severe presentation of the As: amnesia, apraxia, aphasia, agnosia and acalculia (impaired mathematical skills) indicating cortical involvement. **Alzheimer's disease**^{Q} is the prototype of cortical dementia. Others include Creutzfeldt-Jakob disease, Pick's disease and other frontotemporal dementias.

Subcortical dementia: These disorders are characterized by early involvement of subcortical structures like basal ganglia, brain stem nuclei and cerebellum. These disorders are characterized by early presentation of motor symptoms (abnormal movements like tics, chorea, dysarthria, etc.), significant disturbances of executive functioning and prominent behavioral and psychological symptoms like apathy, depression, bradyphrenia (slowness of thinking). The examples include Parkinson's disease, Wilson's disease, Huntington's disease, multiple sclerosis, progressive supra nuclear palsy, normal pressure hydrocephalus.

Some dementias such as vascular dementia, dementia with lewy body have mixed presentation.

Alzheimer's Disease (Dementia of Alzheimer's Type)

It is the **most common**^{Q} cause of dementia. The prevalence of Alzheimer's disease increases with age, the rates are around 5% for all those aged 65 years and older, increasing to around **20-30%** for all those aged above 85 years. The Alzheimer's disease can be divided into early onset (presenile), if the age of onset is 65 years or earlier; or late onset (senile), if the age of onset is after 65 years. At all ages, females out number males by a ratio of 2 or 3:1 except in early onset familial forms (inherited as autosomal dominant disorder) in which sex ratio is 1. The onset is usually insidious and progression is gradual. The **insight**^{Q} (awareness of illness) is lost relatively early in the course of illness. In the initial phase symptoms include memory disturbances, gradually apraxia, agnosia, aphasia and acalculia develop and executive functions are lost. In the later stages neurological disabilities like tremors, rigidity and spasticity may develop.

Pathophysiology: The classical gross neuroanatomical finding in Alzheimers disease is **diffuse atrophy** with flattened cortical sulci and enlarged cerebral ventricles.

Typically, atrophy behind in medial temporal lobes before spreading to lateral and medial parietal and temporal lobes and lateral frontal cortex. At autopsy, the earliest and most severe degeneration is found in medial temporal lobe (**entorhinal/perirhinal cortex**^{Q} and hippocampus), lateral temporal cortex and nucleus basalis of meynert.

The classical microscopic findings are **neuritic (senile) plaques**^{Q} and **neurofibrillary tangles**^{Q}. Senile plaques, also referred to as amyloid plaques are composed of a particular protein Aβ. This protein is derived from **amyloid precursor protein (APP)** by the action of β and γ-secretase enzymes. The Aβ protein combines to form fibrils. The senile plaques are **extracellular** deposits of Aβ and are found in all cortical areas and also in striatum and cerebellum. The amyloid β-peptide not only deposits in the brain parenchyma in the form of amyloid plaques but also in the vessel walls in the form of **cerebral amyloid angiopathy (CAA)**^{Q}.

The senile plaques can also be seen in elderlies who do not have Alzheimer's and their number increases with age. Hence senile plaques are **not specific** for Alzheimer disease. The amyloid plaques are not correlated with the severity of dementia.

The neurofibrillary tangles (NFTs) are **intraneuronal** aggregates of tau protein. The tau protein present in tangles is in a highly phosphorylated form and has abnormal functioning. Normally, tau protein binds and stabilizes microtubules, which are essential for axonal transport, however in Alzheimer's this function is deranged. The neurofibrillary tangles are widely distributed in cortical structures and hippocampus, but always spare **cerebellum**^{Q}. Multiple studies have established that **amount and distribution of NFTs correlates with the duration and severity of dementia**^{Q}. The levels of phosphorylated tau protein are also increased in CSF, and it is being studied as a possible biomarker for Alzheimer disease.

Both senile plaques and neurofibrillary tangles can be present in elderlies without any dementia. However in patients with dementia, these findings are extensive and wide spread. The neuropathological diagnosis of Alzheimer disease requires extensive presence of both senile plaques (extracellular deposits) and neurofibrillary tangles (intracellular inclusions).

Granulovacuolar degeneration (GVD)^Q and **Hirano bodies^Q** (eosinophilic inclusions) are abnormalities seen in the cytoplasm of hippocampal neurons in patients with Alzheimer disease. Both of them are present in elderlies without dementia, however they are much more severe and widespread in Alzheimer's disease.

Amyloid cascade hypothesis: According to this hypothesis, mutation in APP gene near cleavage site favor the cleavage by β and γ-secretase, resulting in the production of Aβ. The Aβ peptides form Aβ oligomers which in turn induce tau phosphorylation, producing neurofibrillary tangles. The tau protein in this highly phosphorylated form is not able to stabilize microtubules, resulting in granulovascular degeneration of neurons, neuronal loss and synaptic loss.

Neurochemistry: Alzheimer's disease is predominantly a disorder of **cholinergic neurons^Q** and loss of cholinergic neurons in nucleus basalis of meynert is a consistent finding. Apart from acetylcholine, norepinephrine and serotonin have also been implicated in some cases.

NINCDS-ADRDA

The diagnostic criterion for Alzheimer's disease put by National Institute of Neurological and Communicative Disorders and Stroke and the Alzheimer's Disease and Related Disorders Association **(NINCDS-ADRDA criteria)** are usually used for the diagnosis

Genetics: Alzheimer's disease has shown linkage to chromosome **1, 14 and 21**. A small number of cases of Alzheimer disease are early onset and familial and are inherited in autosomal dominant fashion. Mutations in three genes, **amyloid precursor protein^Q** (chromosome 21), **presenilin-1^Q** (chromosome 14) and **presenilin-2^Q** (chromosome 1) have been found in most cases with familial Alzheimer's disease. The majority of cases are however sporadic and late onset. *Apo E4 gene^Q* is associated with the risk of development of Alzheimer's disease, however its testing is not recommended as it is neither sensitive nor specific for Alzheimer's disease.

The patients with **Down's syndrome^Q** have significantly higher risk for development of Alzheimer's disease. The gene for APP (amyloid precursor protein) is located on chromosome 21.

Risk factors: Age is the most important risk factors. Other risk factors include head injury, hypertension, insulin resistance, depression. Few studies have claimed that **smoking^Q** is a protective factor against Alzheimer's but this finding has been contradicted by other studies. High education levels and remaining physically and mentally active till late in life are protective factors against Alzheimer's disease.

Vascular Dementia or Multi-infarct Dementia

This is the second most common type of dementia. Occurrence of **multiple cerebral infarctions** (caused by occlusion of cerebral vessels by arteriosclerotic plaques or thromboemboli) results in progressive deterioration of brain functions, finally resulting in dementia. There are acute exacerbations which correspond to the new infarcts, and result is step-wise deterioration of symptoms (**stepladder pattern**). The general symptoms of dementia are present. In addition patient has focal neurological deficits which correspond to site of infarction. There is usually history of previous stroke or transient ischemic attacks. The patients usually have hypertension and other cardiovascular risk factors. The treatment involves management of risk factors and cholinesterase inhibitors.

NINDS-AIREN

NINDS-AIREN^Q criterion are used for the diagnosis of vascular dementia (National Institute of Neurological Disorders and Stroke (NINDS) and the Association Internationale pour la Recherche et l'Enseignement en Neurosciences (AIREN)

Binswanger's disease^Q: It is also known as subcortical arteriosclerotic encephalopathy, and is characterized by multiple small white matter infarctions and can produce symptoms of subcortical dementia.

Lewy Body Disease (Dementia with Lewy Body)

The clinical signs and symptoms are similar to Alzheimer disease. Apart these patients also have fluctuating levels of attention and alertness, recurrent visual hallucinations and Parkinsonian features (tremors, rigidity and bradykinesia). Antipsychotic medications should be avoided as these patients are extremely sensitive to antipsychotics and can develop drug induced Parkinsonism.

Huntington's Disease, Parkinson's Disease, Wilson's Disease and Multiple Sclerosis

These predominantly motor diseases are associated with the development of dementia. The dementia seen is of subcortical type with more motor abnormalities and less of amnesia, apraxia, aphasia and agnosia.

HIV Related Dementia

The diagnosis of HIV dementia (AIDS dementia complex) is made by lab evidence of systemic HIV infection, cognitive deficits, presence of motor abnormalities or personality changes. Personality changes are characterized by apathy, emotional lability or disinhibition.

Head Trauma Related Dementia

Dementia can develop as a sequelae of head trauma. Dementia pugilistica (punch drunk syndrome) can develop in boxers after repeated head trauma.

Frontotemporal Dementia (FTD)

Frontotemporal dementias are a group which have similar presentation but may be caused by a variety of neuropathological substrates. **Pick's disease**^{Q} is one pathological variant of FTD, and is characterized by presence of **Pick's bodies**. The frontotemporal dementia's have an **earlier onset**^{Q}, around 45-65 years and mainly present with behavioral symptoms and change in personality with **relative preservation of memory**^{Q}. Three distinctive forms of FTD have been described on the basis of clinical presentation.

A. *Frontal variant FTD*: The symptoms are primarily of loss of frontal lobe function. The classical feature is stereotyped behavior, disinhibition and apathy.
B. *Semantic dementia*: The symptoms are primarily of loss of temporal lobe functions and is characterized by complaints of loss of memory for words.
C. *Progressive nonfluent aphasia*: It presents with speech dysfluency and word finding difficulties.

Pseudodementia

The depression in elderly patients may mimic symptoms of dementia and hence is known as **pseudodementia**^{Q}. A depressed patient may get a low score on MMSE, as depressed individual lacks motivation to solve the questions. Hence low score on MMSE should be carefully interpreted, if depression is suspected.

Management of Dementia

The evaluation of cognitive functions is usually done using the screening test of **mini mental status examination (MMSE)**^{Q}. A score of less than 24 (out of a maximum 30) is suggestive of dementia. In accordance with the cholinergic hypothesis, **cholinesterase inhibitors** are widely used for treatment of cognitive deficits in Alzheimer's disease. Donepezil, rivastigmine, galantamine and tacrine are few of the drugs belonging to this category.

Memantine, a **NMDA receptor antagonist**^{Q} has also been approved for the treatment. For behavioral and psychological symptoms of dementia, symptomatic treatment is used and may include antidepressants, antipsychotics and benzodiazepines. Please note that antipsychotics can **increase mortality rate**^{Q} in patients with dementia by increasing the incidence of congestive heart failure, sudden death and infections such as pneumonia^Q.

AMNESTIC DISORDERS

Amnestic disorder is a broad category that includes a variety of conditions which present with amnestic syndrome. Amnestic syndrome is characterized by inability to form new memories (anterograde amnesia) and the inability to recall previously remembered knowledge (retrograde amnesia). Short-term and recent memory are usually impaired with preservation of remote and immediate memory. The **major causes**^{Q} of amnestic disorders are:

A. Thiamine deficiency (Korsakoff syndrome)
B. Hypoglycemia
C. Primary brain conditions (head trauma, seizures, cerebral tumors, cerebrovascular disease, hypoxia, electro-convulsive therapy, multiple sclerosis)
D. Substance related disorders (alcohol, benzodiazepines).

Frontal Lobe Syndrome

Frontal lobe syndrome or frontal lobe personality is the broad term used to describe the abnormalities (usually of higher mental functions) that develop due to disturbances of frontal lobe. Three types have been described:

a. **Orbitofrontal syndrome**: It is caused by disorders of orbitofrontal cortex (which is a part of frontal lobe) and presents with:
   1. Behavioural disinhibition (including inappropriate behaviours such as sexually inappropriate behaviours)
   2. Impulsivity
   3. Lack of insight and poor judgement

b. **Dorsolateral syndrome**: It is caused by disorders of dorsolateral prefrontal cortex and presents with:
   1. Apathy, lack of motivation
   2. Psychomotor retardation, impaired attention and concentration
   3. The symptoms are similar to depression and often a wrong diagnosis is made initially

c. **Anterior cingulate syndrome**: It presents with executive function abnormalities primarily.

Multiple Choice Questions

Organic Mental Disorders

1. Which of the following behavioral problems would suggest an organic brain lesion? *(SGPGI 2005, DNB 2006)*
   A. Formal thought disorder
   B. Auditory hallucinations
   C. Visual hallucinations
   D. Depression

2. Organic mental disease is indicated by:
   A. Incoherence *(AIIMS 1991, DNB 1993)*
   B. Delusion
   C. Flight of idea
   D. Perseveration of speech

3. Mini mental status examination is: *(AIIMS 2016, DNB 2004)*
   A. Thought
   B. Cognition
   C. Mood and affect
   D. Insight

4. MMSE is used for diagnosis of: *(NEET 2016)*
   A. Alzheimers
   B. Schizophrenia
   C. Depression
   D. Anxiety disorders

5. While doing MMSE, maximum score is given to: *(NIMHANS 2017)*
   A. Orientation   B. Recall
   C. Registration   D. Language

6. What is the total score of items in MMSE? *(PGI May 2017)*
   A. 10   B. 20
   C. 30   D. 40
   E. 15

7. Cognitive disorders are: *(PGI June 2006, 2007)*
   A. Intellectualization
   B. Depersonalization
   C. Dementia
   D. Delirium
   E. Hallucination
   F. Secondary gain

8. Disorientation occurs in: *(AI 1993)*
   A. Schizophrenia
   B. Organic brain syndrome
   C. Depression
   D. Mania

9. Which of the following suggest a psychotic rather than an organic disorder? *(DNB June 2009)*
   A. Confusion
   B. Complex delusions
   C. Impairment of consciousness
   D. Lack of insight

10. Feature(s) suggestive of schizophrenia rather than organic psychosis is/are: *(PGI June 2009)*
    A. Third person hallucination
    B. Split personality
    C. Visual hallucination
    D. Altered sensorium
    E. Systematized delusion

11. In India psychiatric disorder in people above 60-year of age is mostly due to: *(DNB 2003, Calcutta 2000)*
    A. Depression
    B. Dementia
    C. Hysteria
    D. Schizophrenia

12. Oneiroid state is: *(JIPMER 2017)*
    A. Same as torpor
    B. Dream like state
    C. Characterised by heightened state of consciousness
    D. Same as stupor

13. Pointers to organic disease include all *except*: *(NIMHANS 2019)*
    A. Early age of onset
    B. Absence of family history of psychiatric disorders
    C. Absence of previous history of psychiatric illness
    D. Absence of any apparent psychological precipitant

Delirium

Controversial Question

14. Most important feature of delirium is: *(DNB NEET 2014-15)*
    A. Impaired attention
    B. Anxiety
    C. Hyperactivity
    D. Clouding of consciousness

15. Delirium is defined as: *(DNB NEET 2014-15)*
    A. Acute onset of disturbed consciousness
    B. Chronic onset of disturbed consciousness
    C. Progressive generalized impairment of intellectual functions and memory without impairment of consciousness.
    D. Disorientation without clouding of consciousness

16. Features of delirium: *(NIMHANS 2016, PGI Nov 2010, June 2008)*
    A. Deficit of attention (attention deficit)
    B. Autonomic instability (dysfunction)
    C. Altered sleep wake pattern
    D. Visual hallucination and clouding of consciousness
    E. Delirium cannot be diagnosed clinically

17. **Delirium and schizophrenia differ from each other by:**
    (DNB 2003, WB 2001, KA 2004)
    A. Change in mood
    B. Clouding of consciousness
    C. Tangential thinking
    D. All of the above

18. **Slow waves in EEG activity are seen in:** *(PGI 1998)*
    A. Depression   B. Delirium
    C. Schizophrenia   D. Mania

19. **A patient with pneumonia for 5 days is admitted to the hospital in altered sensorium. He suddenly ceases to recognize the doctor and staff. He thinks that he is in jail and complains of scorpion attacking him. His probable diagnosis is:** *(AI 2001)*
    A. Acute dementia
    B. Acute delirium
    C. Acute schizophrenia
    D. Acute paranoia

20. **A 60-year man had undergone cardiac bypass surgery 2 days back. Now he started forgetting things and was not able to recall names and phone numbers of his relatives. What is the probable diagnosis?** *(AI 2010)*
    A. Depression
    B. Post-traumatic psychosis
    C. Cognitive dysfunction
    D. Alzheimer's disease

21. **Confusional assessment method is used for which of the following:** *(NEET 2019)*
    A. Delirium   B. Schizophrenia
    C. Dementia   D. Depression

Amnestic Syndrome

22. **Anterograde amnesia is seen in:** *(AIIMS Nov 2010)*
    A. Head injury
    B. Stroke
    C. Spinal cord injury (traumatic paraplegia)
    D. Alzheimer's disease

23. **Cause of organic amnestic syndrome include(s):**
    (PGI May 2013)
    A. Multiple sclerosis   B. Hypoglycemia
    C. Hyperglycemia   D. Hypoxia
    E. Hypercapnia

24. **Not diagnostic/defining criteria for amnestic disorder:**
    (PGI Nov 2009)
    A. Visual hallucination
    B. Transient delusion
    C. Impaired concentration/attention
    D. Good recall of recent events
    E. Ability to form new memories

25. **All are true except:** *(PGI Feb 2008)*
    A. Procedural learning is from past experiences
    B. Implicit learning is procedural skill acquirement
    C. Amnestic syndromes, loss of semantic memory is first
    D. Implicit memory is declarative
    E. Anterograde amnesia affects long term memory more in amnestic syndrome

Dementia

26. **What differentiates delirium from dementia?**
    A. Confusion   *(NEET 2018)*
    B. Difficulty in communication
    C. Hallucination
    D. Memory loss

27. **Delirium can be differentiated from dementia by the presence of:** *(NEET 2016)*
    A. Disturbance of memory   B. Hallucinations
    C. Delusions   D. Fluctuating course

28. **Most common cause of dementia is:** *(DNB NEET 2014-15)*
    A. Alzheimer's disease   B. Vascular dementia
    C. Wilson's disease   D. Pick's disease

29. **True about dementia is all except:** *(AI 1994)*
    A. Often irreversible
    B. Hallucinations are not common
    C. Clouding of consciousness is common
    D. Nootropics have limited role

30. **Catastrophic reaction is a feature of:** *(MH 2011)*
    A. Dementia   B. Delirium
    C. Schizophrenia   D. Anxiety

31. **All are causes of subcortical dementia except:**
    (AIIMS May 2009)
    A. Alzheimer's disease   B. Parkinson's disease
    C. Supranuclear palsy   D. HIV associated dementia

32. **Dementia is/are present in all except:**
    A. Alzheimer's disease   B. Pick's disease
    C. Lewy body   D. Binswanger's disease
    E. Ganser's syndrome

33. **Reversible causes of dementia:**
    A. Hypothyroidism   *(JIPMER 2018, PGI June 2004)*
    B. Alzheimer's disease
    C. Vitamin B12 deficiency
    D. Vitamin A deficiency

34. **Treatable causes of dementia are:** *(PGI 2001)*
    A. Alzheimer's disease   B. Hypothyroidism
    C. Multi-infarct dementia D. Subdural hematoma (SDH)
    E. Hydrocephalus

35. **Vascular dementia is characterized by:** *(PGI 2003)*
    A. Disorientation   B. Memory deficit
    C. Emotional lability D. Visual hallucination
    E. Personality deterioration

36. **Visual hallucinations are commonly seen in:**
    A. Alzheimer's disease   *(NIMHANS 2017)*
    B. Lewy body dementia
    C. Frontotemporal dementia
    D. Vascular dementia

37. **A 65-year-old male is brought to the outpatient clinic with one year illness characterized by marked forgetfulness, visual hallucinations, suspiciousness, personality decline, poor self care and progressive deterioration in his condition. His Mini Mental Status Examination (MMSE) score is 21. His most likely diagnosis is:** *(AIIMS Nov 2002)*
    A. Dementia   B. Schizophrenia
    C. Mania   D. Depression

38. Which of the following neurotransmitters are decreased in Alzheimer's disease? *(DNB NEET 2014-15)*
    A. Acetylcholine
    B. Norepinephrine
    C. Corticotropin
    D. All of the above

39. Which of the following is associated with Alzheimer disease: *(NEET 2019)*
    A. Apo E1
    B. Apo E2
    C. Apo E3
    D. Apo E4

40. Following are predispositions to Alzheimer's disease except: *(DNB 1996, AI 1999)*
    A. Down's syndrome
    B. Head trauma
    C. Smoking
    D. Low education group

41. Dementia of Alzheimer's type is not associated with one of the following: *(AIIMS Nov 2005)*
    A. Depressive symptoms
    B. Delusions
    C. Apraxia and aphasia
    D. Cerebral infarcts

Controversial Question

42. Which of the following statements about Alzheimer's disease are true? *(PGI Nov 2016)*
    A. Onset before 45 years of age is rare
    B. Long-term memory is affected before short term memory
    C. Staining shows Tau protein in senile plaques
    D. MRI shows atrophy in frontal and parietal lobes

43. Which of the following statements about Alzheimer's disease are true? *(PGI May 2016)*
    A. Remarkable loss of past events
    B. Definitive diagnosis can be made on MRI
    C. Plaques mostly develop in frontoparietal cortex
    D. Activity of choline acetyl transferase is reduced in cerebral cortex
    E. Levels of phosphorylated tau in CSF are elevated

44. All the following are features of Alzheimer's disease except: *(DNB 1994, WB 2002)*
    A. Cerebellar atrophy
    B. Common in 5th and 6th decade
    C. Atrophied gyri widened sulci
    D. Progressive dementia

45. In Alzheimer's disease (AD) which of the following is not seen? *(AIIMS Nov 2011)*
    A. Aphasia
    B. Acalculia
    C. Agnosia
    D. Apraxia

46. False regarding Alzheimer's disease (AD) is:
    A. Number of senile neural plaques correlates (increases) with age
    B. Presence of tau protein suggest neurodegeneration
    C. Number of neurofibrillary tangles is associated with the severity of dementia
    D. Extracellular inclusions (lesions) can occur in the absence of intracellular inclusions to make pathological diagnosis of AD

47. Part of the brain which is most commonly affected in Alzheimer's disease? *(NIMHANS 2017)*
    A. Locus ceruleus
    B. Entorhinal cortex
    C. Frontal cortex
    D. Cerebellum

48. Area of brain resistant to neurofibrillary tangles in Alzheimer's disease: *(AI 2012)*
    A. Visual association area
    B. Entorhinal cortex
    C. Lateral geniculate body
    D. Cuneal gyrus area VI/temporal lobe

49. Regarding Alzheimer's disease which is/are not true? *(PGI Dec 2008, June 2009) (AIIMS Nov 2011)*
    A. Initial loss of long-term memory
    B. Delayed loss of short-term memory
    C. Step ladder pattern
    D. Cognitive impairment
    E. Judgment impaired

50. All are true regarding Alzheimer's disease except:
    A. Gradually progressive *(PGI Feb 2008)*
    B. Abrupt onset and acute exacerbations
    C. Episodic memory can be affected
    D. Frontotemporal disorder
    E. Ubiquitin Lewy bodies

51. Frontotemporal dementias include all except: *(DNB 2003, UP 2007)*
    A. Pick's disease
    B. Nonfluent aphasia
    C. Semantic dementia
    D. Alzheimer's disease

Controversial Question

52. A 70-year-old man presents with h/o prosopagnosia, loss of memory, 3rd person hallucinations since 1 month. On examination deep tendon reflexes are increased, mini-mental examination score is 20/30. What is most likely diagnosis? *(AIIMS 2001)*
    A. Dissociated dementia
    B. Schizophrenia
    C. Alzheimer's disease
    D. Psychotic disorder

53. Not a feature of Alzheimer's disease:
    A. Hirano bodies *(PGI May 2013)*
    B. Amyloid angiopathy
    C. Granulovacuolar degeneration of neurons
    D. Senile plaque
    E. Cerebellar atrophy

54. Which of the following medications acts as NMDA antagonist? *(NIMHANS 2017)*
    A. Entacapone
    B. Amantadine
    C. Memantine
    D. Donepezil

55. True regarding FTD are all except:
    A. Semantic dementia *(AIIMS 2011, NEET 2013)*
    B. Nonfluent aphasia
    C. Apathetic, disinhibited personality
    D. Rapid onset static course

56. All are true regarding frontotemporal dementia: *(AIIMS Nov 2012)*
    A. Stereotypic behavior
    B. Insight present
    C. Age less than 65 years
    D. Affective symptoms

57. The following are the psychiatric sequelae after stroke in elderly: *(PGI 2003)*
    A. Depression
    B. Post-traumatic stress disorder
    C. Dementia
    D. Anxiety

58. **The psychiatric disorder most commonly associated with myxedema:**
    A. Depression
    B. Mania
    C. Phobia
    D. Psychosis

59. **Myxedema madness includes:** *(DNB NEET 2014-15)*
    A. Auditory hallucinations and paranoia
    B. Visual hallucinations and depression
    C. Auditory hallucinations and depression
    D. Paranoia and depression

60. **A 20-year-old female has thoughts of cutting her fingers, and imagines doing it but never actually does it. She says she is not having any guilt of having such thought. And also says the thoughts are distressing her and she is unable to control them. The thoughts vanish either by ending with a seizure or automatically subside on their own. Which of the following is the likely cause?**
    (AIIMS May 2017)
    A. Obsession
    B. Thought insertion
    C. Forced thinking
    D. Crowding of thoughts

61. **A patient presents with habit of urinating in public and doesn't have any feelings of guilt or remorse for the same? Which of the following lobes involvement could cause these symptoms?** *(AIIMS Nov 2018)*
    A. Frontal
    B. Parietal
    C. Temporal
    D. Occipital

62. **Which of the following is more prevalent in Down's syndrome:** *(NEET 2019)*
    A. Alzheimers disease
    B. Parkinson's disease
    C. Lewy body dementia
    D. Frontotemporal dementia

63. **Criteria for vascular dementia?** *(NIMHANS 2019)*
    A. NINDS-AIREN criteria
    B. NINCDS-ADRDA criteria
    C. Roman criteria
    D. MDS criterion

64. **Regarding frontotemporal dementia, false statement is:** *(NIMHANS 2019)*
    A. Memory is affected early in the illness
    B. Repetitive behaviour are seen
    C. Personality changes are seen
    D. Apathy is usually present

Answers With Explanations

Organic Mental Disorders

1. **C.** If a patient presents with prominent visual hallucinations, organic mental disorders (organic brain lesions) should always be looked for.
2. **D.** Perseveration of speech is suggestive of organic mental disorders. Few books are giving the answer as delusion which is completely wrong.
3. **B.** Mini mental status examination is used to evaluate cognitive functions in illnesses like dementia and delirium.
4. **A.** Alzheimers disease.
5. **A.** Orientation.
6. **C.** 30
7. **C, D.**
   As organic mental disorders commonly have disturbances of cognition, they are also known as cognitive disorders.
8. **B.** Presence of disturbances of consciousness and disorientation is suggestive of organic mental disorders.
9. **B.** The complex delusions are frequently seen in psychotic disorder. In organic mental disorders, the delusions are usually transient and fragmented. Presence of complex delusions in organic mental disorder is very rare. The lack of insight is a feature of both whereas confusion and impairment of consciousness is seen in organic mental disorders.
10. **A, E.**
    Third person hallucinations are quite suggestive of schizophrenia. Also systematized delusions (elaborate delusions) are much more likely in schizophrenia. Please remember that schizophrenia is not a disorder of personality and hence there is no "split personality" in schizophrenia. Visual hallucinations and altered sensorium are more suggestive of organic mental disorders although visual hallucinations can also be seen in schizophrenia.
11. **B.** In older age (>60 years) dementia is the most common psychiatric disorder followed by depression.
12. **B.** Dream like state
13. **A.** Early age of onset usually goes against the diagnosis of organic disorders. They are more common in old age. Rest all the options are favourable for diagnosis of organic disorders.

Delirium

14. **D.** Please remember that the hallmark symptom of delirium is clouding of consciousness, which is associated with impairment of global cognitive functions, most importantly attention.
15. **A.** Acute onset of disturbed consciousness
16. **A, B, C, D.**
17. **B.** Delirium presents with clouding of consciousness whereas in schizophrenia consciousness is intact. The mood changes and tangential thinking cannot be used for differentiation.
18. **B.** Delirium.
19. **B.** History of a medical disorder (pneumonia) followed by disturbances in consciousness (altered sensorium), disorientation (failure to recognize doctor and staff and thinking that he is in jail) and hallucinations (scorpions attacking) is suggestive of delirium.
20. **C.** The history of cardiac surgery 2 days prior followed by behavioral changes is suggestive of delirium. The question here is stressing on "disturbances of memory" which can be seen in delirium, however are usually restricted to short term memory loss. The other important features such as clouding of consciousness and attention impairment has not been provided. Nonetheless, the most likely diagnosis appears to be delirium. As delirium has prominent cognitive dysfunction, that is the correct answer. Alzheimer disease does not have such sudden onset.
21. **A.**

Amnestic Syndrome

22. **B.** Anterograde amnesia is seen in stroke.
23. **A, B, D.**
    See text for explanation.
24. **A, B, C, D, E.**
    None of the options are included in diagnostic criterion for amnestic disorder. Amnestic syndrome is characterized by inability to form new memories (anterograde amnesia) and the inability to recall previously remembered knowledge (retrograde amnesia). Short-term and recent memory are usually impaired with preservation of remote and immediate memory.
25. **C, D, E.**
    Explicit memory (declarative memory) is the memory which is associated with awareness, whereas implicit memory (nondeclarative memory) does not involve awareness. For example, if you have to choose the correct option for a particular MCQ, you first try to remember the correct answer, i.e. you try to bring the memory associated with MCQ into awareness, hence its an example of explicit memory. However, when you drive a car, you do not really try to remember everything every time. Changing clutches, pressing breaks and accelerator happens automatically and you do not have to remember anything, its an example of implicit memory.
    Explicit memory is further divided into **episodic memory** for events (e.g. the memory of your first day in medical college) and **semantic memory** for facts (e.g. memory for the most common, least common type of questions).

Procedural memory (for procedures like driving) is a type of implicit memory. Now, looking at options. Option A is true, procedural learning depends on past experience. Initially we have to remember every detail about how to use clutch, break and accelerator, however, with repeated experience it becomes implicit. Option B is also correct as procedure learning is a type of implicit memory. Option C is wrong, in amnestic syndrome, episodic memory is lost more and not the semantic memory. Option D is wrong as implicit memory is nondeclarative. Option E is also wrong, in amnestic syndrome short-term and recent memory are more affected and not the long-term memory.

Dementia

26. A. Confusion. Confusional state which is basically a disturbance of consciousness is a feature of delirium and is never seen in dementia.
27. D. Fluctuating course. Delirium tends to have a fluctuating course whereas dementia has a chronic and downhill course.
28. A. Alzheimer's disease
29. C. There is no disturbance of consciousness in dementia. It is often irreversible. The hallucinations can be present but are not common. Nootropics (or cognitive enhancers) have very limited role in the management of dementia.
30. A. *See* text for explanation.
31. A. Alzheimer's disease is a cortical dementia.
32. E. Ganser's syndrome is a type of dissociative disorder. The other options are examples of dementia.
33. A, C.
34. B, D, E.
    Perhaps the use of word "treatable" is in appropriate here since all the types of dementia can be "treated". The examiner most likely wants to ask the types which can be "reversed" or "cured".
35. A, B, C, D.
    Vascular dementia presents with memory loss, mood changes (depression, irritability, emotional lability), delusions and hallucinations, confusion and disorientation.
36. B. Lewy body dementia
37. A. Old age with history suggestive of a progressive impairment in memory, presence of behavioral and psychological symptoms (hallucinations, suspiciousness), poor self care and personality decline and a MMSE score <24, are all suggestive of dementia.
38. A. Acetylcholine.
39. D. ApoE 4
40. C. Smoking is considered to be one of the protective factors in Alzheimer's disease, however this finding has been inconsistent across the studies.
41. D. Cerebral infarcts are a feature of vascular dementia and not dementia of Alzheimer's type (Alzheimer's disease).
42. A. The first statement is correct. Onset is usually after 65 years of age. Second statement is incorrect, long-term memory gets affected in advanced stages only. Third statement is also incorrect as senile plaques contain amyloid beta (A®) and not tau proteins. The last statement can be argued upon. Alzheimer's disease is usually described as a disease of temporal and parietal lobe and MRI usually shows atrophy in temporal and parietal lobe. Although we must remember that frontal cortex does get involved in the advanced phases.
43. A, D, E.
    In Alzheimers disease patient mostly present with loss of recent memory, particularly episodic memory. Options D and E are also correct. Please remember definitive diagnosis of Alzheimer can be made only on brain biopsy (usually post death). Plaques mostly develop in temporal and parietal lobe.
44. A. In Alzheimer's, the disease process usually spares cerebellum. Especially neurofibrillary tangles are never seen in cerebellum.
45. B. The best answer here is B. In reality, all four options given here are seen in Alzheimer's however, the DSM criterion for Alzheimer's disease does not include acalculia as a symptom, while other three, aphasia, apraxia and agnosia have been included.
46. D. Please remember that the neuropathological diagnosis of Alzheimer's disease requires extensive presence of both senile plaques (extra cellular deposits) and neurofibrillary tangles (intracellular inclusions).
47. B. Entorhinal cortex
48. C. Lateral geniculate body.
49. A, B, C.
    Short-term memory is lost first, long-term memory gets lost only in the later stages of illness. Step ladder pattern is typical of vascular dementia.
50. B, D, E.
    Alzheimer's has an insidious onset and gradual progression. In the course of disease episodic memory does get disturbed. Alzheimer's disease primarily involves parietal and temporal lobe.
51. D. Alzheimer's disease
52. C. The presence of loss of memory, prosopagnosia (difficulty in identifying face) in a 70 year old man is quite suggestive of Alzheimer's disease. Third person auditory hallucinations are usually seen in schizophrenia, however they can be present in Alzheimer's disease too. Further on examination, deep tendon reflexes are increased, which again can be seen in late stages of Alzheimer's disease. Finally MMSE score below 24 seals the diagnosis.
53. E. *See* text for explanation.
54. C. Memantine
55. D. The frontotemporal dementias have a progressive course and not static course.
56. B. Insight is usually lost.
57. A, C, D.
    The psychiatric sequelae of stroke includes dementia, depression, mania, apathy, psychosis, emotional instability.
58. A. The most common psychiatric disorder associated with hypothyroidism is cognitive slowing followed by depression.
59. A. Myxedematous madness has been described in a small number of patients with hypothyroidism. The

characteristic symptoms include auditory hallucinations and paranoia (persecutory ideas).

60. C. Forced thinking
    Focal seizures can present with psychic symptoms without impairment of cognition. These may later progress to generalised seizures, usually of tonic clonic type. Forced thinking is a type of 'psychic symptoms' in which patient feels compelled to think about a specific topic or word again and again. Another psychic symptoms is 'crowding of thoughts' in which patient has a feeling of racing, disorganised thoughts. In this question, the phenomenon described ends with a seizure and is consistent with description of 'forced thinking'

61. A. The patient has disinhibition and lack of insight for the same, usually seen in orbitofrontal syndromes.
62. A. Alzheimer's disease
63. A. NINDS-AIREN criterion
64. A. Memory is usually affected late in frontotemporal dementia

CHAPTER 7

Personality Disorders

Personality is defined as the dynamic organization within the individual that determines his/her unique adjustment to his/her environment. The personality can be described under five broad dimensions. These five dimensions, also called **personality traits**[Q] can be remembered with the pneumonic, OCEAN.
1. *Openness to experience*: It reflects the curiosity, **novelty seeking**[Q], **sensation seeking**[Q] and desire to have new experiences. Individuals with high openness to experience may indulge in activities such as skydiving, bungee jumping, gambling, etc.
2. *Conscientiousness*: It reflects the tendency to be organized, disciplined and dutiful.
3. *Extraversion*: It reflects the sociability, talkativeness and preference for group activities over solitary activities.
4. *Agreeableness*: It reflects compassion and cooperation for others and a trusting and helpful nature.
5. *Neuroticism*: It reflects the tendency to experience unpleasant emotions easily. It also refers to the degree of emotional stability.

If the personality of an individual deviates from social norms and is a cause of unhappiness and impairment, the individual is diagnosed with a personality disorder.

Personality disorder is defined as presence of abnormal behavior and subjective experiences which causes significant impairment. The prevalence of personality disorder is around 10–20% in the general population. The onset is in **adolescence or early adulthood**[Q], the symptoms remain stable throughout the adult life and **maturing**[Q] occurs by around **40 years**. Maturing means the resolution of abnormal patterns of behavior. The personality disorder is **"ego syntonic"**[Q] (**agreeable to self**).

In other words, the individual with a personality disorder does not find anything wrong with himself and hence is often unwilling to take any treatment. DSM-5 has classified the personality disorders into three clusters.

Cluster A Personality Disorders

The following personality disorders are included in cluster A:
A. *Paranoid personality disorder*: The characteristic feature is **excessive suspiciousness** and distrust of others. These patients may be **excessively sensitive**[Q] and may be quick to react angrily. They give **excessive importance to themselves** and believe in conspiracy theories. Psychotherapy is the treatment of choice. Medications like benzodiazepines and antipsychotics may be used for agitation and paranoia (excessive suspiciousness).
B. *Schizoid personality disorder*: These patients are **detached**[Q] from social relationships and **prefer solitary activities**. They are **emotionally cold**[Q] and are indifferent to praise or criticism. They appear self-absorbed and lost in day dreams and may be preoccupied with fantasies. Since they are uncomfortable with human interaction, they have little interest in sexual activities. The management revolves around psychotherapy. The medications which are occasionally used include antipsychotics, antidepressants and benzodiazepines.
C. *Schizotypal personality disorder*: These patients have disturbances of thinking and communication. They frequently exhibit **odd beliefs or magical thinking**[Q] (e.g. superstitiousness, belief in telepathy or "sixth sense"). Their inner world may be like that of a child, filled with fears and fantasies. They may have strange ways of communication making it difficult to understand. They may also report illusions and other perceptual disturbances.

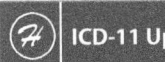 **ICD-11 Update**
Schizotypal disorder is not considered as a personality disorder, instead it is classified as a psychotic disorder along with schizophrenia.

They usually do not have any close relationships and appear "odd and eccentric" to others. When in severe stress, they may decompensate and have psychotic symptoms, but these are usually brief. The management revolves around psychotherapy. The medications which are occasionally used include antipsychotics, antidepressants and benzodiazepines. The "cluster A" personality disorders (especially schizotypal personality disorder) are considered to be on a "schizophrenia continuum" which means that they lie somewhere in between the "normal" and "schizophrenia".

Cluster B Personality Disorders

The following personality disorders are included in cluster B:

A. *Histrionic personality disorder*: These patients are excitable and overtly emotional and behave in a dramatic and extroverted way. They want to be the center of attention and exaggerate everything, making it sound more important than it really is. They tend to behave in a sexually seductive manner and use physical appearance to draw attention towards self. Management usually involves psychotherapy. Medications like antidepressants are occasionally useful.

B. *Narcissistic personality disorder*: These patients have a heightened sense of **self-importance**^{Q}. They believe that they are special and very talented. They are preoccupied with fantasies of unlimited success and power. They want to be admired by others. If condemned, they may become very angry or they may show complete indifference to criticism. They have a fragile self-esteem and are susceptible to development of depression, when faced with rejection. Management usually involves psychotherapy. Medications like antidepressants are occasionally useful.

C. *Antisocial personality disorder (dissocial personality disorder)*: These patients do not have regard for rights of others and frequently violate them. They frequently get involved in unlawful behaviors such as theft, lying, truancy and conning. They have a lack of remorse or guilt for their actions. Substance use disorders are frequently present in these patients. Treatment usually is psychotherapy. Medications like carbamazepine, beta blockers are occasionally used.

D. *Borderline personality disorder*: These patients are almost always in a state of crisis. They have significant **mood swings**. They may start feeling angry, anxious or frustrated without any reason. Their interpersonal relationships are intense and tumultuous. They swing from being excessively dependent to being hostile to persons close to them. Hence, they have a history of **unstable relationships**^{Q}. Another characteristic feature is the repetitive **self-destructive acts**^{Q} such as slashing of wrists, or over dosage of medications. The patients indulge in these behaviors to elicit help from others, to express the anger or just to numb themselves to the overwhelming painful feelings they have. These patients are also **impulsive**^{Q} in areas such as spending, sex and substance use. These patients have **identity disturbances**^{Q} and have **unstable self image**^{Q} (they have sudden changes in life goals, values, career plans, sexual identity etc).

Finally, these patients excessively use the defense mechanism of **splitting** (wherein they consider each person to be either "all good" or "all bad"). Management involves psychotherapy. **"Dialectical behavior therapy"** is a therapy which has been designed for treatment of borderline personality disorder. Medications used include antipsychotics, antidepressant and mood stabilizers like carbamazepine. In ICD-10, the borderline personality disorder has been described as a subtype of a broader diagnosis of "emotionally unstable personality disorder".

Cluster C Personality Disorders

The following personality disorders are included in cluster C:

A. *Avoidant personality disorder*: These patients are excessively **sensitive to rejection**. They are afraid that they would be criticized or rejected in social situations. Hence, they tend to remain socially withdrawn. These persons are usually unwilling to enter into a relationship unless they are given a strong guarantee of uncritical acceptance. The ICD-10, uses the diagnosis of anxious personality disorder for such patients. Management mostly involves psychotherapy. Beta blockers and selective serotonin reuptake inhibitors (SSRIs) are also useful.

B. *Dependent personality disorder*: These patients are **dependent** on others for everyday decisions. All the major decisions in their lives are taken by someone else. They ask for excessive amount of advice and reassurance from others. They also have difficulty expressing disagreement with others because of fear of loss of support. They get very uncomfortable and helpless when alone and fear that they would not be able to take care of themselves. Management usually involves psychotherapy. Benzodiazepines and SSRIs can be used for symptomatic relief.

C. *Obsessive-compulsive personality disorder*: These patients are preoccupied with rules and regulations. They give excessive importance to details and show perfectionism that interferes with task completion (since they want everything to be perfect, it often results in significant delays). They are inflexible and insist that others agree to their demands. They are excessively devoted to work and may not have any time for leisure activities. They are formal and serious and often lack a sense of humor. The ICD-10, used the diagnosis of "anankastic personality disorder" for these patients. Management usually involves psychotherapy.

> **ICD-11 Update**
>
> The older classification of personality disorders (e.g. schizoid, paranoid, narcissistic etc) has been removed. According to ICD-11, personality disorders have been divided according to severity of symptoms into:
> - Mild personality disorder
> - Moderate personality disorder
> - Severe personality disorder
>
> According to ICD-11, depending on the specific symptoms present, a specifier of 'prominent personality trait' can be added after the diagnosis, e.g. a person who does not follow rules, doesn't care for feelings of others, does not have any guilt feeling will get a diagnosis of moderate personality disorder (dissociality in personality disorder). This patient according to ICD-10 would have received a diagnosis of Dissocial Personality disorder.

Types A and B Personality

Another way of classifying personality is what is known as Type A and Type B personality. **Type A personality** is characterized by **competitiveness^Q, time urgency, hostility^Q** and **anger**. The people with Type A personality are ambitious, impatient and hard working workaholics. Many studies have suggested that Type A personality (especially the hostility and anger traits) is a risk factor for **coronary heart disease^Q**.

In comparison individuals with Type B personality are easy going and relaxed, they are not excessively competitive and may focus more on enjoyment and less on winning or losing. Recent studies have suggested a new personality type, **Type D personality^Q** which is characterized by negative affectivity (a tendency to experience negative emotions) and social inhibition (tendency to inhibit expression of emotions). Individuals with Type D personality are predisposed to development of **coronary heart disease^Q**.

IMPULSE CONTROL DISORDERS

These disorders are characterized by irresistible impulses or temptations to perform a particular act which is harmful to self or others. Impulse is described by patients as a feeling of increasing tension and arousal that leads to performance of a certain behavior. The performance of the behavior gives a sense of relief and also gratification. After some time, however the person feels guilty or remorseful. The following are described as impulse control disorders. All of them are preceded by the irresistible impulses:

1. *Pyromania:* Recurrent and purposeful setting of fires.
2. *Kleptomania^Q*: Recurrent stealing of objects which are not needed for personal use or are of no monetary value.
3. *Intermittent explosive disorder*: It is characterized by episodes of aggression resulting in serious assault or destruction of properties.
4. *Compulsive sexual behavior disorder*: This diagnosis has been included as an impulse control disorder in ICD-11. It is characterized by failure to control strong, repetitive, sexual impulses that result in repetitive sexual behaviors. The repetitive sexual activity becomes the focus of life and results in adverse consequences.
5. *Others*: These include, **Oniomania^Q** or compulsive buying: Recurrent episodes of buying or shopping despite the buying behavior causing significant monetary and socio-occupational distress.

Multiple Choice Questions

1. Which of the following is not a personality trait? *(AIIMS Nov 2009)*
   A. Sensation seeking
   B. Neuroticism
   C. Openness to experience
   D. Problem solving

2. True about personality disorder: *(PGI June 2007)*
   A. Onset in early childhood and adolescence
   B. Matures around adulthood
   C. Not associated with social norms
   D. Direct result of disease or damage

3. Which of the following is a Type B Personality disorder? *(NEET 2016)*
   A. Anxious PD
   B. Narcissistic PD
   C. Dependent PD
   D. Anankastic PD

4. Characteristic disorder that appears in late childhood and continues in adulthood: *(DNB NEET 2014-15)*
   A. Somatoform disorder
   B. Personality disorder
   C. Anxiety disorder
   D. Mood disorder

5. True about personality disorder: *(PGI 2003)*
   A. Typically onset at early childhood and adolescence
   B. Mature around at 30-40 years
   C. Ego dystonic
   D. Dramatic, emotional and erratic behavior in paranoid PD
   E. Pervasive and maladaptive behavior

6. True about personality disorder: *(PGI June 2008)*
   A. Onset in early childhood and adolescence
   B. Matures around adulthood
   C. Suspiciousness is seen in paranoid personality disorder
   D. Excessive preoccupation with fantasy is seen in schizoid personality disorder

7. Odd beliefs, oddities of speech, fantasies mannerism, odd clothing with magical thinking is seen in which type of personality disorder: *(NEET 2016, NIMHANS 2013, DNB 2003)*
   A. Schizoid
   B. Paranoid
   C. Schizotypal
   D. Borderline

8. Shy, self oriented and relationship problems are seen in which personality disorder: *(AIIMS May, 2018)*
   A. Schizoid PD
   B. Paranoid PD
   C. Emotionally unstable PD
   D. Antisocial PD

9. Characteristic feature of schizoid personality disorder is: *(AIIMS 1999)*
   A. Conversion reaction
   B. Not concerned with disease
   C. Check details of all things
   D. Emotional coldness

10. Which personality disorder can be considered a part of autistic spectrum disorders? *(DNB NEET 2014-15)*
    A. Schizoid
    B. Schizotypal
    C. Borderline
    D. All of the above

11. Markedly inappropriate sensitivity, self-importance and suspiciousness are clinical features of: *(DNB NEET 2014-15, DNB 2001, TN 1999, AMU 2002)*
    A. Antisocial PD
    B. Histrionic PD
    C. Schizoid PD
    D. Paranoid PD

12. Antisocial personality is associated with: *(PGI 1999)*
    A. Drug abuse
    B. Paranoid schizophrenia
    C. Obsessive compulsive disorder
    D. None

13. Which of the following is not seen in a case of borderline personality disorder? *(JIPMER Nov, 2018)*
    A. Identity crisis
    B. Dissociative events
    C. Risk taking behavior
    D. Strong interpersonal relationships

14. Antisocial personality disorder, which of the following statements are correct: *(PGI May, 2018)*
    A. Disrupted self image or internal environment
    B. Lack of concern for feelings of others
    C. Inability to feel guilt
    D. Delusion of Grandiosity
    E. Intense but unstable relationships

15. A 16-year-old girl was brought to psychiatric emergency after she slashed her wrist in an attempt to commit suicide. On enquiry her father revealed that she had made several such attempts of wrist slashing in past, mostly in response to trivial fights in her house. Further she has marked fluctuations in her mood with a pervasive pattern of unstable interpersonal relationships. The most probable diagnosis is: *(AIIMS Nov 2002)*
    A. Borderline personality disorder
    B. Major depression
    C. Histrionic personality disorder
    D. Adjustment disorder

16. Patients who are grandiose and require admiration from others, have which type of personality? *(DNB NEET 2014-15)*
    A. Narcissistic
    B. Histrionic
    C. Borderline
    D. Antisocial

17. A young lady was admitted with h/o taking over dose of diazepam after broken affair. She has history of slitting her wrist previously. Most likely diagnosis is: *(AIIMS 2000)*
    A. Narcissistic PD
    B. Dependent PD
    C. Borderline PD
    D. Histrionic PD

18. A person has the habit of inflicting repeated injuries to self, what is the type of personality?
    (NEET 2016, PGI June 2004)
    A. Borderline
    B. Schizoid
    C. Histrionic
    D. Narcissistic
    E. Depressive

Controversial Question

19. Egocentric and magical thinking, excessive emotionality and attention seeking pattern is associated with which type of personality? *(NIMHANS 2015)*
    A. Schizoid
    B. Schizotypal
    C. Avoidant
    D. Narcissistic

20. Pervasive pattern of instability of interpersonal relationships, self-image and affect, with marked impulsivity that begins at early adulthood and present in varieties of context is characteristics of: *(Bihar 2006)*
    A. Bipolar disorder
    B. Schizoaffective disorder
    C. Borderline personality disorder
    D. Schizotypal personality disorder

21. A lady has changed multiple boyfriends in last 6 months, she keeps breaking her relationships, and she also has attempted suicide many times. Most likely diagnosis is:
    (MP 2006)
    A. Borderline personality disorder
    B. Post-traumatic stress
    C. Acute depression
    D. Acute panic attack

22. Which of the following therapy is used in treatment of Borderline Personality Disorder? *(NEET 2016)*
    A. Modelling
    B. Cognitive behavioral therapy
    C. Dialectical behavior therapy
    D. Exposure and response prevention

23. A person with shy, anxious and avoidant personality comes under which cluster? *(AIIMS May 2015)*
    A. Cluster A
    B. Cluster B
    C. Cluster C
    D. Cluster D

24. Obsessive personality disorder is also called:
    (DNB NEET 2014-15)
    A. Anankastic personality disorder
    B. Dissocial personality disorder
    C. Eccentric personality disorder
    D. Histrionic personality disorder

25. True about treatment of personality disorder:
    (PGI May 2010)
    A. Antipsychotics are used
    B. SSRIs' are used
    C. Behavior therapy is used
    D. No need for treatment

26. False regarding Type A personality:
    A. Hostile *(NEET 2016, AIIMS Nov 2007)*
    B. Time pressure
    C. Competitiveness
    D. Mood fluctuations

27. A person is very impatient, competitive and works like a perfectionist. He/she can be best described as:
    (DNB 2017)
    A. Type A personality
    B. Type B personality
    C. Type C personality
    D. Type D personality

28. Individual with Type D personality are recently found to be at risk of developing: *(AIIMS Nov 2011)*
    A. Coronary artery disease
    B. Depression
    C. Schizophrenia
    D. Mania

29. Which of the following personalities have high risk of development of Coronary artery disease?
    (PGI Nov 2016)
    A. Type A
    B. Type B
    C. Type C
    D. Type D

30. Which of the following is false: *(NIMHANS 2019)*
    A. Cluster B: Antisocial personality disorder
    B. Cluster C: Borderline personality disorder
    C. Cluster C: Obsessive compulsive personality disorder
    D. Cluster B: Histrionic personality disorder

Impulse Control Disorder

31. Kleptomania is: *(PGI May 2011, 2007)*
    A. Delusional disorder
    B. Obsession
    C. Impulse disorder
    D. Compulsion seclusion
    E. Hallucination

32. One of the following is not a compulsive and habit forming disorder: *(KA 1995)*
    A. Kleptomania
    B. Pyromania
    C. Nymphomania
    D. Pathological gambling

Answers With Explanations

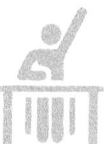

1. D. Sensation seeking is apart of "openness to experience". Problem solving is not a personality trait.
2. A, B, C.
   Personality disorders have onset in early childhood and adolescence and maturing occur in adulthood by 30-40 years of age. People with personality disorders tend to have conflicts with the societal norms (e.g. patients with antisocial personality disorders tend to break societal rules and regulations).
3. B. Narcissistic PD.
4. B. Personality disorder.
5. A, B, E.
   Personality disorders are "ego syntonic" and not "ego dystonic". Option D is description of histrionic personality disorder.
6. A, B, C, D.
   See text for explanation.
7. C. Odd behavior including odd speech, mannerisms and magical thinking is seen in schizotypal personality disorder.
8. A. Schizoid Personality Disorder.
9. D. *See* text for explanation.
10. A. The characteristic feature of autistic spectrum disorder (ASD) is impairment in social interaction and communication. These features are also seen in schizoid personality disorder. There can be significant difficulty differentiating between schizoid PD and milder forms of ASD. It must be remembered that patients with ASD have more severe social impairment and also have stereotypical behaviors and interests.
11. D. *See* text for explanation.
12. A. Antisocial PD is frequently associated with substance use disorders.
13. D. Patients with borderline personality do not have strong, stable interpersonal relationship. When under extreme stress, they may have dissociative episodes.
14. B, C. People with antisocial PD characteristically disregards rights of others, have lack of concern for others and are unable to feel guilt.
15. A. This patient has history suggestive of self-harming behavior with mood fluctuations and pervasive unstable pattern of interpersonal relationships, all of which are features of borderline PD.
16. A. Narcissistic.
17. C. The repetitive episodes of self-harming behavior after stressors is suggestive of borderline personality disorder.
18. A. Borderline.
19. D. Narcissistic PD. This question best describes Histrionic PD, which is not given in the option. Hence, Narcissistic PD would be the best option as question describes egocentricity. Attention seeking pattern totally goes against schizoid, schizotypal and anxious PD as all three avoid social activities.
20. C. Borderline personality disorder.
21. A. Borderline personality disorder.
22. C. Dialectical behavior therapy is most effective in treatment of Borderline PD.
23. C. Cluster C.
24. A. Anankastic personality disorder.
25. A, B, C.
    The mainstay of treatment in personality disorders is psychotherapy. Medications used include SSRIs, antipsychotics and mood stabilizers.
26. D. Mood fluctuations.
27. A. Type A Personality.
28. A. Coronary artery disease.
29. A. and D.
30. B.

Impulse Control Disorder

31. C. Kleptomania is an impulse control disorder in which the patient has recurrent irresistible desire to steal objects, which he/she does not need for personal use or for monetary value.
32. C. Nymphomania is the condition of excessive sexual desire in females. It is not an impulse control disorder. According to ICD-11 and DSM-5, even pathological gambling is no longer an impulse control disorder, it has been classified as an addictive disorder.

8 Eating Disorders

ANOREXIA NERVOSA

Anorexia nervosa is most commonly seen in **adolescent females**. Initially, it was reported to be more common in upper class, however recent data doesn't support that fact. It must be noted that anorexia nervosa is a misnomer since the **appetite of these patients** is **usually normal**^{Q} and hence there is no symptom of anorexia in anorexia nervosa.

It is characterized by the following signs and symptoms:
1. Disturbance of body image (patient perceives that she is fat despite being quite thin in reality).
2. Excessive fear of fatness and excessive emphasis on thinness.
3. Restriction of energy intake resulting in a **significantly less weight**^{Q} than normal (According to ICD-11, the BMI should be less than 18.5 kg/m^2 to make the diagnosis in adults & BMI-for-age should be under fifth percentile in children and adolescents)
4. Medical symptoms secondary to starvation such as **amenorrhea**^{Q}, lanugo (appearance of neonatal hairs), hypothermia, dependent edema and bradycardia. The adolescent patients often have **poor sexual development**^{Q} whereas the adult patients usually report **low**^{Q} **interest** in sexual activities. Patients often exhibit **peculiar behavior**^{Q} about food such as hiding food in the house, trying to dispose food in napkins, cutting food into very small pieces and rearranging the food repeatedly around the plate. These patients are preoccupied with the thoughts about food and may spend a large amount of time collecting recipes or cooking food for others.

Patients are usually **secretive and deny any symptoms**^{Q} and refuse the treatment.

Subtypes

Anorexia nervosa has the following two subtypes:
1. *Restricting type*: This type is seen in around 50% of patients and is characterized by highly restricted food intake.
2. *Binge eating/purging subtype*: It is seen in 25-50% of patients. In this type, patient alternates attempts at rigorous dieting with intermittent binging and purging episodes. The binging involves intake of a large amount of food in a short duration with an associated feeling of lack of self-control during binge episode. The purging is a compensatory mechanism wherein patient tries to compensate for excess calories by self-induced vomiting, laxative use, diuretic use or emetic use. The repeated vomiting episodes may cause **dental caries**, **parotitis**, and hypokalemic alkalosis.

Treatment

The treatment may include hospitalization to restore patients nutritional status and manage complications like dehydration and electrolyte imbalances.

The **hospitalisation**^{Q} is advised if weight for height is **less than 20%** of expected. Long-term psychiatric hospitalisation is recommended if, weight for height is less than 30% of expected.

The treatment focuses on a combination of behavioral management (praise for healthy eating habits, restriction of self-induce vomiting), individual psychotherapy and family education.

 DSM-5 & ICD-11 Update

In DSM-4 & ICD-10 amenorrhea was a necessary symptom for diagnosis of anorexia nervosa in females, however in DSM-5 & ICD-11 this criterion has been removed and anorexia nervosa can be diagnosed in the absence of amenorrhea now.

Medications such as cyproheptadine, tricyclic antidepressants (TCAs) and selective serotonin reuptake inhibitors (SSRIs) have been tried with varied success.

BULIMIA NERVOSA

Bulimia nervosa is characterized by **episodes of binge eating** combined with **inappropriate ways of preventing weight gain**. Bulimia nervosa is more common than anorexia nervosa, is usually seen in **females**^{Q}, and the age of onset is mostly **late adolescence**^Q. The following are the clinical features:

1. Episodes of binge eating in which large amount of food is usually consumed in a small duration with an associated feeling of lack of self-control during binge episode.
2. Compensatory behavior after binge eating to prevent weight gain. These measures usually include purging behaviors like self-induced vomiting, laxatives or diuretics abuse, use of emetics and in few patients excessive exercising (hypergymnasia) and dieting.
3. Like patients of anorexia nervosa, the patients with bulimia nervosa too have a morbid fear of gaining weight and give excessive emphasis to thinness.
4. Weight is usually **normal**^Q, and is an important differentiating factor between bulimia nervosa and anorexia nervosa.

The patients with bulimia nervosa usually tend to have features secondary to purging such as **enamel erosion**^Q and **dental caries**^Q, salivary gland inflammations, **callus on knuckles**^Q (as knuckles get injured against teeth during episodes of self-induced vomiting). The patient may develop hypokalemia and hypochloremic alkalosis and rarely gastric and esophageal tear during forceful vomiting.

Patients have **normal sexual functioning**^Q and are usually not secretive about their symptoms as patients with anorexia nervosa.

Treatment

It is usually outpatient and involves psychotherapeutic techniques like cognitive behavioral therapy (first line) and dynamic psychotherapy. The medications mostly used are antidepressants like selective serotonin reuptake inhibitors.

Binge Eating Disorder

It is the **most common** eating disorder. It is characterised by episodes of binge eating, however, unlike bulimia nervosa, there are no compensatory behaviours. Binge eating disorder is associated with overweight and obesity. Treatment is similar to bulimia nervosa.

Avoidant Restrictive Food Intake Disorder

It is a new diagnosis that has been included in both ICD-11 and DSM-5. It is characterised by the following:

1. Insufficient intake of quantity or variety of food, that results in weight loss (or inability to gain weight) and nutritional deficiencies. The patient may report lack of interest in eating or may avoid food due to sensory characteristics (e.g not liking the smell or taste of food).
2. There are no disturbance of body image (This characteristic helps in differentiating from anorexia nervosa, restrictive type).

Multiple Choice Questions

1. **Which of the following is not a common feature of anorexia nervosa?** *(DNB 2007, AI 2006)*
   A. Binge eating
   B. Amenorrhea
   C. Self-perception of being fat
   D. Under weight

2. **Which of the following eating disorder is more common?** *(NEET 2016)*
   A. Anorexia nervosa
   B. Bulimia nervosa
   C. Same prevalence
   D. Last option not available

3. **Anorexia nervosa can be differentiated from bulimia by:** *(AIIMS Nov 2008)*
   A. Intense fear of weight gain
   B. Disturbance of body image
   C. Adolescent age
   D. Peculiar patterns of food handling

4. **Which of the following is not true about bulimia nervosa?** *(UPSC 2009)*
   A. Recurrent bouts of binge eating
   B. Lack of self-control over eating during binge
   C. Self-induced vomiting or dieting after binge
   D. Weight gain

5. **With regard to anorexia nervosa all of the following are true *except*:** *(DNB NEET 2014-15, DNB 03, Kerala 2K)*
   A. Phobic avoidance of normal weight
   B. Over perception of body image
   C. Self-induced vomiting
   D. Menorrhagia
   E. Excessive exercise

6. **Not true about anorexia nervosa:** *(NIMHANS 2015)*
   A. Loss of 10% of body weight
   B. Amenorrhea
   C. Over consciousness about body structure
   D. Loss of weight according to patient

7. **A young lady presents with h/o repeated episodes of over eating (binge) followed by purging using laxatives, she is probably suffering from:** *(AI 2002, UP 2004, AIIMS 10, 07, DNB 2009)*
   A. Bulimia nervosa
   B. Schizophrenia
   C. Anorexia nervosa
   D. Benign eating disorder

8. **Which of the following is not true about bulimia nervosa?** *(UPSC-1 08)*
   A. Invariable weight loss with endocrine disorder
   B. Occurrence of both binge eating and inappropriate compensatory behaviors at least twice weekly on an average for 3 months
   C. Recurrent episodes of binge eating
   D. Recurrent self-induced vomiting

Controversial Question

9. **False regarding anorexia nervosa:** *(DNB 2008, AI 2006)*
   A. Evident psychosis
   B. Vigor exceeding physical well-being
   C. Weight loss
   D. Decreased appetite

10. **False regarding anorexia nervosa:** *(DNB NEET 2014-15)*
    A. Psychiatric symptoms such as depression may be associated
    B. Excessive exercising can be a feature
    C. Weight loss is a feature
    D. Decreased appetite is a feature

11. **Following are true about bulimia nervosa *except*:** *(DNB NEET 2014-15)*
    A. Uncontrolled eating episodes
    B. Overweight individuals
    C. Depressive symptoms are present
    D. Patients are sexually active

12. **Not true about bulimia nervosa is:** *(DNB NEET 2014-15)*
    A. Onset is in late adolescence
    B. Dental caries/tooth decay is a finding
    C. Amenorrhea is a common finding
    D. Normal weight is usually seen

13. **Which of the following disorders is more common in females?** *(NIMHANS 2017)*
    A. Eating disorders   B. ADHD
    C. Autism   D. Conduct disorder

14. **Not true about bulimia nervosa:** *(NIMHANS 2017)*
    A. Seen in 20 to 40 yrs age group
    B. More common in males
    C. Characterised by episodes of binge eating followed by compensatory behaviours
    D. Serotonin has been implicated in pathophysiology

15. **An 18-year-old girl was brought to the psychiatrist with the complaints of excessive exercising and dieting. Which of the following will help in differentiation between anorexia nervosa and bulimia nervosa?** *(NIMHANS 2019)*
    A. Significantly lesser weight for height
    B. Binge eating
    C. Fear of becoming fat
    D. Purging epsiodes

16. **Indoor management of anorexia nervosa is done on priority in patients with:** *(FMGE 2017)*
    A. Binging episodes
    B. Weight for height less than 75% of normal
    C. Amenorrhea
    D. Depression

Answers With Explanations

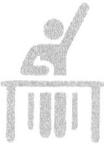

1. A. All the four options are features of anorexia nervosa. However, if one has to chose, the best answer would be binge eating. Though binge eating is seen in almost 50% of patients with anorexia nervosa, however it's not a core symptom of anorexia nervosa.
2. B. According to DSM-5, 12 month prevalence of bulimia nervosa is higher than anorexia nervosa.
3. D. Unlike patients with bulimia, patients with anorexia remain preoccupied with food and show peculiar behavior like hiding food in the house, trying to dispose food in napkins, cutting food into very small pieces and rearranging the food repeatedly around the plate.
4. D. The patients with bulimia nervosa usually have normal weight.
5. D. Amenorrhea and not menorrhagia is the menstrual disturbance seen in anorexia.
6. D. Patients are secretive about their symptoms and deny that they have any problem.
7. A. Bulimia nervosa.
8. A. Weight loss and endocrine abnormality are seen in anorexia not bulimia nervosa.
9. A. There are no psychotic symptoms in anorexia nervosa. Option D is also false, however if one has to chose, option A would be the better answer as Anorexia nervosa and psychotic disorders are entirely different disorders.
10. D. The appetite of patients with anorexia is normal and as such there is no anorexia in anorexia nervosa.
11. B. Overweight individuals.
12. C. Presence of amenorrhea is a differentiating feature between anorexia and bulimia. It is seen only in patients with anorexia.
13. A. Eating disorders.
14. B. Bulimia nervosa is much more common in females than males.
15. A. Binge eating, purging and fear of becoming fat are features of both. Patients with anorexia nervosa have significantly lesser weight for height, weight in bulimia nervosa is usually normal.
16. B. Weight for height less than 80% of expected is an indication for admission.

9 CHAPTER

Sleep Disorders

ELECTROENCEPHALOGRAM

It is the recording of electrical activity of the brain. It is recorded by placing electrodes on the scalp and recording the potential difference between various electrodes. A normal EEG has following types of rhythm.

Stages of Sleep

Sleep can be divided into two stages:
A. **Nonrapid eye movement sleep (NREM) or slow wave sleep** and
B. **Rapid eye movement (REM) sleep or paradoxical sleep.**

A. *Nonrapid eye movement sleep*: It is further divided into following four stages:
- *Stage 1, NREM*: It is the first stage and the sleep is light (person can be easily aroused). The EEG shows, **loss of alpha waves** (which predominate when person has eyes closed but is still awake) and **predominance of theta waves**.
- *Stage 2, NREM*: It is the stage with **maximum duration**^{Q}. It is characterized by two typical findings on electroencephalogram:
   a. *Sleep spindles*^{Q}: These are bursts of regular waves (frequency of 13–15 Hz, 50 microvolt) and
   b. *K-complexes*^{Q}: These are high voltage spikes which are seen intermittently.
- *Stage 3, NREM*: The sleep deepens and there is appearance of delta waves.
- *Stage 4, NREM*: This is deep sleep and is characterized by predominance of delta waves on EEG.

During the NREM sleep, there is pulsatile release of **gonadotropins** and **growth hormones**. Further, the blood pressure, heart rate and respiratory rate also decreases.

B. *Rapid eye movement sleep*: It follows the NREM sleep. It is characterized by the following:
- The EEG shows increased activity similar to awake state (**beta activity**) along with return of **alpha activity.**
- Presence of **rapid eye movements.**
- There is generalized **loss of muscle tone**.

Table 1: EEG rhythms.				
EEG rhythm	**Frequency (Hz)**	**Amplitude (microvolt)**	**Salient points**	**Region**
Alpha (α)	8–12	50–100	Seen when individual is awake, at rest, eyes closed and mind wandering	Present maximally in occipital and parieto-occipital area
Beta (β)	14–30	5–10	Normal awake pattern, when attention is focussed beta waves appear	Predominantly in frontal area
Theta (θ)	4–7	10	Transition from wakefulness to sleep, early sleep	Parietal region and temporal region (hippocampus)
Delta (δ)	1–4	20–200	Deep sleep	

- **Increased rate**^{Q} of metabolism in brain
- **Penile erection**^{Q}, autonomic hyperactivity (increase in pulse rate, respiratory rate and blood pressure)
- **Dreams**^{Q}, which can be recalled are seen during REM sleep.

Ponto-geniculo-occipital spikes^Q (large phasic potentials that originate from cholinergic neurons in pons and pass rapidly to lateral geniculate body and then to occipital cortex) are a characteristic feature.

REM sleep is called **paradoxical sleep**^{Q} because though the EEG is quite similar to awake state, it is quite difficult to awaken the patient.

In an 8-hour sleep, maximum time (around 6 to 6.5 hours) is spent in NREM sleep and the rest (around 1.5 hours) in REM sleep. Most of the stage 4, NREM occurs in the first one-third of the night whereas most of REM sleep occurs in the last one-third of the night. The REM sleep occurs regularly after every 90–100 minutes with a total of around 4 to 5 REM sleeps in the entire night.

SLEEP DISORDERS

The various sleep disorders can be divided into two categories:
1. Dyssomnias
2. Parasomnias

Dyssomnias

These disorders are characterized by abnormality in the duration or quality of sleep. They include:

A. **Insomnia:** Primary Insomnia is diagnosed when no cause can be found for decreased sleep and may present with difficulty in initiation of sleep, difficulty in maintenance of sleep (frequent awakening during night or early morning awakening) or non-restorative sleep (not feeling refreshed in the morning due to poor quality of sleep). The management usually involves use of benzodiazepines, zolpidem and other hypnotics.

Few other disorders which can present with insomnia include:

- **Periodic limb movement disorder:** It is characterized by sudden contraction of muscle groups (usually leg) while sleeping. This results in partial or complete awakening, repeatedly in the night. The patient is usually not aware of these sudden contractions, however the bed partner frequently gets disturbed. The patient may report non-restorative sleep and day time sleepiness. The treatment usually involves benzodiazepines.
- *Restless leg syndrome (Ekbom syndrome):* It is characterized by uncomfortable sensation in legs (such as insect crawling on the skin) which get relieved by **moving** the leg or **walking around**. This can cause difficulty in initiation of sleep as patient keeps on moving the leg. The only approved drug for treatment is **ropinirole**[Q] (a dopamine agonist).

B. **Hypersomnia:** Primary hypersomnia is diagnosed when no cause can be found for excessive sleepiness which can present with either prolonged sleep episodes or excessive day time sleep episodes.

Few other disorders which can present with hypersomnia include:

- *Narcolepsy:* This disorder is characterized by the following symptoms:

  a. **Sleep attacks:** The patient has irresistible urge for sleep which can occur at any time during the day.
  b. **Cataplexy**[Q]: It is sudden loss of muscle tone, due to which patient can even have a fall.
  c. **Hypnagogic hallucinations**[Q]: These are the hallucinations, which occur while going to sleep. Patient may also have **hypnopompic hallucinations**[Q] (hallucinations while getting up from sleep).
  d. **Sleep paralysis:** It usually occurs when the patient gets up in the morning. Though he has woken up, he is not able to move his body.

  The hallmark of narcolepsy is reduced latency of REM sleep[Q]. Normally, it takes around 90 minutes to reach REM sleep (after crossing all the stages of NREM sleep) however in patients with narcolepsy, patient reaches REM sleep much earlier. Narcolepsy is caused by deficiency of **hypocretin**[Q], a neurotransmitter which promotes appetite and alertness. Hypocretin neurons project from **hypothalamus** to other parts of brain.

  There is a strong association with **human leucocyte antigens class II**[Q] (HLA-DR2 and HLA-DQB1*0602). It has been hypothesized that narcolepsy in an immune mediated disorder, and is caused by destruction of hypothalamic neurons that secret hypocretin.

  The management includes a regimen of forced naps at regular time. The medications used are **modafinil** and other stimulants like amphetamines.

- *Kleine-Levin syndrome:* This is a rare disorder which is characterized by episodes of **hypersomnia**[Q], hyperphagia and **hypersexuality**[Q] (increased sexual activity). In between the episodes patient is essentially asymptomatic.

Parasomnias

These disorders are characterized by dysfunctional events associated with the sleep. These include:

A. **Stage 4, NREM sleep disorders:** These disorders occur during stage 4, NREM (also stage 3, NREM). Since most of the stage 4, NREM is present in first third of the sleep, these disorders are also seen in the same period. Also, the patient is not able to recall the events in the morning. These disorders are usually seen in children[Q] and include:

- ***Night terror or sleep terror (pavor nocturnus^Q)***: The patient suddenly gets up screaming and has symptoms of intense anxiety such as tachycardia and sweating. The patient is not able to recall any dream or reasons for feeling scared.
- ***Sleep walking (somnambulism^Q)***: The patients may carry out a range of activities for which he doesn't have any memory later on. It may include leaving the bed and walking about and also activities like dressing, moving around or even driving. The person who is having sleep walking is **difficult to awake^Q**, and if awakened, appears confused.
- ***Sleep related enuresis***: The enuresis which is defined as voiding of urine at inappropriate places, is nocturnal in around 80% of cases. The most common cause of bed wetting are psychosocial such as sibling rivalry. The treatment of choice is **bed alarms^Q**, which start ringing, as soon as child passes urine. The medications which can be used include tricyclic antidepressants such as **imipramine^Q**, although their use is associated with severe side effects. Intranasal **desmopressin^Q** is a better alternative.
- ***Bruxism (teeth grinding^Q)***: The patient grinds his teeth making loud sounds and there may be damage to the enamel of teeth.
- ***Sleep talking (somniloquy)***: Patient talks during stages 3 and 4, NREM and is unable to recall the same in the morning.

In most cases these disorders do not require any treatment and the parents must be reassured. In some cases, **benzodiazepines^Q** are prescribed. As benzodiazepines decrease the duration of stage 4, NREM, they also decrease these episodes.

B. ***Other sleep disorders***:
- ***Nightmare***: It occurs during REM sleep, wherein patient has a bad dream and gets up scared and has behavioral signs of anxiety such as tachycardia and hypertension. In contrast to night terror, in nightmare, the patient is able to recall the dream.

Multiple Choice Questions

1. **Maximum duration of time spent is in which of the following NREM stage?** *(NEET/DNB)*
   A. I
   B. II
   C. III
   D. IV

2. **A middle-aged man complains of lack of sleep during the night time. The duration of the time he is truly asleep or awake can be ascertained by which of the following?** *(AIIMS Nov 2012)*
   A. Barograph
   B. Kymograph
   C. Actigraphy
   D. Plethysmography

3. **Not a feature of paradoxical sleep is:** *(PGI 1999)*
   A. Decreased muscle tone
   B. Rapid eye movements
   C. Brain shows increased metabolism
   D. EEG shows decreased activity

4. **Slow wave in hippocampal area is:** *(MP 2000)*
   A. Delta
   B. Theta
   C. Beta
   D. Alpha

5. **Alpha-rhythm is seen in:** *(PGI 1997)*
   A. Sleep with eyes closed with mind wandering
   B. Mental activity
   C. Awake with eyes open
   D. REM sleep

6. **Pontogeniculo-occipital spike is characteristic of which of the following sleep stage?** *(DNB NEET 2014-15)*
   A. Stage 1 NREM
   B. Stage 2 NREM
   C. Stage 3 NREM
   D. REM

7. **The EEG recorded shown below is normally recordable during which stage of sleep?** *(AI 2003)*

   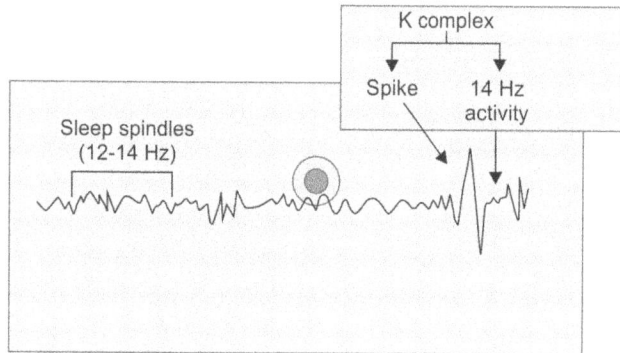

   A. Stage I
   B. Stage II
   C. Stage III
   D. Stage IV

8. **What are the EEG waves recorded for parieto-occipital region with subject awake and eyes closed?** *(Kerala 1997)*
   A. Alpha waves
   B. Beta waves
   C. Delta waves
   D. Theta waves

9. **Which one of the following phenomenon is closely associated with slow wave sleep?** *(AIIMS Nov 2004)*
   A. Dreaming
   B. Sleep walking
   C. Atonia
   D. Irregular heart rate

10. **Not true about nocturnal penile tumescence is:**
    A. Totals about 100 min/night *(AIIMS 1995)*
    B. Normal phenomenon
    C. Occurs in NREM sleep
    D. Can be used to distinguish between psychological or organic impotence

11. **Which of the following conditions are seen during NREM sleep?** *(DNB NEET 2014-15)*
    A. Teeth grinding
    B. Nightmares
    C. Narcolepsy
    D. Sleep paralysis

12. **Somnambulism is mostly seen in which age group?** *(NEET 2016)*
    A. Children
    B. Adolescents
    C. Adults
    D. All age group

13. **Pavor nocturnus is:** *(NEET 2016, JIPMER 2016)*
    A. Sleep terror
    B. Sleep apnea
    C. Sleep bruxism
    D. Somnambulism

14. **Antidepressant drug used in nocturnal enuresis is:** *(AI 2011)*
    A. Imipramine
    B. Fluoxetine
    C. Trazodone
    D. Sertraline

15. **Drug of choice for night terrors:** *(PGI 1998)*
    A. Meprobamate
    B. Tricyclic antidepressant
    C. Clonazepam
    D. Diazepam

16. **Sleep paralysis is seen in:** *(NEET 2016)*
    A. NREM I
    B. NREM II
    C. NREM III and IV
    D. REM

17. **Feature of narcolepsy include(s) all except:** *(PGI May 2013)*
    A. Disorder of REM sleep regulation
    B. Disorder of NREM sleep regulation
    C. Hypnagogic hallucination
    D. Hypnopompic hallucinations
    E. Cataplexy

18. **Not true about narcolepsy:** *(PGI Dec 2006)*
    A. Sudden sleep
    B. Long duration (>3 hours) of sleep
    C. Cataplexy
    D. Presents in IInd decade

19. **A 30-year-old female has history of sudden falls while standing, gets naps of sleep while at work and also has episodes of hallucinations while going to sleep. What is the most likely diagnosis?** *(NIMHANS 2017)*

A. Narcolepsy
B. Obstructive sleep apnea
C. Restless leg syndrome
D. Kleine-Levin syndrome

20. **All of the followings are true about narcolepsy except:**
    (DNB 2018)
    A. Strong association with HLA class II
    B. Sudden loss of voluntary muscle tone
    C. NREM abnormality
    D. Irresistible desire to sleep

21. **Modafinil is approved by FDA for treatment of all except:**
    (DNB 2006, AI 2009)
    A. Obstructive sleep apnea syndrome (OSAS)
    B. Shift work syndrome (SWS)
    C. Narcolepsy
    D. Lethargy in depression

22. **Following is true about ropinirole:** *(DNB NEET 2014-15)*
    A. Selective D2/3 receptor agonist
    B. It is used in restless leg syndrome
    C. Both A and B
    D. None of the above

23. **Regarding, Kleine-Levin syndrome which of the following is not true?** *(DNB NEET 2014-15)*
    A. Hypersomnia
    B. Hyposexuality
    C. Spontaneous resolution
    D. Also called sleeping beauty syndrome

24. **Treatment of Insomnia includes all except?**
    (NIMHANS 2018)
    A. Recollecting and reviewing the events of the day just before sleep
    B. Warm water bath just before going to bed
    C. Going to bed and waking up at the same time
    D. Avoiding caffeine before sleep

25. **Which is the most common symptom of Narcolepsy?**
    A. Sleep paralysis *(NIMHANS 2018)*
    B. Hypnagogic hallucinations
    C. Cataplexy
    D. Sleep attacks

26. **Not seen in narcolepsy:** *(NIMHANS 2018)*
    A. Catalepsy
    B. Cataplexy
    C. Sleep paralysis
    D. Sleep attack

27. **All of the following are true about somnambulism except:**
    (NEET 2019)
    A. Also called as sleep walking
    B. Disorder of sleep arousal
    C. Patient remains conscious throughout the episode
    D. Patient can do low skill motor movements

Answers With Explanations

1. B. II
2. C. Actigraphy is the procedure which is used for studying the sleep patterns. It usually involves wearing a small sensor on the wrist, which detects the movements. However, the gold standard technique for studying sleep disorder is polysomnography.
3. D. In paradoxical sleep or REM sleep, the EEG shows increased activity, similar to awake state.
4. B. Theta
5. B, D.
   Alpha rhythm is seen when a person is awake with eyes closed and his mind is wandering (having mental activity) and not when a person is sleeping with eyes closed. Also, alpha rhythm is seen in REM sleep.
6. D. *See* text for explanation.
7. B. The sleep spindles and K complexes are seen in stage II, NREM.
8. A. Alpha waves
9. B. Somnambulism is usually seen in NREM III and IV (slow wave sleep).
10. C. Nocturnal penile erections are a feature of REM sleep.
11. A. Teeth grinding or bruxism is seen in NREM III and IV.
12. A. Somnambulism is mostly seen in children and is mostly prevalent in ages 4 to 8 years.
13. A. Sleep terror.
14. A. Remember it is not the drug of choice. Desmopressin is the drug of choice and bed alarms are the treatment of choice.
15. C, D.
    Benzodiazepines can be used in night terrors though usually no treatment is required.
16. D. Sleep paralysis most oftenly occurs while awakening in the morning. During the episode patient gets up and is awake but is not able to move at all. It occurs due to disruption of REM sleep. It can be seen in narcolepsy and isolated episodes in normal persons also.
17. B. Disorder of NREM sleep regulation.
18. B. The onset of narcolepsy is mostly in adolescence or young adulthood. There are sudden sleep attacks which last for 10–20 minutes (and not more than 3 hours) and cataplexy is a feature.
19. A. Narcolepsy
20. C. Narcolepsy is a disorder of REM sleep. Rest statements are correct.
21. D. Modafinil is FDA approved for narcolepsy, shift work sleep disorder and as an adjunct in obstructive sleep apnea.
22. C. Ropinirole is a dopamine agonist (D2, D3 receptors) and is approved for restless leg syndrome.
23. B. There is hypersexuality and not hyposexuality.
24. A. Recollecting and reviewing events may cause emotional arousal that would interfere with sleep.
    "Sleep hygiene" refers to changes in behaviors and lifestyle that help in improving quality of sleep. It includes:
    1. Going to bed and getting up at the same time, everyday.
    2. Avoiding heavy meals before bed time.
    3. Avoiding stimulants like caffeine and nicotine before bed time.
    4. Maintaining regular exercise schedule (exercising just before going to bed should be strictly avoided).
    5. Not thinking about problems of life immediately before bedtime.
    6. Establishing a relaxing bedtime routine such as taking warm shower or reading a book.
    7. Keeping the bedroom cool, dark and quiet.
25. D. Sleep attacks are the most common symptom of narcolepsy.
26. A. Catalepsy is a feature of catatonia
27. C. Somnambulism. Patient is not conscious, and is difficult to awake while sleep walking. Patients have been found to do semi purposeful activities like dressing etc, during episodes of somnambulism.

10 CHAPTER

Sexual Disorders

GENDER IDENTITY DISORDERS

Gender is the sense of being a male or a female. Mostly the gender corresponds to the anatomical sex (i.e. a man with male body organs, also psychologically considers himself as a male). However, there might be a mismatch resulting in gender identity disorder. The following are types of gender identity disorders:

A. *Gender identity disorder of childhood*: It usually manifests in preschool years. The child shows preoccupation with the dress and activities of the opposite sex (e.g. the male child insists on wearing skirts and frocks and may play exclusively with dolls and reject the cars and other toys which are usually preferred by boys). The child expresses the desire to be of the opposite sex and rejects behaviors, attire and attributes of his anatomical sex. Usually, there is no feeling of rejection of the anatomical structures. However, in a small minority it may be present (e.g. the male child may repeatedly assert that the penis and testicles are disgusting and will disappear in due course of time).

B. *Transsexualism*: In adolescents and adults, the symptoms are quite similar to gender identity disorder of childhood. The patients manifest a **desire to live**^{Q} and be treated as the other sex, usually accompanied by a **discomfort with one's anatomical sex**^{Q} and a **desire to change**^{Q} it with the help of a surgery or some other form of treatment. The patient frequently uses the phrases like "I am a man trapped in body of woman". The homosexual orientation is frequently present.

C. *Dual-role transvestism*: The patient wears the clothes of opposite sex, to enjoy the **temporary feeling**^{Q} of belonging to the other sex. Unlike transsexualism, there is **no desire to permanently change the sex**^{Q}. There is **no sexual arousal**^{Q} associated with cross-dressing. (Remember, in fetishistic transvestism, which is a type of paraphilia, the cross-dressing is associated with sexual arousal).

Treatment: In patients who insist for sex change, **sex reassignment surgery** can be done. In a person born anatomically male, removal of penis, scrotum and testes and construction of labia and vagina is done.

> DSM-5 Update: In DSM-5, the diagnosis of "gender dysphoria" is used in place of DSM-4 diagnosis of "gender identity disorder".

In a person born anatomically female, bilateral mastectomy, hysterectomy, removal of ovaries and construction of a neophallus (penis) is done. The hormonal treatment usually accompanies with it.

Disorders of Sexual Orientation

It must be remembered that homosexuality is not a psychiatric disorder (homosexuality is considered as a normal variant, if it is egosyntonic, i.e. the individual accepts his sexual orientation). However, egodystonic homosexuality (wherein the individual does not accept his sexual orientation and wants to change it) has been classified as a disorder.

Disorders of Sexual Response

Phases of Sexual Response Cycle

Normally, sexual response has been divided into four phases:

1. *Desire*: It is characterized by a desire to have sex (hypoactive sexual desire disorder is a disorder of this phase).
2. *Excitement (arousal)*: This phase is characterized by penile erection and vaginal lubrication. Other changes such as nipple erection, enlargement of size of testes and elevation of testes, engorgement and thickening of labia minora and clitoris, and physiological changes like increased heart rate, blood pressure and respiratory rate are also seen. There is an associated subjective sense of pleasure (erectile dysfunction is a disorder of this phase). Another phase called **Plateau phase** is at times described as a separate phase, and is characterized by intensified sexual tensions before orgasm. Excitement phase lasts for several minutes to several hours.
3. *Orgasm*: There is a peaking of sexual pleasure, followed by release of sexual tension and ejaculation of semen.

In females, orgasm is characterized by involuntary contraction of lower third of vagina and contractions from fundus downward to cervix (premature ejaculation and anorgasmia are disorders of this phase). Orgasm phase lasts for 3 to 15 seconds. It is the **shortest phase**[Q] of sexual response cycle.

4. *Resolution*: The body goes back to the resting state. This phase lasts for 10 to 15 minutes. If there is no orgasm, it may last from half to full day.

There are disorders specific to each phase of sexual cycle as described below:

1. *Sexual desire disorders*: It has been further subdivided into two categories: hypoactive sexual desire disorder, characterized by lack of desire for sexual activity and sexual aversion disorder, characterized by active aversion and avoidance of sexual activity. The only FDA-approved drug for treatment of hypoactive sexual desire disorder in females is **flibanserin**, which got approval in August 2015. Due to risk of severe hypotension, flibanserin should not be taken concomitantly with alcohol.

   > **DSM-5 Update:** In DSM-5, the diagnosis of sexual aversion disorder has been removed.

2. *Disorders of excitement (arousal) phase*:
   – *Male erectile disorder (erectile dysfunction)*: It is characterized by recurrent or persistent inability to attain or to maintain the erection required for satisfactory sexual intercourse. Erectile dysfunction is usually caused by psychological factors, such as anxiety and poor marital relation.

   The presence of **early morning erections** and erections during REM sleep (**nocturnal erections**[Q]) are suggestive of psychogenic erectile dysfunction.

   Investigation such as penile plethysmography and **nocturnal penile intumescence (NPT)**[Q] are used to record nocturnal erections.

   The physical causes include vascular and neurological disorders like arteriolosclerosis and autonomic neuropathy.

   Treatment: The medications with best evidence include **PDE-5 inhibitors**[Q] (phosphodiesterase-5 inhibitors like **sildenafil**, tadalafil and vardenafil, which facilitate blood flow into penis and enhance erection. The other medications which can be used include oral phentolamine (decreases sympathetic tone and relaxes smooth muscles of corpora cavernosa) and injectable and transurethral alprostadil. **Alprostadil**[Q] contains naturally occurring prostaglandin E and, hence has vasodilator action. It can be injected into corpora cavernosa or administered intraurethrally.

   Apart from medications, psychotherapy also plays an important role. The most successful is **dual-sex therapy**[Q] (or simply sex therapy) which was developed by Masters and Johnson. This therapy treats the **"couple"**[Q] and **not the individual**[Q]. The couple is taught ways to improve their communication. The couple is also taught exercises which increases the sensory awareness. These exercises are called sensate focus exercises. Initially, the couple is asked to touch, rub, kiss on each others body parts, excluding breasts and genitals (this stage is called nongenital sensate focus). In the next stage, the same activities are done on breasts and genitals (called genital sensate focus). The whole purpose is to make the couple aware that pleasure can be given and received by methods other than sexual intercourse. The sex therapy is effective not only for erectile dysfunction but other sexual disorders like premature ejaculation.

   Other techniques, such as behavioral therapy, hypnotherapy and psychoanalysis have also been used.
   – *Female sexual arousal disorder*: It is characterized by inability to achieve adequate vaginal lubrication required for sexual intercourse. The management involves use of lubricants during the intercourse.

3. *Disorders of orgasm phase*[Q]
   – *Premature ejaculation*: It is characterized by a pattern of persistent or recurrent ejaculation with minimal sexual stimulation before or immediately after the vaginal penetration.

   > In DSM-5, the criterion for premature ejaculation has been defined more clearly, and states that premature ejaculation is a pattern of ejaculation within approximately one minute following vaginal penetration.

   The cause of premature ejaculation is usually psychogenic.

   Treatment: Specific techniques have been described for the management of premature ejaculation. These include:

   a. *Squeeze technique*[Q]: When the man gets the feeling of impending ejaculation, the female partner (or the man himself) squeezes the coronal ridge of glans, which results in inhibition of ejaculation.
   b. *Stop-start technique (Semans technique)*: Here, when the man gets the feeling of impending ejaculation, the sex is stopped for some time and once excitement has decreased, it is restarted.

   Apart from these techniques, sex therapy (as described earlier) is also an effective method of treating premature ejaculation.

   SSRIs (selective serotonin reuptake inhibitors) are also frequently used as they can delay the ejaculation.

- *Female orgasmic disorder (anorgasmia)*: It is characterized by recurrent delay or absence of orgasm in females. It is a common sexual disorder in females and the treatment involves psychotherapy.
- *Male orgasmic disorder (retarded ejaculation)*: It is characterized by recurrent delay or absence of orgasm in males. It is less common than premature ejaculation and is treated with psychotherapy.

4. **Other disorders**:
   - *Dyspareunia*: It is recurrent or persistent genital pain in either men or women, before, during or after sexual intercourse.
   - *Vaginismus*: It is involuntary muscle constriction of outer third of vagina which makes penile insertion difficult. Vaginismus and dyspareunia frequently coexist.
   - *Nymphomania*[Q]: It is the term used to describe excessive sexual desire in females.

   > DSM-5 Update: Genitopelvic pain/ penetration disorder is a new diagnosis in DSM-5 and represents a merging of the DSM-4 categories of vaginismus and dyspareunia, which were highly comorbid and difficult to distinguish.

   - *Satyriasis*[Q]: It is the term used to describe excessive sexual desire in males.

Multiple Choice Questions

1. **Most accurate treatment of erectile dysfunction is:**
   A. Sildenafil   *(PGI 2002)*
   B. Master and Johnson technique
   C. β-blockers
   D. Papaverine

2. **Excessive sexual desire in males is known as:**
                                                    (AIIMS May 2008)
   A. Nymphomania   B. Satyriasis
   C. Tribadism   D. Sadism

3. **A homosexual person feels that "he is a woman trapped in a man's body" and has persistent discomfort with his sex. Most likely diagnosis is:** *(NEET 2016, PGI 2003)*
   A. Transsexualism   B. Transvestism
   C. Voyeurism   D. Paraphilias

4. **How to differentiate between psychological and organic erectile dysfunction?** *(NEET/DNB)*
   A. Nocturnal penile tumescence
   B. PIPE test
   C. Sildenafil-induced erection
   D. Squeeze technique

5. **Squeeze technique is used for:** *(NEET 2018, DNB 2017)*
   A. Impotence   B. Premature ejaculation
   C. Infertility   D. Priapism

6. **SSRIs are useful in treatment of:** *(NEET 2016)*
   A. Erectile dysfunction
   B. Premature ejaculation
   C. Retrograde ejaculation
   D. Infertility

7. **Which drug is used in intracavernous injection for erectile dysfunction?** *(NEET 2016)*
   A. Epoprostrenol   B. Alprostadil
   C. Sildenafil   D. Tadalafil

8. **A 30-year-old male presents to OPD with erectile dysfunction. Basic screening evaluation is unremarkable. The next step in evaluation/management should be:** *(AI 2008)*
   A. Oral sildenafil titrate trial   B. Cavernosometry
   C. Doppler study   D. Neurological testing

9. **A 20-year-old girl Neelu enjoys wearing male clothes. Wearing male clothes gives her a feeling of more confidence and after these episodes she is an absolutely normal girl. The likely diagnosis is:** *(AIIMS 1997)*
   A. Transsexualism   B. Fetishism
   C. Dual role transvestism   D. Fetishistic transvestism

10. **True about dual sex therapy is:** *(DNB June 2011)*
    A. Patient alone is not treated
    B. Uses sildenafil
    C. It treats sexual perversion
    D. It is used for people with dual gender identities

11. **Which is the shortest in sex cycle:** *(NEET 2016)*
    A. Excitement   B. Resolution
    C. Orgasm   D. Desire phase

12. **Premature ejaculation is a disorder of which of the stage of sexual response:** *(NEET 2019)*
    A. Excitement   B. Plateau
    C. Orgasm   D. Resolution

Answers With Explanations

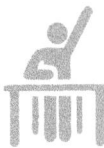

1. A, B.
   The pharmacological treatment with best evidence in erectile dysfunction is phosphodiesterase-5 inhibitors like sildenafil. The psychotherapeutic technique which is most commonly used is Master and Johnson technique.
2. B. Satyriasis is the condition of excessive sexual desire in males while the same in females is known as nymphomania.
3. A. As mentioned in the question, the person is uncomfortable with his sex and feels that he is imposed by a female body (i.e. he is of another sex). Both are characteristics of gender identity disorder. Most of the patients with gender identity disorder have homosexual orientation.
4. A. Presence of early morning erections and erections during REM sleep (nocturnal erections) are suggestive of psychogenic erectile dysfunction. As during sleep, there is no anxiety, hence, a patient with psychogenic erectile dysfunction is able to have erections. Whereas, a patient with organic erectile dysfunction (due to vascular or neurological causes) would not have erections even during sleep. Investigations, such as penile plethysmography and nocturnal penile intumescence (NPT) can be used to record nocturnal erections.
5. B. Squeeze technique and stop-start technique are used for treatment of premature ejaculation.
6. B. Premature ejaculation. See text for explanation.
7. B. Alprostadil. See text for explanation.
8. A. In a young patient with negative screening, the most likely cause of erectile dysfunction is psychogenic erectile dysfunction. He should be given a trial of oral sildenafil.
9. C. Here the person only enjoys wearing clothes of opposite sex and there is no discomfort with her own sex and there is no desire to be of other sex. Hence, it is a case of dual role transvestism.
10. A. In dual sex therapy, the couple is treated and not an individual.
11. C. Orgasm
12. C. Orgasm

11 CHAPTER

Child Psychiatry

ATTENTION DEFICIT HYPERACTIVITY DISORDER (ADHD) (HYPERKINETIC DISORDER)

The DSM-5 & ICD-11, both use the diagnosis of ADHD. The older name of ADHD was **minimal brain dysfunction**^{Q}. It is a common **neuropsychiatric** disorder of child-hood, which is more prevalent in **boys** in comparison to girls. The predominant symptoms and signs in the ADHD are as follows:

- *Inattention*: The child has **difficulty in giving close attention** to details, makes **frequent mistakes** in school work and other activities. The child is **distractible**^{Q} and frequently shifts from one activity to another as he loses interest in one task quickly.
- *Hyperactivity and Impulsivity*: The child is **hyperactive** and appears restless. Teacher frequently complains that child keeps on roaming in the class and is **excessively talkative** and **disturbs other students**^{Q}. The child is also **impulsive**^{Q} and often blurts out answer before question has been completed. He also has **difficulty in waiting for his turn** and often interrupts others or intrudes in others conversation.

Along with the core symptoms of inattention and hyperactivity/impulsivity, children with ADHD frequently show destructive and aggressive behavior and are irritable. Neurological examination may reveal **soft neurological signs**^{Q} (the neurological soft signs are fine abnormalities found during detailed neurological examination such as difficulty in copying age appropriate figures, difficulty in performing rapid alternating movements, difficulty in right left discrimination, etc.).

Depending on the predominant symptoms, three subtypes have been defined.
- Combined presentation
- Predominantly inattentive presentation
- Predominantly hyperactive/impulsive presentation.

Course

Around 50% of patients achieve remission before puberty and early adulthood. Others achieve only partial remission and are at risk of developing **substance use disorders**^{Q} (particularly alcoholism), **antisocial personality disorder** and **mood disorders**.

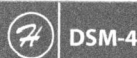
DSM-4

Required the presence of symptoms before age of 7 years, however according to DSM-5 the onset of symptoms should be before **12 yrs**^{Q} of age to make a diagnosis of ADHD.

Treatment

ADHD is a **serious medical illness**^{Q} and must be promptly treated. The pharmacological treatment is the mainstay of the treatment. The following medications are used:

- *Stimulant medications*: CNS stimulants are the first line drugs in the treatment of ADHD. **Methylphenidate**^{Q} is the drug of choice. **Dexmethylphenidate** (containing only the d-enantiomer) has also been used recently. Other stimulant medications used are dextroamphetamine, lisdexamfetamine and "**dextroamphetamine and amphetamine salt**" combinations. Modafinil has also been used with varied success.
- *Nonstimulant medications*: The nonstimulant medications are used, if stimulants are not effective or contraindicated. They include **atomoxetine** (norepinephrine reuptake inhibitor), **clonidine**, guanfacine, venlafaxine and bupropion.

Apart from medications, psychosocial interventions such as social skill training, psychoeducation for parents, behavioral therapy and cognitive behavioral therapy are also effective in the management.

PERVASIVE DEVELOPMENTAL DISORDERS (AUTISM SPECTRUM DISORDER)

These are group of neurodevelopmental or **neurobehavioral disorders**^{Q}, which are characterized by disturbance of social interaction, abnormalities of communication and restricted behaviors. The following are the subtypes of pervasive developmental disorders:

- *Autism (Childhood autism, autistic disorder)*: It is a neurodevelopmental disorder (neurobehavioral disorder) with a strong genetic basis. The onset is before the age of 3 years. Chromosome 7, 2, 4, 15 and 19 have been found to contribute to the disorder. **Fragile X syndrome**[Q], tuberous sclerosis, congenital rubella and phenylketonuria are associated with autism and are found with high frequency in children with autistic disorders. Around **30%**[Q] of children with autism have comorbid mental retardation. Out of these, around 30% have mild to moderate MR and 45-50% have severe to profound MR. The prevalence of perinatal insults like birth asphyxia has also been found to be higher in children with autism. Following are the symptoms:
  - *Impairment in social interaction*: The patients with autism have impaired reciprocal social skills. As infants they have **poor eye contact**[Q], **lack social smile**[Q] and anticipatory posture (the posture which the kid assumes when he wants to be picked up). They may have poor attachment to their parents and other important persons and may not acknowledge their presence (e.g. they won't come running to meet when the father returns to home after office). However, if the routine of these children is disturbed (e.g. if someone rearranges the furniture in their room), they may show **excessive reaction**[Q]. When they grow up, they may have difficulty in making friends and getting into a romantic relationship.
  - *Impairment of communication and language*: These children usually have **significant delay in language milestones**[Q], whereas the motor milestones are usually normally achieved. The patients also have development of abnormal language such as difficulty in making sentences properly (articulation difficulties) and pronoun reversals (using "me" instead of "you").
  - *Restricted, repetitive and stereotyped behavior*: The activities and play of these children tend to be **repetitive**[Q] and boring. They may show stereotyped behaviors like **hand wringing**[Q], spinning and **banging**. These children are quite resistant to changes and may become extremely upset if their routines are disturbed (e.g. bathing routine is changed or furnitures are rearranged in the room). These restrictive behaviors usually result from a lack of **imagination**[Q] and creativity.

  Apart from these three characteristic features, the patients with autism also have abnormal responses to stimuli. They may have a higher threshold for pain and may show intense interest in some sounds (like that of a ticking watch) and may totally ignore other sounds. They may also have self destructive behaviors like head banging, biting, scratching, etc. *Associated physical abnormalities*: Children with autism have many minor physical anomalies such as ear malformations. Also they have a high incidence of **abnormal dermatoglyphics (fingerprints)**[Q]. A greater than expected number of children with autism have late development of handedness and lateralization (i.e. do not become clearly right handed or left handed) and may remain ambidextrous.

  Precocious skills or islets of precocity: Some individuals with autism may have skills in certain areas, which are much higher than their normal peers. For example, hyperlexia (early ability to read very well), extremely good rote memory or calculating ability, etc.

  A fraudulent research paper published in 1998, claimed a link between administration of MMR vaccine and development of autism, but this claim was found to be untrue. **MMR vaccine is not associated with the development of autism**[Q].

  Treatment: Educational interventions such as a structured classroom teaching along with use of behavioral therapy is the recommended treatment. The role of medications is limited. Atypical antipsychotics such as risperidone and aripiprazole have been used to reduce aggressive and self injurious behavior.

- *Rett's disorder (Rett's syndrome)*: Earlier it was believed that Rett's disorder occurs exclusively in **females**[Q], however of late males with similar presentation have been described. It is characterized by normal development till the age of 5 months. Between 5-48 months, the child starts to lose acquired hand skills (such as fine motor skills) and there is loss of acquired speech. Also, there is deceleration of head circumference producing **microcephaly**[Q]. The child gradually develops stereotyped hand movements such as hand wringing, licking or biting of fingers. The language function remains impaired and there is also loss of social interaction. The child also develops **poorly coordinated gait** or trunk movements.

  Along with these symptoms around 75% of children have seizures. The disorder is usually progressive and treatment is symptomatic.

- *Childhood disintegrative disorder (Heller's syndome)*: It is characterized by normal development till the age of 2 years. Between 2-10 years, there is loss of acquired motor skills, social skills, language skill and bowel or bladder control. The child develops the three core symptoms of impaired communication, impaired social interaction and repetitive, stereotyped behavior. The course is usually progressive though some patients may show improvement. The treatment is symptomatic.

ICD-11 & DSM-5 Update

In both ICD-11 & DSM-5, the term pervasive developmental disorder has been replaced by autism spectrum disorder. Also, all the subtypes, such as autism, Rett's disorder, Asperger's syndrome have been removed. Now, autism spectrum disorder is considered as a continuum with difference in severity, rather than presence of subtypes.

ICD-11 & DSM-5 Update

In both ICD-11 & DSM-5, in autism spectrum disorders, language dysfunction has been removed as a core criterion. Only impaired social interaction and repetitive, restrictive behaviors form the core criterion now.

- *Asperger's syndrome*: It is characterized by impairment of social interaction and restricted, repetitive and stereotyped behavior. However, no language delay or disturbance is seen. The treatment is usually supportive.

CONDUCT DISORDER AND OPPOSITIONAL DEFIANT DISORDER

- *Conduct disorder*: It is characterized by repetitive and persistent pattern of **disregard for rights of others**^{Q} and **aggressive**^{Q} and **dissocial behavior**^{Q}, such as excessive levels of fighting or bullying, cruelty to animals or other people, severe destruction of property, fire setting, stealing, truancy from school, **repeated lying**^{Q}, frequent running from school and home, defiance of authority figures and a pattern of disobedience. Boys are more likely to indulge in physical aggression as well as relational aggression (aggression in social relationships), girls tend to show more of relational aggression. Conduct disorder is frequently associated with unsatisfactory family relationships and failure at school. These children may later on develop **antisocial personality disorder**^{Q} (dissocial personality disorder). **Low resting heart rate**^{Q} is a strong and consistent predictor of conduct disorder and chronic aggression
- *Oppositional defiant disorder*: It is less severe than conduct disorder and is characterized by persistently negativistic and defiant behavior such as frequent arguing with adults, refusal to comply with adults' requests and rules, frequent loss of temper and often deliberately annoying adults. However, unlike conduct disorder, there are no serious violations like theft, fire setting, destruction, etc.

The management for both involves family intervention and behavioral therapy. In some cases, low dose antipsychotics have been found to be effective.

LEARNING DISORDERS (SPECIFIC DEVELOPMENTAL DISORDERS OF SCHOLASTIC SKILLS)

These developmental disorders are characterized by **significant impairment** in one or more of the **scholastic skills**^{Q} which are out of proportion to the intellectual functioning of the child. For example, a child may present with significant difficulty in reading while having normal writing and arithmetic skills and a **normal IQ**^{Q}. Depending on the symptoms, the subtypes have been described.

- *Specific reading disorder (Dyslexia)*: The child's reading performance is significantly impaired and he may make errors while reading, may have slow reading speed or may have difficulty in comprehension.
- *Disorder of written expression (specific spelling disorder)*: The child may make frequent spelling mistakes, errors in grammar and punctuations and may have poor hand writing.
- *Specific disorder of arithmetic skills*: The area of impairment is arithmetics.
- *Mixed disorders of scholastic skills*: There is impairment in reading, writing and arithmetics combined.

Apart from the above-mentioned symptoms, the child may have associated problems such as inattention, hyperactivity and emotional disturbances.

MENTAL RETARDATION

Mental retardation is a condition characterized by incomplete development of intellectual functions and adaptive skills (skills which help an individual live a successful life). The intelligence is usually measured by calculating the Intelligence Quotient (IQ).

$$IQ = Mental\ age/Chronological\ age \times 100^Q$$

In this formula, the maximum denominator is 15, even if assessment of an older individual is being performed. Mental retardation is diagnosed, if the IQ is less than 70.

Category	IQ
Normal	90-109
Borderline	70-89
Mild mental retardation	50-69
Moderate mental retardation	35-49
Severe mental retardation	20-34
Profound mental retardation	< 20

The level of functioning varies in different severity of mental retardation. The following table summarizes the same.

Category	Class	Mental age as adults	Educational achievement	Life	Work
Mild MR	Educable	9–12 yrs	Up to 6th class	Independent living	Unskilled or semi-skilled work
Moderate MR	Trainable	6–8 yrs	Up to 2nd class	Needs support	Unskilled or semi-skilled work
Severe MR	Dependent	3–6 yrs	No formal education	Needs attention	Simple task-under supervision
Profound MR	Needs life support	< 3 yrs	No formal education	Needs continuous supervision	None

An earlier classification of retardation used the words "idiots, imbecile, and moron".

Term	IQ range
Moron	51–70
Imbecile	26–50
Idiot	0–25

The most common chromosomal cause of mental retardation is **Down syndrome**^{Q} followed by **fragile X syndrome**^{Q}.

Behavioral problems in mental retardation: The patients with mental retardation may have maladaptive behavior such as aggression, self-injurious behaviors, hyperactivity, etc. These behaviors can usually be modified using behavioral therapy techniques like **contingency management**^{Q}, in which the desired behaviors are rewarded and undesired behaviors are punished.

DSM-5 & ICD 11 Update

DSM-5 Update: In DSM-5, the diagnosis of mental retardation has been replaced with "intellectual disability^Q".
ICD-11 Update: In ICD-11, the diagnosis of mental retardation has been replaced with 'Disorders of Intellectual Development'

TIC DISORDERS

Tics are brief, rapid, recurrent motor movements (motor tics) or vocalizations (vocal tics) that are performed in response to internal urges. Though, often patient experience these movements as irresistible and involuntary, but they can be suppressed for varying periods of time.

Motor tics can be simple motor tics (involving contractions of functionally similar muscle groups) such as eye blinking, head jerking, shoulder shrugging or face grimacing or complex motor tics, which appear purposeful and are more complicated movements such as jumping, echopraxia (repetition of observed behavior), copropraxia (displaying obscene gestures). Similarly, vocal tics can be simple (coughing, throat clearing, grunting, etc.) or complex (echolalia which is repetition of words or coprolalia which is use of obscene words or phrases).

Tourette's syndrome is a form of tic disorder in which there are multiple motor tics and one or more vocal tics. The most common comorbidity with Tourette's syndrome (Tourette's disorder) is ADHD followed by OCD. Another common comorbidity is Depression.

The onset is usually between 4 and 6 years of age, symptoms peak between 10 and 12 years of age and between half to two third of children achieve remission or are much improved by adolescence or young adulthood. It is morecommon in **males**^{Q} than females.

Treatment

Combination of behavioral therapy and pharmacotherapy are used with behavioral therapy being the first line treatment. Amongst behavioral therapy, the first line therapy is **Habit Reversal**. In habit reversal, patient learns to identify the urge that happens before tics. And when he senses the urge, he follows it with a voluntary behavior (such as slow rhythmic breathing) instead of the tic. Other behavioral therapy that can be used is Exposure and Response Prevention.

In pharmacotherapy, noradrenergic agents such as clonidine and guanfacine are often used as first line agent due to better side effect profile. Atypical antipsychotics, particularly risperidone have been found to be efficient in the treatment. Haloperidol and Pimozide, which are typical antipsychotics, are FDA approved for treatment of Tourette's disorder, but can cause significant side effects.

Multiple Choice Questions

1. **Which of the following is not seen in a hyperkinetic child?** *(DNB 1993, AI 1991)*
   A. Aggressive outbursts
   B. Decreased attention span
   C. Left to right disorientation
   D. Soft neurological signs

2. **Minimal brain dysfunction syndrome is the older name of:** *(NEET 2018)*
   A. Dyslexia
   B. ADHD
   C. Mental retardation
   D. Down's syndrome

3. **The preferred drug for treating attention deficit hyperactivity disorder in a 6-year-old boy, whose father has a history of substance abuse:** *(JIPMER May, 2018)*
   A. Methylphenidate
   B. Atomoxetine
   C. Clonidine
   D. Dexamphetamine

4. **A 9-year-old child disturbs other people, is destructive, interferes when two people are talking, does not follow instructions and cannot wait for his turn while playing a game. He is likely to be suffering from:** *(AIIMS Nov 2005)*
   A. Emotional disorders
   B. Behavioral problems
   C. No disorder
   D. Attention deficit hyperactivity disorder

5. **A 10-year-old child presents with hyperactivity and inattention. Parents are extremely worried, what would you say to the parents?** *(AIIMS Nov 2008)*
   A. It is a normal behavior
   B. Child has a behavioral problem and should receive behavioral therapy
   C. Child has a serious problem and should receive medical therapy
   D. There should be a change in environment

6. **According to DSM 5 criteria, all are true about ADHD except:** *(JIPMER 2017)*
   A. Adult ADHD symptoms are similar to children
   B. For diagnoses, symptoms should be present before 7 years
   C. For diagnoses, symptoms should be present before 12 years
   D. Symptoms should be present in more than one setting

7. **ADHD in childhood can lead to what in future:** *(JIPMER 2018, PGI 2000)*
   A. Schizophrenia
   B. Alcoholism
   C. Intellectual changes
   D. Antisocial behavior

8. **Drugs not given in ADHD:** *(JIPMER 2016)*
   A. Clonidine
   B. Atomoxetine
   C. Methylphenidate
   D. Barbiturate

9. **Which of the following drug is not given in ADHD?** *(NEET 2016)*
   A. Clonidine
   B. Methylphenidate
   C. Atomoxetine
   D. Phenobarbitone

10. **Drug(s) used in treatment of attention deficit hyperactivity disorder:** *(PGI Dec 2008)*
    A. Atomoxetine
    B. Methylphenidate
    C. Dexmethylphenidate
    D. Quetiapine
    E. Dextroamphetamine

11. **Not an associated comorbid condition in children with hyperkinetic attention deficit disorder is:** *(DNB Dec 2010)*
    A. Elimination disorder
    B. Anxiety disorder
    C. Sleep disorder
    D. Language disorder

12. **A neurodevelopmental disorder which is characterized by impaired social interaction, impaired verbal and nonverbal communication, and restricted and repetitive behavior is description for:** *(DNB NEET 2014-15)*
    A. Autism
    B. Anxiety disorder
    C. Antisocial personality disorder
    D. Paranoid schizophrenia

13. **A 10-year-old child presents with impaired social interaction, impaired communication and stereotyped behavior. He has normal IQ and language skills. What is the most probable diagnosis?** *(DNB NEET 2014-15)*
    A. Asperger's syndrome
    B. Autism
    C. Rett syndrome
    D. Childhood depression

14. **A 3-year-old child has normal developmental milestones except delayed language development (poor speech development). He has difficulty in concentration, communication, and making friends (i.e. he has no friends) and spends time seeing his own hands. The most probable diagnosis is:** *(AI 2012, AIIMS Nov 2006)*
    A. Autism
    B. ADHD
    C. Specific learning disability
    D. Mental retardation

15. **Infantile autism is characterized by:** *(PGI Dec 2004)*
    A. Impaired vision
    B. Impaired neurobehavioral development
    C. Impaired folate level
    D. A socioeconomic hazard
    E. Result of wrong parenting

16. **Autism is:** *(PGI 2000)*
    A. Neurodevelopmental disorder
    B. Social and language communication problem
    C. Metabolic disease
    D. Mainly due to hypothalamus damage

17. **A 6-year-old child with history of birth asphyxia does not communicate well, has slow mental and physical growth, does not mix with people, has limited interests and gets widely agitated, if disturbed. Diagnosis is:** *(AIIMS 2001)*
    A. Hyperkinetic child
    B. Autistic disorder
    C. Attention deficit disorder
    D. Mixed receptive–expressive language disorder

18. **A girl with normal milestones spend her time seeing her own hand and does not interact with others. What is the likely diagnosis:** *(FMGE 2018, AIIMS 2008)*
    A. ADHD   B. Autism
    C. Asperger's syndrome D. Rett's disorder

19. **A 2-year-old girl child is brought to the outpatient with features of handwringing stereotyped movements, impaired language and communication development, breath holding spells, poor social skills and deceleration of head growth after six months of age. The most likely diagnosis is:** *(NEET 2016, AIIMS Nov 2003)*
    A. Asperger syndrome B. Rett's syndrome
    C. Fragile X-syndrome D. Cotard syndrome

20. **Which of the following is not seen in autism?** *(AIIMS Nov 2014)*
    A. 2/3rd patients are mentally retarded
    B. Poor eye contact
    C. Language is impaired
    D. Abnormal dermatoglyphics

21. **MMR vaccine has been controversially associated with the development of the following psychiatric disorder?** *(NIMHANS 2017)*
    A. Autism   B. ADHD
    C. Mental retardation D. Schizophrenia

22. **A child with pervasive developmental disorder will have all except:** *(AIIMS Nov 2015)*
    A. Stereotyped behavior B. Reduced social interaction
    C. Poor language skills D. Impaired cognition

23. **Which of the following disease is seen only in females?** *(DNB Dec 2011)*
    A. Autism   B. Asperger's syndrome
    C. Rett's disease   D. Cotard disease

24. **Rett's syndrome is characterized by all except:** *(DNB NEET 2014-15, AIIMS 2013)*
    A. Regression of acquired skills
    B. Breath holding spells
    C. Autistic behavior
    D. Macrocephaly

25. **Following statements are true about Rett's syndrome** *(PGI Nov 2017)*
    A. Loss of acquired motor skills between 5 to 48 months
    B. Language impairment
    C. Poorly coordinated gait
    D. More common in males

26. **IQ is:** *(DNB NEET 2014-15)*
    A. Mental age/chronological age × 100
    B. Chronological age/mental age × 100
    C. Mental age + chronological age × 100
    D. Mental age – chronological age × 100

27. **According to Wechsler intelligence scale scoring, average IQ of a normal child is:** *(AIIMS 2013)*
    A. 50   B. 75
    C. 90   D. 111

28. **A 16-year-old male is found to have a mental age of 9 years on IQ testing. He has:** *(AIIMS May 2005)*
    A. Mild mental retardation
    B. Moderate mental retardation
    C. Severe mental retardation
    D. Profound mental retardation

29. **Which of the following score is not included in mild mental retardation?** *(NIMHANS 2012, PGI May 2012)*
    A. 85   B. 50
    C. 45   D. 75
    E. 65

30. **A patient with IQ 30 will be diagnosed with:** *(DNB NEET 2014-15)*
    A. Mild mental retardation
    B. Moderate mental retardation
    C. Severe mental retardation
    D. Profound mental retardation

31. **True about mental retardation:** *(PGI Nov 2011)*
    A. More common in females than males
    B. Severe MR is IQ < 20
    C. Antenatal factor can cause mental retardation
    D. Common cause is Down's syndrome
    E. Life-long inability to learn and progress

32. **In a child with IQ 50, which of the following is true:** *(PGI 2001)*
    A. Can look after himself independently
    B. Can study up to 8th standard
    C. Can follow simple verbal commands
    D. Can handle money
    E. Recognize family members

33. **All of the following statements about 'Imbecile' are true, except:** *(AI 2011)*
    A. IQ is 50–60
    B. Intellectual capacity is equivalent to a child of 3–7 years of age
    C. Impaired self care
    D. Condition usually congenital or acquired at an early age

34. **X-linked disease leading to mental retardation is:** *(PGI 2000)*
    A. Myotonic dystrophy   B. Fragile X-syndrome
    C. Tuberous sclerosis   D. Phenylketonuria

35. **What is the new name for mental retardation according to DSM-5?** *(NEET 2018)*
    A. Mental handicap   B. Intellectual disability
    C. Subnormal intelligence   D. Lunatic person

36. **Best therapy suited to teach daily life skill to a mentally challenged child:** *(AIIMS May 2011, 2009)*
    A. CBT (Cognitive behavior therapy)
    B. Contingency management
    C. Cognitive reconstruction
    D. Self instruction

37. A 14-year-old boy is not able to get good grades in 9th standard exam. But he is very sharp and intelligent. Best test to diagnose his problem: *(AIIMS 2012)*
    A. Child behavior checklist
    B. Bhatia's battery
    C. Specific learning disability test
    D. Child behavior battery

38. A child finds difficulty to spell and read, otherwise his IQ is normal, interacts well with parents and friends. Vision is normal. Most probable diagnosis of the condition is: *(DNB June 2011)*
    A. ADHD
    B. Dyslexia
    C. Autism
    D. Asperger syndrome

39. A 14-year-old boy has difficulty in expressing himself in writing and makes frequent spelling mistakes. He passes his examination with poor marks. However his mathematical ability and social adjustment are appropriate for his age. Which of the following is the most likely diagnosis? *(AIIMS Nov 2004)*
    A. Mental retardation
    B. Specific learning disability
    C. Lack of interest in studies
    D. Examination anxiety

40. A boy presents with history of abnormal excessive blinking and grunting. He says he has no control over his symptoms which have risen in frequency of late. This has started affecting his social life and is making him depressed. Which of the following medications should be used in the management? *(AIIMS May 2015)*
    A. Carbamazepine
    B. Imipramine
    C. Risperidone
    D. Methylphenidate

41. Appetite for non-nutritive substances is called: *(DNB NEET 2014-15)*
    A. Pica   B. Anorexia
    C. Bulimia   D. Binge

42. Scholastic performance is impaired in all of the following except: *(AI 2012)*
    A. Attention deficit hyperactivity disorder
    B. Specific learning disorder
    C. Anxiety
    D. Pica

43. Conduct disorder in a child manifests with: *(PGI 2001)*
    A. Disregard for right of others
    B. Doesn't care for authority
    C. Backward in studies
    D. Decreased head circumference
    E. Steals things

44. Most uncommon in childhood is: *(NEET 2016)*
    A. Panic disorder
    B. ADHD
    C. Autistic spectrum disorder
    D. Separation anxiety disorder

Controversial Question

45. A 6-year-old child presents with bed wetting at night. There is no history of any day time symptoms. The urine microscopy is normal, the specific gravity of urine is 1.020 and other investigations are normal. What should be advised: *(AIIMS May 16)*
    A. Reassurance and revisit after 6 months
    B. CT pelvis   C. USG kidney and bladder
    D. Refer to child psychiatrist

46. Most common cause of death in Rett's syndrome is: *(JIPMER 2016)*
    A. Hypoglycemia   B. Cardiac arrhythmias
    C. Seizures   D. Respiratory failure

47. M-CHAT is used for screening of:
    A. ADHD   B. Autism
    C. Separation anxiety disorder
    D. Schizophrenia

48. Tourette's syndrome is associated with all of the following except: *(NIMHANS 2015)*
    A. Depression
    B. Obsessive compulsive disorder
    C. ADHD
    D. Parkinson's disease

49. Tics, hair pulling, nail biting can be treated by:
    A. Mind fullness   B. Social habit treating
    C. Habit reversal training   D. No intervention required

50. All are rue about Tourette syndrome except: *(DNB 2017)*
    A. Motor tics
    B. More common in females
    C. Associated with OCD
    D. Neuroleptics are useful in the treatment

51. Transitional objects appear at the age of: *(NIMHANS 2017)*
    A. 2-5 yrs   B. 5-10 yrs
    C. 6 months-2 years D. Less than 6 months

52. Habit disorder is all except: *(NEET 2018)*
    A. Thumb sucking   B. Nail biting
    C. Temper tantrums   D. Tics

53. Regarding Rett's syndrome, false is: *(NIMHANS 2018)*
    A. Microcephaly at birth   B. X-lined
    C. Poor social interaction
    D. Stereotypical hand movements

54. Least commonly present in conduct disorder seen in girls, in comparison to boys: *((JIPMER May 2018)*
    A. Run away from home   B. High risk sexual behavior
    C. Physical aggression   D. Emotional bullying

55. Biological marker for antisocial behavior in boys: *(JIPMER May 2018)*
    A. Low serum testosterone   B. Low resting pulse rate
    C. Increased urinary dopamine levels
    D. Shortened REM latency

56. All of the followings disruptive and impulse control disorders except: *(DNB 2018)*
    A. Munchausen syndrome   B. Conduct disorder
    C. Intermittent explosive disorder
    D. Oppositional disorder

Answers With Explanations

1. C. The best answer here would be left to right disorientation. Please remember, in ADHD, "left to right discrimination" difficulties can be found. However, the term "left to right disorientation" is used for describing gross inability to distinguish left from right and is usually a feature of Gerstmann's syndrome.
2. B. ADHD.
3. B. Usually stimulants are the preferred drugs in the treatment of ADHD. In this question, history of substance abuse in child's father has been given to indicate genetic predisposition to substance abuse. Since stimulants carry the risk of development of dependence, in this case, nonstimulants would be the preferred drug. Hence atomoxetine is the better answer (atomoxetine is preferred over clonidine).
4. D. This child has symptoms of hyperactivity and impulsivity and the most likely diagnosis would be attention deficit hyperactivity disorder.
5. C. The symptoms are suggestive of ADHD. ADHD is a serious medical problem and should be treated properly. The symptoms of ADHD interfere with education of child, and if not treated child's education may suffer greatly and will adversely affect his future life. Also, medications like methylphenidate are the first line treatment.
6. B. According to DSM-5, symptoms should be present before 12 yrs of age to make a diagnosis of ADHD.
7. B, D.
   Kindly note, that few books have also mentioned intellectual changes as an answer. This is not true. Though children with ADHD tend to have lower educational achievements, however it is not because of any intellectual impairment but because of poor attention and hyperactivity.
8. D. Barbiturate.
9. D. Phenobarbitone. See text for explanation.
10. A, B, C, E
    See text for explanation.
11. A. Elimination disorders are not a common comorbiity in ADHD.
12. A. Autism.
13. A. Asperger's syndrome.
14. A. The child has all the three core features of autism, impairment in social interaction (difficulty in making friends), impaired communication and repetitive, stereotyped behavior (spends most time seeing own hands).
15. B, D.
    Autism is a neurodevelopmental or neurobehavioral disorder. It causes socioeconomic problems as a majority of autistic patients remain dependent on others however use of term "hazard" is a bit insensitive here.
16. A, B.

17. B. The history of poor social interaction and restricted behaviors along with history of agitation when disturbed supports the diagnosis of autism. Around 30% of children with autism have comorbid mental retardation. The prevalence of perinatal insults like birth asphyxia has been found to be higher in children with autism.
18. B. The history of restricted behaviors and poor social interaction is suggestive of autism.
19. B. The deceleration of head growth after 6 months of age followed by repetitive, stereotyped behavior (wringing hand movements), impaired communication and poor social interaction is suggestive of Rett's syndrome.
20. A. Around 30% of children with autism have comorbid mental retardation.
21. A. Autism.
22. D. Impaired cognition.
23. C. Rett's syndrome was earlier believed to occur exclusively in females, however of late males with similar presentation have been described.
24. D. Macrocephaly.
25. A, B, C.
26. A. Mental age/chronological age × 100.
27. C. According to Wechsler intelligence scale, the following is the classification.

IQ range	IQ classification
130 and above	Very superior
120–129	Superior high
110–119	Above average
90–109	Average
80–89	Low average
70–79	Borderline
69 and below	Extremely low

28. A. The formula for IQ is mental age/chronological × 100. However, please remember that the maximum denominator can be 15. In this case 9/15 × 100 = 60. Hence, it will come under the category of mild mental retardation.
29. A, C, D.
    The range for mild mental retardation is IQ from 50-69.
30. C. Severe mental retardation.
31. C, D.
    Mental retardation is more common in boys, severe MR is IQ < 35 and patients with mild and moderate MR can learn.
32. A, C, D, E.
    IQ of 50 corresponds to mild mental retardation. People with mild mental retardation can handle money, can have an independent living, study till 6th class.

Child Psychiatry

33. A. The IQ of imbeciles is between 26-50. Hence, most of their features would correspond to that of moderate mental retardation.
34. B. Fragile X-syndrome.
35. B. Intellectual disability.
36. B. Contingeney management. See text for explanation.
37. C. The history of poor academic performance despite good intelligence should raise suspicion of learning disorders (specific learning disability). Hence, he should take a specific learning disability test to rule out the same.
38. B. The history of difficulty in reading and spelling mistakes in presence of normal IQ is suggestive of learning disorders (specific learning disability).
39. B. Scholastic difficulty in a particular skill (written expression) is suggestive of specific learning disability.
40. C. The history of motor tics (abnormal excessive blinking) and vocal tics (grunting) is suggestive of tics disorder (possibly Tourette syndrome). Antipsychotics like risperidone would be the best choice amongst the options.
41. A. Pica.
42. D. Pica.
43. A, B, C, E.
    See text for explanation.
44. A. Panic disorder. Panic disorder median age at onset is 20-24 years and is very rare in childhood.
45. D. Refer to child psychiatrist. Lets solve this question step by step. First of all, the age of child is 6 years and he is still not continent, so we can make a diagnosis of enuresis (remember the diagnosis of enuresis can be made only after 5 years of age). Since, enuresis can have a significant impact of child's self esteem and may be associated with psychiatric disorders, we must treat it, hence the option of reassurance is easily ruled out.

    The question arises should we investigate the child further or not. Please remember that you cannot presume the enuresis of child to be of psychological origin unless organic causes (medical causes) have been ruled out. Also, remember we do not go on doing investigations in children unless we have reasons to investigate the child. So, lets analyse the symptoms to decide whether to investigate or not.

    Here, there are no day time symptoms. This history is extremely important as absence of day time symptoms goes against the common causes like UTI, obstructions and anatomical conditions.

    Further, the question says that routine microscopy is normal (suggests that there are no infections), the specific gravity is normal (to rule out diabetes insipidus) and the question further says "other investigations are normal" without specifying them. The examiner is of course giving all these hints for us to rule out the organic causes of enuresis.

    Since the treatment of choice is to review toilet training and use bed alarms, the best answer here is option D, refer to a child psychiatrist/psychologist.

    I know you guys will be a bit confused as different faculties are giving different answers so I am adding few references

    Kaplan's psychiatry says "To make the diagnosis of enuresis, organic causes of bladder dysfunction must be investigated and ruled out. Organic syndromes, such as urinary tract infections, obstructions, or anatomical conditions, are found most often in children who experience both nocturnal and diurnal enuresis combined with urinary frequency and urgency".

    Kaplan's psychiatry says "Sophisticated radiographic studies are usually deferred in simple cases of enuresis with no signs of repeated infections or other medical problems".
46. B. Cardiac arrhythmias.
47. B. The **Modified Checklist for Autism in Toddlers (M-CHAT)** is a questionnaire that evaluates risk for autism spectrum disorder in toddlers.
48. D. Parkinson's disease. See text for explanation.
49. C. Habit reversal training. See text for explanation.
50. B. Tourette syndrome is more common in males than females.
51. C. Transitional objects are the objects that provide comfort to the infants, in the absence of mothers. Different type of objects can act as transitional objects, with 'blankets' being the most common one. Trasitional objects usually develop around six months, though different authors differ about the exact age of their appearance.
52. C. Temper tantrums. The term 'habit disorder' is used to describe a class of disorder that is characterized by repetitive and unwanted behaviors. Two types have been described: (1) Tic disorders, (2) Body focused repetitive behaviors such as hair pulling, skin picking, nail biting, thumb sucking, and cheek chewing.
53. A. In Rett's syndrome, the head circumference is normal at birth.
54. C. According to DSM-5, Boys are more likely to indulge in physical aggression as well as relational aggression (aggresion in social rleationships), girls tend to show more of relational aggression.
55. B. Low resting heart rate is a strong and consistent predictor of conduct disorder and chronic aggression.
56. A. Munchausen syndrome is not a disruptive disorder, the rest all are.

12 CHAPTER

Psychoanalysis

The term "psychoanalysis" was coined by **Sigmund Freud**^{Q} who is also known as **"father of psychoanalysis"**^{Q}. **Freud (1856-1939)**^{Q} was born in Freiburg, Moravia (now in Czech Republic) and lived most of his life in **Vienna**^{Q}. He died in London in 1939.

Psychoanalysis is a theory which states that the childhood experiences and memories and unconscious mental activity (activity of mind which we are not aware of) plays an important role in determining human behavior and emotions and also in the development of psychiatric disorders. The term "psychoanalysis" is used not only to refer to this theory but also for the treatment method which is based on this theory.

The theory of psychoanalysis was developed by Freud while working with patients of hysteria **(the term hysteria is no longer used, these patients will get a diagnosis of "dissociative disorder" according to current classification)**. In particular Freud came to know about a patient Anna O, who had developed multiple unexplained neurological symptoms including paralysis of limbs, after the death of her father. Whenever she was able to recall how a particular symptom originated, that symptom would improve. For example, once she was able to recall that on one occasion while she was sitting at her sick father's bedside, she had a daydream that a snake was crawling towards her father and while she wanted to ward off the snake she couldn't do it as her arm had gone into sleep. As soon as Anna O, was able to recall this event, the paralysis of her arm improved. This case provided Freud a strong demonstration, that unconscious memories (memories which an individual has forgotten, but which are still present in the unconscious mind) can result in development of symptoms.

Freud started treating hysterical patients, wherein he would try to retrieve the unconscious memories during the treatment procedure. Initially, Freud used hypnosis and found that patients when in a state of trance (an altered state of consciousness) were able to recall forgotten traumatic events. **Abreaction**^{Q} is a process by which repressed material (forgotten material) is remembered back, relived again along with the expression of associated emotions. Abreaction would help in improvement of symptoms in few patients.

Later Freud developed a technique called **"free association"** in which the patient was asked to say whatever came into their minds without censoring their thoughts. With the help of this technique, Freud was able to gain access to unconscious memories, which would come out as patient would start saying all that came into their minds and would not try to stop any thought. Freud also gave a lot of importance to **slips of the tongue** (which he called **parapraxis**^{Q}). Freud believed that these "slips of tongues" were not simple mistakes, and that these slips actually conveyed **important information**^{Q} about what was going on in the unconscious mind.

The psychoanalytic treatment provided by Freud also used the principles of transference and countertransference.

Transference^Q is the feeling that the patient develops for the doctor. This feeling is a combination of the feelings patient had for figures from the past and the real feeling for the clinician. For example, if the doctor reminds the patient of his dominating and insensitive father, the patient will develop a negative feeling for the doctor, despite the fact that doctor has not done anything to offend him.

Countertransference^Q is the feeling that the clinician develops for the patient.

TOPOGRAPHICAL THEORY OF MIND

In **1900**^{Q}, Freud published a book called **"The interpretation of dreams"**^{Q}. In this book, Freud said that dreams were meaningful and by understanding dreams, one can understand about the unconscious mind of an individual. In this book, Freud proposed a theory of mind, called the **topographical theory of mind**^{Q}. According to this theory the mind can be divided into three regions:

A. The conscious
B. The preconscious
C. The unconscious

A. ***The conscious***: It is the part of mind which is accessible to us. We are aware of the contents of conscious mind. Everything you know about yourself is a part of conscious mind.

B. ***The preconscious***: The content of preconscious mind are not normally available to us, but they can be recalled or brought into awareness by focusing attention. For example, you may not be aware of the appearance of your 5th class teacher, however, if you try to focus and remember hard, you might be able to recall her appearance. The preconscious separates the conscious and unconscious mind. The preconscious mind has a barrier, called **repression**, which normally does not allow the contents of unconscious mind to reach the conscious mind. If any unconscious memory has to reach the conscious awareness, it must find a way to overcome the force of "repression". Freud reported that during sleep, the repression force becomes lax, and many unconscious memories and desires are able to reach the conscious in the form of dreams. That's why Freud believed that the interpretation of dreams can reveal the contents of unconscious memories and desires. Further, when a person indulges in "free association", few unconscious contents are able to cross the barrier of repression and are able to come out in the form of "slips of tongue".

C. ***The unconscious***: The unconscious mind is not accessible to an individual. The unconscious mind contains, **the instinctual drives** (i.e. the drives and desires one is born with) such as sexual instinct and aggressive instinct. Further, distressing childhood memories and distressing desires are also buried inside the unconscious. These contents are not available to the conscious mind due to the barrier of "repression". Freud believed that by not allowing these memories to reach conscious, repression causes development of psychiatric symptoms and disorders.

The unconscious mind is characterized by **"primary process thinking"**^{Q}. This is primitive way of thinking in which the mind wants immediate "wish fulfillment" and instinctual discharge (wants all desires and instincts to be fulfilled immediately without considering the consequences). The primary process thinking is **illogical** and **contradictory.**

In "The Interpretation of dreams", Freud postulated that dreams are a way by which unconscious impulses get expressed consciously. He believed that unacceptable desires and impulses, which are a part of unconscious mind, are normally not allowed to enter in the conscious mind by the barrier of 'repression'. However, during sleep, this barrier allows certain such desires and impulses to enter the conscious mind, after they have been transformed. This transformation is necessary as if allowed to enter the conscious mind in their original form, they will cause lot of distress to the sleeping person and may result in him getting awakened. This process of transformation is called as 'dream work' and it transforms 'latent content' of dream to 'manifest content' of dream.

During this process, the unconscious desires and impulses are attached with certain other images from the dreamer's current experience and hence are transformed in such a way that they no longer remain as unacceptable. E.g. Say, a person has an unconscious impulse of aggression against his father, if he sees a dream in which he is hitting his father, it may result in so much distress that he will wake up. So the process of dream work will attach this aggressive impulse with the image of the teacher who the dreamer met in the morning, and during the dream the dreamer will see himself hitting this teacher. This dream allowed expression of aggressive impulse and it was modified in such a way that the dreamer did not get distressed and didn't wake up. The mechanisms that are involved in dream work are as follows:

A. ***Condensation***^{Q}: This mechanism allows several unconscious desires and impulses to be combined in a single image in manifest dream content. The converse called 'irradiation or diffusion' can also happen and involves breaking a single desire or impulse into various parts.

B. ***Displacement***^{Q}: This involves displacement of impulse from an original object to a substitute of the object. E.g. In example taken above, the aggression was displaced from father to teacher.

C. ***Symbolic representation***^{Q}: Here, a strong or complex emotion towards an individual is symbolised by a simple image. E.g A strong homosexual impulse towards a person may be represented as a snake (snake is symbolising 'penis' here)

STRUCTURAL THEORY OF MIND

Later in his life, Freud replaced the topographical theory of mind with a newer theory, called the structural theory of mind. According to this theory, there are three components of mind: id, ego and superego.

A. **Id**: It is the most primitive part of mind with which an infant is born. Id consists of the instinctual drives. It is that part of mind which wants to have pleasure and that too immediately. Id does not care about the external world or any consequences. Id hence works on **"pleasure principal"**. Id uses the primary process thinking. Id is completely in the **unconscious domain** of mind.

All the defense mechanisms operate at an unconscious level (except, suppression which is a conscious and voluntary defense mechanism).

B. ***Ego***: Ego is that part of mind which deals with the external world. The part of your mind which is reading this book is "ego". Apart from dealing with the external world, another important function of ego is to deal with the "id" and "superego" and maintain a balance between the two and the external world. Since, the ego maintains a balance and helps in dealing with the realities of the outside world, it is said to work on **"reality principal"**. Ego is said to be the **"executive organ"** of the mind. Ego has **both conscious and unconscious** components. The "defense mechanisms" reside in the **unconscious component** of ego.

C. ***Superego***: It is that part of our mind, which wants to follow the moral principles and do the right thing. The voice of conscience, which scolds you, when you are not studying, comes from superego. Superego is **mostly unconscious**, but also has a **conscious component**.

To understand how these components work, an example can be illustrated. While you are studying, your id wants you to throw away the books and instead go out and have fun and indulge in some pleasurable activity. On the other hand, your superego wants you to study very hard without taking many breaks and stay away from all distractions. Finally, your ego does a balancing act and you decide that you will study for two hours and after that you will take a break and will watch a movie. This is how, ego always keeps a balance.

As mentioned in this example, conflicts keep on going in the mind (between id, ego and superego) and these **unconscious conflicts**[Q] in the mind are believed to cause psychiatric disorders according to the psychodynamic (or psychoanalytic) theories.

DEFENSE MECHANISMS

An important function of ego is to prevent a build up of excessive and unbearable anxiety. Many unacceptable urges, if they reach the conscious awareness, can produce excessive anxiety. Defense mechanisms are the tools used by the "ego" to prevent the development of excessive anxiety. The defense mechanisms have been divided into four groups: narcissistic, immature, neurotic and mature defense mechanisms. Following are the important defense mechanisms:

Narcissistic Defenses

A. ***Denial***: It is refusal to acknowledge the reality. The person continues to behave as, if nothing has happened. For example, a mother refused to accept that her 7-year-old son died in an accident and insists that he will be back for dinner.

B. ***Projection***: Projecting "own" unacceptable feeling about others, on to others. For example, a husband with an unacceptable wish of indulging in infidelity, starts accusing his wife of indulging in infidelity. Here, the husband has "projected" his own wish on to the wife. This defense mechanism is responsible for development of **delusions and hallucinations**.

Immature Defenses

C. ***Acting out***: Acting on unconscious desires without becoming aware of them. For example, a person suddenly steals an item from a shop without any prior planning. In this case, this person had an unconscious desire of indulging in stealing. His mind, however, did not allow this feeling to enter his conscious, as that would result in this person feeling bad about himself. Hence, this person resorts to straight away acting on the unconscious desire without even becoming aware of the same. This defense mechanism is involved in development of **impulse control disorders**.

D. ***Passive-aggressive behavior***: Indirectly expressing the anger towards others. For example, a young boy was forced to bring a glass of water for the father, while bringing the water, the child accidentally tripped and dropped the glass. Here, the child was able to express his anger indirectly by dropping the glass.

E. ***Regression***: Attempt to return to an earlier phase of development (i.e. childhood) to avoid the tensions and conflicts of present phase of development (i.e. adulthood). For example, extremely stressed because of an upcoming entrance examination, a medical students goes to a park and starts playing cricket along with the children. Regression is involved in development of **neurosis**[Q].

F. ***Projective identification***: In this defense mechanism, intolerable aspects of self are projected on to another person, that person is induced to play the projected part and the two persons than act in unison. For example, a wife who has lots of aggression can project her aggression on to the husband, and make him behave in an aggressive manner and finally a system develops where the husband indulges in aggression and wife is the recipient of aggression. Please remember all of this happens unconsciously without entering into awareness of either the wife or the husband. Projective identification is seen in patients with **borderline personality disorder**.

Neurotic Defenses

G. *Displacement*: Shifting emotions about one object/individual onto another object/individual. For example, after being scolded by his consultant, a senior resident comes to the ward and started shouting at the intern. Here, actually the senior resident is angry at the consultant but he is displacing his anger on the intern. Displacement is involved in the development of **phobias**[Q].

H. *Intellectualization*: Excessive use of intellectual process to avoid the painful emotions. For example, a doctor who was diagnosed with pancreatic cancer has a long discussion about the pathophysiology of the cancers with his treating physician. Here, the doctor is trying to avoid the painful emotion of being diagnosed with the cancer by discussing excessively about the pathophysiology of cancers.

I. *Isolation of affect*: Removing the feelings associated with a stressful life event. For example, without showing any emotions, a woman tells her family members that she has been diagnosed with advanced stage cholangiocarcinoma.

J. *Repression*: It is one of the most important defense mechanism, often referred to as the "primary" defense mechanism. It is unconsciously forgetting something, which cannot be retrieved later. For example, a young girl who was sexually abused by her father, "forgets" this incidence of sexual abuse. Now, even if she wants to recall it, she cannot do it in normal circumstances.

K. *Rationalization*: Offering rational explanations to justify own unacceptable behavior. For example, an alcoholic blamed his family environment for his habit of excessive drinking. It is a commonly used defense mechanism in **substance use disorders**.

L. *Dissociation*: Splitting of a single (e.g. memory, identity) or group of mental functions from the remaining mental functions. It is seen in disorders like **dissociative identity disorder**, where for example, the identity of an individual gets split from rest of the mental functions.

M. *Reaction formation*: Transformation of feelings into exact opposite. For example, a man who is actually infatuated by an office colleague tells his friend that he really hates her. Here, the actual feeling is that of infatuation but that is being transformed into the feeling of "hatred".

N. *Undoing*: An act which is done to nullify a previous act. For example, a husband brings gifts for wife next day after having a fight with her the previous day. The defense mechanism of undoing is used in **obsessive compulsive disorder**[Q].

O. *Aim inhibition*: Placing a limitation upon instinctual demands, accepting partial or modified fulfillment of desires. For example, a student who wanted to became a doctor but who was not able to clear the pre medical tests takes admission in a veterinary course and becomes a veterinary doctor.

Mature Defenses

P. *Altruism*: Satisfying internal needs by helping others. For example, while driving in a drunk state, a man met an accident and lost his son who was travelling alongside him. Later, he started a campaign against drunk driving and started educating people about ills of drunk driving.

Q. *Anticipation*: Planning in advance to deal with an uncomfortable event. For example, a student plans all his arguments comprehensively before going to home after a bad exam result.

R. *Humor*: Using comedy to deal with unpleasant feeling and situations. For example, two medical students joked and laughed at themselves after getting humiliated by the examiner during the viva.

S. *Sublimation*: Expression of unacceptable feelings in a socially acceptable manner. For example, a middle aged man with unacceptable sexual desire becomes a painter and starts making nude paintings. Here, the sexual desires are getting an outlet and its socially acceptable since painting nudes is considered an art.

T. *Suppression*: It is the only **voluntary or conscious defense mechanism**. It involves a voluntary decision to not think about an event for some time and hence avoid the accompanying emotions. For example, a medical student who is extremely stressed out because of an upcoming entrance exam decides to take a one day break during which he does not think at all about the exam.

Defense mechanisms in psychiatric disorder: All the defense mechanisms are used at times by all of us. However when used excessively, they can result in development of psychiatric disorders. Following is a list of few defense mechanisms and associated disorders:

A. *Obsessive compulsive disorder*: **Reaction formation**[Q], **displacement**[Q], **undoing, isolation of affect**[Q] **and inhibition**[Q]

B. *Phobia*: **Displacement and inhibition**[Q]

C. *Dissociative disorder*: **Dissociation**[Q]

D. *Neurosis*: **Regression**[Q].

PSYCHOSEXUAL STAGES OF DEVELOPMENT

Sigmund Freud[Q] proposed that the sexuality develops in multiple stages. Freud used the term "sexuality" in a broader concept that included others forms of pleasure also and not only genital sexuality. He proposed five stages of development. Freud further proposed that the development may get arrested at a particular stage (called **"fixation"**) and may result in development of psychiatric disorders:

A. *Oral stage (0-1.5 years)*: This is the first stage of development where in the pleasure is derived from the oral cavity. The child derives pleasure in cutting, biting, chewing, etc.

B. *Anal stage (1.5-3 years)*: The site of pleasure is anal region. The child gets a sense of achievement by getting toilet trained. If the psychosexual development gets arrested at this stage (called **fixation at anal stage**), it can result in development of **obsessive compulsive disorder**[Q].

C. *Phallic stage (3-5 years)*: The site of pleasure is the genital area. According to Freud, penis becomes the organ of principal interest to children of both sexes. The male child develops what is known as **oedipus complex**[Q] in which he starts developing sexual feeling towards the mother and wants to replace the father. However, the male child also becomes fearful, that if father finds it out, his father might castrate him (and hence the child develops **castration anxiety**[Q]). The oedipus complex in male child gets resolved once the child shifts his affection away from mother to some other female and starts identifying (starts imitating father and trying to become like him) with the father.

In females, the oedipus stage unfolds differently (at times the term used for female child is **"electra complex"**). The girl child develops sexual desire for the father. At the same time, she becomes aware that she does not have a penis and desires to get one (known as "penis envy"). The female child believes that she was castrated and that's why does not have a penis and holds her mother responsible for it, developing anger against the mother. The stage gets resolved when the female child starts identifying with the mother. Failure to resolve the oedipus and electra complex can result in development of neurotic illnesses (like hysteria). Hence, the **neurotic illness develops due to fixation at phallic stage**[Q].

D. *Latent stage (5-12 years)*: During this stage, there is relative quiescence or inactivity of sexual drive and child focuses on learning and gaining skills.

E. *Genital stage (12 years onward till young adulthood)*: This stage is characterized by maturation of genital functioning and gradual achievement of a mature sexual and adult identity.

Psychoanalysis

Multiple Choice Questions

1. The term 'id' and "superego" were coined by:
   (DNB 2003, DNB 1994, WB 2001)
   A. Freud
   B. Skinner
   C. Erik Erikson
   D. Bleuler

2. Topographic theory of mind was given by: (NEET 2016)
   A. Adler
   B. Carl Jung
   C. Sigmund Freud
   D. Emil Kraepelin

3. Who is the father of psychoanalysis? (NEET 2016)
   A. Adler
   B. Carl Jung
   C. Sigmund Freud
   D. Emil Kraepelin

4. The part of mind which works on reality principle is:
   (DNB 2004, Karnataka 2001)
   A. id
   B. Ego
   C. Super ego
   D. Ego ideal

5. The term "free association" which is a fundamental technique of psychoanalysis was coined by?
   (DNB 2006, JIPMER 2001)
   A. Freud
   B. Adler
   C. Erikson
   D. Jung

6. Theory of "Psychosexual development" was given by:
   (DNB Dec 2010)
   A. Anna Freud
   B. Sigmund Freud
   C. Jean Piaget
   D. Skinner

7. Interpretation of dreams by Freud was published in:
   (UP 2001, KA 2002, DNB 1999)
   A. 1990
   B. 1900
   C. 1956
   D. 1919

8. Counter transference is: (AIIMS Nov 2011)
   A. Type of defense mechanism
   B. Psychic connection between patient and disease with transfer of psychic energy from body parts to brain
   C. Implies doctor's feelings towards patient
   D. Patient's feelings towards doctor during psychotherapy

9. According to Sigmund Freud, primary process thinking is: (JIPMER 2011)
   A. Illogical and bizarre
   B. Rational
   C. Absent during sleep
   D. Logical and unconscious

10. Psychodynamic theory of mental illness is based on:
    (AIIMS Nov 2007)
    A. Unconscious internal conflict
    B. Maladjusted reinforcement
    C. Organic neurological problem
    D. Focuses on teaching patients to restrain absurd thoughts

11. Wrong statement about psychoanalysis is:
    (DNB 2007; J&K 2008; TN 2006)
    A. Parapraxis has meaning
    B. Transference is patient's feeling for therapist
    C. Counter transference is clinician's feelings for patient
    D. Unguided communication has no meaning

12. Oedipus complex (given by Sigmund Freud) is seen in:
    (JIPMER 2017, DNB 2017, NEET 2016)
    A. Boys of 1-3 years of age
    B. Girls of 1-3 years of age
    C. Boys of 3-5 years of age
    D. Girls of 3-5 years of age

13. In psychoanalytic terms, obsessive compulsive disorder is fixed at: (DNB 1998, Delhi 1998, TN 2002, Mah. 2003)
    A. Oedipal stage
    B. Genital stage
    C. Oral stage
    D. Anal stage

14. Expression and consequent release of previously repressed emotion is called as: (NEET 2018)
    A. Regression
    B. Dissociation
    C. Abreaction
    D. All of the above

15. Freud's theory of dream includes all *except*:
    (NEET 2018)
    A. Displacement
    B. Condensation
    C. Symbolisation
    D. Correlation

16. Fixation of hysteria is:
    (DNB 1999, WB 2002, J&K 2004, PGI 2005)
    A. Genital
    B. Anal
    C. Oral
    D. Phallic

17. Following name(s) is/are associated with psychodynamic theory: (PGI Nov 2009)
    A. Carl Jung
    B. Sigmund Freud
    C. Emil Kraepelin
    D. Eugen Bleuler
    E. Kurt Schneider

Defense Mechanisms

18. Defense mechanism in depression: (DNB 2018)
    A. Altruism
    B. Projection
    C. Undoing
    D. Introjection

19. Which of the following is a mature defense mechanism?
    (DNB 2002, JIPMER 1991, UP 2007)
    A. Projection
    B. Reaction formation
    C. Anticipation
    D. Denial

20. Which of the following is not a neurotic defense mechanism? (DNB NEET 2014-15)
    A. Isolation
    B. Regression
    C. Reaction formation
    D. Undoing

21. Which of the following is a neurotic defense mechanism? (DNB NEET 2014-15)
    A. Repression
    B. Anticipation
    C. Projection
    D. Undoing

22. Which of the following excludes painful stimuli from awareness? (AIIMS 1998)
    A. Repression
    B. Reaction formation
    C. Projection
    D. Rationalization

23. Avoiding awareness of pain of reality by negative sensory data is seen in which of the following defense mechanisms? *(MH 2011)*
    A. Distortion   B. Denial
    C. Displacement   D. Dissociation

24. Postponing paying attention to a "conscious impulse" or "conflict" is a mature defense mechanism known as:
    A. Sublimation   B. Suppression
    C. Humor   D. Anticipation

25. A reluctant child forced to bring sugar from a shop spills half of it on the way. This is an example of:
    (JIPMER 1997, Delhi 2002, DNB 2004)
    A. Hysteria
    B. Passive aggression
    C. Disobedience
    D. Active aggression

26. A chronic alcoholic blames the family environment as a cause of his alcoholism. This is phenomenon of:
    (AIIMS 2000)
    A. Projection   B. Denial
    C. Rationalization   D. Sublimation

27. Ego's defense mechanism "Undoing" is typically seen in:
    (PGI 2001, AIIMS 1993, 1995)
    A. Depression
    B. Schizophrenia
    C. Obsessive compulsive neurosis
    D. Hysteria

28. Most important cause of neurotic reaction is the excessive use of: *(DNB 2005, PGI 1998, NIMHANS 2001, Mah. 2004)*
    A. Projection   B. Regression
    C. Suppression   D. Sublimation

29. Displacement reaction is characteristically seen in:
    (DNB 1998, MP 1998)
    A. Mania   B. Phobia
    C. Conversion disorder   D. Depression

30. Defense mechanism in phobia is: *(DNB NEET 2014-15)*
    A. Inhibition   B. Dissociation
    C. Distorsion   D. Conversion

31. Defense mechanisms involved in OCD are:
    (PGI 2016, PGI 2012, PGI 2007)
    A. Isolation of affect   B. Undoing
    C. Rationalization   D. Sublimation
    E. Reaction formation

32. Name the person shown here, who worked in the field of Psychoanalysis? *(NIMHANS 2016)*

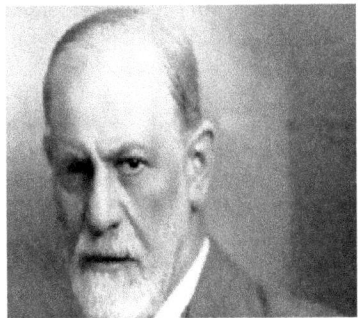

    A. Sigmund Freud   B. Erik Erikson
    C. Carl Jung   D. Erich Fromm

33. Who worked on dreams and wrote a book "Interpretation of Dreams"? *(NIMHANS 2018)*
    A. Sigmund Freud   B. Erik erikson
    C. Carl Jung   D. Adolf Meyer

Answers With Explanations

1. A. Freud
2. C. Sigmund Freud
3. C. Sigmund Freud
4. B. Ego
5. A. Freud
6. B. Sigmund Freud
7. B. 1900
8. C. Implies doctor's feelings towards patient
9. A. The primary process thinking is a characteristic of unconscious mind. It is illogical and aims for immediate wish fulfillment.
10. A. Psychodynamic (or psychoanalytic) theory stresses that unconscious memories and conflicts are responsible for development of psychiatric disorders. The "conflict" may be between different parts of mind such as id and ego or ego and superego.
11. D. According to psychoanalytic theory, "parapraxis" or "slips of tongue" are believed to reveal unconscious content and hence are believed to have meaning. The description of transference and counter transference given in this question is also correct. The last statement is wrong. In psychoanalysis, unguided communication is believed to have meaning. Unguided communication here refers to the technique of "free association" in which patient speaks all that comes into his mind, without any censoring. The "free association" helps in understanding the unconscious contents of mind and hence is meaningful.
12. C. Sigmund Freud described oedipus complex for both sexes, however, that term is mostly associated with male sex now a days.
13. D. Anal stage
    See text for explanation.
14. C. Abreaction
15. D. Correlation
16. D. Phallic
    See text for explanation.
17. A, B. Apart from Sigmund Freud, other big names associated with psychoanalysis include Carl Jung and Alfred Adler. Initially Jung and Adler worked along with Freud, however, later they separated and gave their own theories.

Defense Mechanisms

18. D. Introjection is a defense mechanism in which the person internalises the idea of another person. E.g. A person who is distressed at losing his mother, may create an internal image of the mother in his mind, this is introjection. If the person introjects an image towards whom he has mixture of love and hate, the person may end up hating self, and this results in development of depression.
19. C. Anticipation
20. B. Regression is an immature defense mechanism. Rest all are neurotic defense mechanism.
21. A, D. However, if you have to chose, go for repression. It is one of the most important neurotic defense mechanism.
22. A. Repression is the defense mechanism which removes painful memories or unacceptable desires away from the consciousness or awareness.
23. B. Denial is the defense mechanism which helps a person to avoid (or refuse to accept) the reality. Do not get confused by the phrase "negative sensory data".
24. B. Postponing or delaying action on a conscious impulse (a conscious wish) and its accompanying emotions is known as suppression.
25. B. passive aggression
    See text for explanation.
26. C. Rationalization
    See text for explanation.
27. C. Undoing is typically seen in obsessive compulsive disorder.
28. B. Excessive use of regression causes neurotic illnesses.
29. B. Displacement and Inhibition are the defense mechanisms involved in phobia.
30. A. Inhibition
31. A, B, E.
    This is one of the favorite question of PGI.
32. A. Sigmund Freud.
    It is unfortunate that students are being asked to identify the photographs in entrance examination, but we can not do anything about it. So, remember this photo. He is the father of psychoanalysis "Sigmund Freud"
33. A. Sigmund Freud.

13 CHAPTER

Miscellaneous

ELECTROCONVULSIVE THERAPY (ECT)

The convulsive therapies have long been used for treatment of psychiatric disorders. Initially, intramuscular injections of camphor were used to produce convulsions in patients with psychosis, with good therapeutic results. Later, electricity was used as an agent to induce convulsions and it was called "electroconvulsive therapy."

Types

A. *Direct ECT*: In this technique, anesthetic agents and muscle relaxants are not used. The generalized convulsions produced can result in **fractures^Q or teeth dislocations**. Due to higher incidence of side effects this technique is rarely used now.

B. *Modified ECT (Indirect ECT)*: Here, **anesthetic agents and muscle relaxants** are administered before giving ECT. As muscles are relaxed, the risk of bone fractures and other injuries from the motor activity during the seizures gets minimized.

Electrode Placement

Various configurations have been developed for electrode placement. These include:

A. *Bilateral ECT*: This is used most commonly and it involves placement of electrodes on both sides of the skull. In bilateral ECTs, various configurations of electrode placement have been devised. The **bifronto-temporal electrode placement** is deployed most commonly. Other commonly used configuration uses **bifrontal electrode placement**.

B. *Unilateral ECTs*: In an attempt to decrease the side effects of ECTs, the unilateral electrode placements have been introduced. The **right unilateral** ECT has been found to have better side effect profile in comparison to the bilateral ECTs and is being increasingly used.

Mechanism of Action

The induction of a bilateral generalized seizure is considered necessary for the beneficial effect of ECTs. Earlier it was considered that the response to ECTs was an "all or none" phenomenon, however of late it has been found that at least in right unilateral ECTs, a dose response relation is present. The mechanism of action of ECTs is still not completely understood. Various hypotheses include changes in the neurotransmitters (especially downregulation of postsynaptic β-adrenergic receptors), changes in growth factors and molecular mechanisms (latest research suggests increase in brain derived neurotrophic factor, **BDNF^Q** as an important mechanism) and neurogenesis in areas like hippocampus.

Indications

A. *Depression (Major depressive disorder)*: The ECT was initially invented for the treatment of schizophrenia and other psychotic illnesses, however currently it is mostly used for treatment of **depression^Q**. ECT is effective for depression in both major depressive disorder as well as bipolar disorder. The clearest indication for ECT is depression with **suicide risk^Q**. The indications of ECT in depression include the following:
   - Depression with suicide risk (**ECT is treatment of choice** in **acutely suicidal patients^Q** due to immediate onset of action)
   - Depression with stupor^Q
   - Depression with psychotic symptoms (psychotic depression or delusional depression)
   - In case of failed medication trials or intolerance to medications.

A. *Manic episode*: Electroconvulsive therapy can be used in the treatment of acute mania, however since effective pharmacotherapy is available for mania, ECT is not the first line treatment. The ECT is used in only those patients who are either intolerant/unresponsive to pharmacotherapy or when mania is so severe that there is a risk of homicide/suicide or danger of physical violence and immediate control of symptoms is required.

B. *Schizophrenia*: Electroconvulsive therapy is the first line treatment in **catatonic schizophrenia^Q**. It is also effective in other types of schizophrenia however since the advent of antipsychotics, is used only if patient is unresponsive/intolerant to medications. Electroconvulsive therapy is not effective in **chronic schizophrenia**^{Q}.

C. Other indications where ECT is occasionally used include **intractable seizures**^{Q}, **neuroleptic malignant syndrome**^{Q}, delirium, on-off phenomenon of Parkinson's disease, etc.

Adverse Effects

A. *Memory disturbances*: It is the most common side effect of ECT. Both retrograde and anterograde amnesia is seen, however, **retrograde amnesia**^{Q} is much more common. It is however mild and recovery occurs usually within 1-6 months after treatment.

B. Other side effects include delirium, headache, muscle aches, fractures (very rare with modified ECT), nausea and vomiting.

C. *Prolonged seizures*: After administration of ECT, if the seizure continues for more than **180 seconds**^{Q}, it is called as a prolonged seizure and must be terminated to prevent progression to status epilepticus.

Contraindications

There are **no absolute contraindications**^{Q} of ECT. Earlier raised intracranial tension was considered as an absolute contraindication, however it is now regarded as a relative contraindication. Pregnancy is not a contraindication for ECT. The following are the relative contraindications of ECT:

A. **Raised intracranial tension**^{Q} **(space occupying lesion in CNS**^{Q}**)**
B. Recent myocardial infarction
C. Severe hypertension
D. Cerebrovascular disease
E. Severe pulmonary disease
F. Retinal detachment.

COGNITIVE DEVELOPMENT STAGES

The thinking process undergoes a series of changes as the child grows up into an adult. **Jean Piaget**^{Q}, described four stages of development of thinking processes, also known as cognitive developmental stages. These are described below:

A. *Sensorimotor stage (Birth to 2 years)*: This is the first stage. During this stage, child learns through sensory observations and gradually gains control of his motor functions. Initially, the child thinks that if he cannot see an object, it means that the object has ceased to exist. For example, if a rattle with which child is playing, is taken away from the child and is covered, so that the child can no longer see it, the child will think that the rattle no longer exists and will not try to look for it. This type of thinking is also described as **"out of sight, out of mind"**^{Q} and **"here and now"**^{Q} type of thinking. In the end of the sensorimotor stage the child develops **"object permanence"**, which is the development of the concept that object continue to exist even if they are not visible currently. In the above example, once the child develops object permanence, he will try to search for the rattle by removing the covering cloth as he now knows that the rattle continues to exist though he is not able to see it. Another important development at around 18 months, is a process known as **"symbolization"**. It means that the infants now start developing mental symbols and using words for objects. For example, they make a mental symbol to represent a ball and use a word for it. The development of "object permanence" indicates the transition to the next stage of development, i.e. stage of preoperational thought.

B. *Stage of preoperational thought (2-7 years)*: In this stage, use of symbols and language becomes more extensive. The thinking process is characterized by **"intuitive thought"**,^{Q} which refers to thinking without use of reasoning and an inability to use logicality. The children are also **"egocentric"** in this stage, which means that they are only concerned about their own needs and cannot think from others perspective.

C. *Stage of concrete operations (7-11 years)*: In this stage, the egocentric thought is replaced by "operational thought" and hence the children start to see things from others perspective also. The thinking is concrete (concrete thinking is the literal thinking). For example, when asked, the meaning of proverb "people who live in glasshouses should not throw stones" the child will say that "if my house is of glass, I should not throw stones as it will break my house". The child is not able to understand the deeper meaning. The logical thinking starts to develop and children are able to understand and follow rules and regulations. Two important developments in this stage are attainment of **"conservation"** and **"reversibility"**. Conservation is the ability to understand that despite changes in shape, the object remains the same. For example, water may be transferred from a cup to a glass, and may appear different in shape, however the amount will remain the same. Reversibility is the capacity to understand that one thing can turn into another and back again, e.g. water and ice.

D. *Stage of formal operations (11 to end of adolescence)*: This stage is characterized by development of **abstract thinking**^{Q}, which is ability to understand the deeper meaning and deduce the larger meanings. For example, when asked to explain the meaning of phrase "pen is mightier than sword", a child with concrete thinking will say that the pen is heavier and stronger than the sword, whereas a child who has achieved abstract thinking will say that "power of knowledge is stronger than power of brute force". The thinking becomes logical, the child understands the concept of permutation and combination and probability. There is development of "hypothetico deductive thinking". Hypothetico deductive thinking is ability to make hypothesis and use deductive reasoning (ability to deduce, e.g. a child while playing a video game observes that whenever he breaks a banana, apple or cherry, he loses point, and hence is able to deduce that in this game to win he should avoid breaking the fruits).

LEARNING THEORY

Learning is acquiring of new behavioral patterns. The two types of learning are:

A. Classical conditioning
B. Operant conditioning

A. **Classical conditioning**: Classical conditioning (also called respondent conditioning) results from the repeated pairing of a neutral stimulus with one that naturally produces a response. The concepts of classical conditioning emerged from the experiments of Russian physiologist, Ivan Pavlov. The Pavlovian experiment included the following:

Under normal circumstances, a dog would salivate to the smell of food. The ringing of bell would not produce any salivation response. In the experiment, a bell was rung everytime before the presentation of food. The dog ultimately paired the bell with the food. Eventually the ringing of bell alone started to produce salivation, even if no food was presented to the dog. The following are the elements of classical conditioning:

- *Unconditioned stimulus*: It is a stimulus that naturally without any learning, produces a response. For example, smell of food, which produces a response of salivation.
- *Unconditioned response*: It is the natural response to an unconditioned stimulus. For example, salivation is the unconditioned response to smell of food.
- *Conditioned stimulus*: It is a stimulus which when paired with unconditioned stimulus, starts producing a response. For example, ringing of bell usually does not produce any response. However, when it is repeatedly paired with food (unconditioned stimulus), it also starts to produce a response.
- *Conditioned response*: The response which results from pairing of conditioned stimulus to the unconditioned stimulus. For example, the salivation which results secondary to ringing of bell is a conditioned response.
- *Extinction*: If the conditioned stimulus (ringing of bell) is presented repeatedly without the unconditioned stimulus (smell of food), the response (salivation) will decrease and eventually disappear. This is called extinction.
- **Stimulus generalization**[Q]: Here, a conditioned response gets transferred from one stimulus to other. For example, apart from the bell, ringing of a tuning fork also starts resulting in salivation.

B. *Operant conditioning (Instrumental conditioning)*: The principles of operant conditioning were given by BF Skinner. According to this theory, a behavior is determined by its **consequences**[Q] for the individual. Hence, according to this theory any behavior can be learned or unlearned and its frequency can be changed by modifying the consequences of that behavior. If a behavior is followed by pleasant consequence (called reward), that behavior will get reinforced, i.e. its frequency will increase. For example, if a child is given a chocolate on studying for a particular amount of time, the frequency of studying will increase. Similarly, if the consequence is negative, the frequency of behavior will decrease. For example, if a child is slapped on using a bad word, the frequency of using bad words will decrease.

Types: The frequency of a behavior is increased by positive or negative reinforcement and decreased by punishment or extinction.

Table 1: Types of operant conditioning.

Type	Effect	Example
Positive reinforcement[Q]	Behavior is increased by a positive consequence (reward)	A child increases his study hours as every study session is rewarded with a chocolate
Negative reinforcement[Q]	Behavior is increased to avoid a negative consequence	A child increases cleaning of his room to avoid scolding by the mother
Punishment[Q]	Behavior is decreased by a negative consequence	A child stops using foul language after getting slapped for the same
Extinction	Behavior is decreased due to lack of reinforcement	An intern who used to work very hard in the ward, becomes inefficient as he was never praised by his seniors.

Psychotherapy

Psychotherapy is treatment of psychiatric disorders by using psychological methods. The following are important kinds of psychotherapy:

Behavior Therapy

According to learning theory, the maladaptive behaviors are learned by either classical conditioning or operant conditioning and hence can be unlearnt. A large number of psychiatric disorders can be treated, if the psychiatric symptoms are considered as learned maladaptive behaviors. Behavior therapy is a psychological treatment in which the maladaptive behaviors of patients are changed to improve the quality of life. Behavior therapy is a generic term and is used to describe a variety of specific techniques, which intend to remove maladaptive behaviors. The techniques of behavior therapy include.

A. *Systematic desensitization*: This technique was developed according to the principle of **"reciprocal inhibition"**^{Q}. According to this principle if an anxiety provoking stimulus is provided while a person is in a relaxed state, the anxiety gets inhibited. For example, if a person who is phobic to spiders is first made to relax and then is exposed to a spider, he may develop much lesser anxiety. In systematic desensitization, the patient is first taught relaxation techniques (usually progressive muscle relaxation) and then a hierarchy is made of anxiety provoking stimuli. For example, if a person is afraid of heights, the list may have "standing at the roof of a ten-storey building" at the top, "standing on the balcony at second floor" in the middle and "standing on third stair" at the bottom of list. The patient is then exposed (or asked to imagine that exposure) to a series of anxiety provoking stimuli, starting with the least anxiety provoking stimulus while he is also using relaxation techniques. As the patient masters the technique of relaxation in the presence of an anxiety provoking stimuli, he moves up to the next stimulus. Systematic desensitization is used in the treatment of **phobias**^{Q}, **obsessive compulsive disorders**^{Q} and certain sexual disorders.

B. *Therapeutic graded exposure or in vivo exposure (or exposure and response prevention)*: It is similar to systematic desensitization except that no relaxation techniques are used and that real life situations are used. For example, if a patient is afraid of dogs, the exposure will start with looking at a picture of dog, then looking at a video of dog, followed by looking at a dog from a distance and finally holding a dog in arms. The patient learns to get habituated to anxiety (i.e. he learns that anxiety gradually decreases by itself). It is used in **phobias**^{Q} and obsessive compulsive disorder.

C. *Flooding (Implosion)*: Here, the patient is made to confront the feared situation directly, without any hierarchy, as in systematic desensitization or graded exposure. No relaxation exercises are used either. The patient is exposed to the feared situation, experiences fear and anxiety which gradually subsides, and the patient is not allowed to escape.

D. *Modeling (Participant modeling)*: Here, therapist himself makes the contact with phobic stimulus and demonstrates this to the patient. Patient learns by imitation and observation. For example, a therapist himself took a dog in his arms while a patient who had phobia of dogs observed him. This technique is used in phobias as well as obsessive compulsive disorders.

E. *Assertiveness training*: Here a person is taught to be assertive while asking for his rights and while refusing unjust demands of others.

F. *Social skills training*: Usually used in patients with schizophrenia, it involves imparting skills required for dealing with others and living a social life.

G. *Aversive conditioning (Aversion therapy)*: It is the clinical use of principles of classical conditioning. It is used for treatment of unwanted behaviors (such as **paraphilias**^{Q}). Here, the patient is asked to imagine that he is indulging into an unwanted behavior and immediately a painful stimulus (such as an electric shock) is given. An association gets created between the unwanted behavior and **painful stimuli**^{Q} and the unwanted behavior ceases. It is now rarely used due to ethical considerations.

Uses: The various technique of behavior therapy are used primarily in treatment of anxiety disorders (like phobia, panic disorders). Behavior therapy can also be used in depression, dissociative disorders, eating disorders, sexual disorders, personality disorders, substance used disorders and schizophrenia.

Biofeedback

It is a treatment technique that uses the principles of operant conditioning. The biofeedback is based on the idea that autonomic nervous system (which is usually involuntary) can be brought under voluntary control with the help of operant conditioning. It is used for treatment of disorders, which are caused by dysfunction in autonomic control such as asthma, tension headaches, arrhythmias, etc. The technique uses a feedback instrument, the choice of which depends on the patient's problem. This instrument gives patient a feedback about the current status of a specific autonomic function. For example, an electromyogram (EMG) may be used to give patient feedback about muscle tension in a particular muscle group. When the muscle tension is high, the EMG will emit a higher tone and when muscle tension is low (i.e. when muscle is relaxed), the EMG will emit a lower tone. Using feedback, patient learns to control his muscle tone and hence is able to control symptoms caused by increased muscle tone (e.g. bruxism).

Cognitive Therapy

The cognitive theory assumes that the cognitions (thoughts) are at the core of psychiatric symptoms. On the basis of early experiences, an individual may develop wrong patterns of thinking, known as cognitive distortions (or maladaptive assumptions). For example, a child who was praised when he came first and was scolded when he got second rank, may develop a cognitive distortion that "To be successful it is necessary to get first rank, otherwise I would be considered as a failure". These cognitive distortions (or maladaptive assumptions) give rise to "negative automatic thoughts", which are thoughts with a negative connotation and appear automatically. For example, in the above example, when the child with the above mentioned cognitive distortion has a below expectation performance in the exam, he may start having "negative automatic thoughts" like " I am a failure", "I performed badly in exams, I will perform badly in every other exam" "I will never get a postgraduation seat", etc. The cognitive therapy aims to correct these "negative automatic thoughts" and "cognitive distortions". When along with these, behavioral techniques are also used, the therapy method is known as "cognitive behavioral therapy". Cognitive therapy and cognitive behavioral therapy are used in the treatment of depression, panic disorder, obsessive compulsive disorder, personality disorder and somatoform disorder.

Cognitive Distortions: Following is the list of common **cognitive distortions^Q** (maladaptive assumptions):
A. *All or nothing thinking*: Seeing things in black and white. For example, if I failed to get a particular job, it means that I would never ever get any job.
B. *Approval seeking*: Belief that you should always be liked and loved by others, otherwise life would be terrible.
C. *Disqualifying positive*: It is a tendency of refusal to acknowledge the positive events in life and insisting that they "don't count". For example, a housewife was praised by her husband, however she thought that "he is praising me just to make me feel better, in reality I don't deserve to be praised".
D. *Emotional reasoning*: Belief that your emotions reflect the reality. For example, if I am having a bad feeling about a person, it means that the person in reality is a bad human being even if I have no evidences for the same.
E. *Fallacy of fairness*: Tendency to judge a random negative event as an issue of justice. For example, you missed the flight due to heavy traffic and you believe "life is always unfair to me".
F. *Jumping to conclusions*: Making an interpretation with minimal evidence. For example, a friend did not reply to your message and you made a conclusion that the friend hates you.
G. *Labeling mislabeling*: Giving labels to self or others. For example, if your room-mate did not clean room once, you label him as a "lazy slob".
H. *Magnification (catastrophizing) and minimization*: Focusing on worst possible outcome is maximization and in its extreme form, it is called catastrophizing. For example, if you lose a hundred rupee note and you say that its one of the biggest losses I ever had, its maximization. If you say that now there is nothing left in my life, its catastrophization. Minimization is trying to minimize the importance of events. For example, an alcoholic when criticized about his heavy drinking says that "I don't really drink much, just a peg here and there".
I. *Mental filtering/selective perception*: Picking a single negative detail while ignoring the rest. For example, in a party, everybody gave you a complement for your looks, however a single person said that "have you gained weight" and you give all the importance to that one person's remark and ignore all the praise.
J. *Overgeneralization*: Considering a single negative event and making a general rule out of it. For example, you made a mistake at work and then you start thinking "I always mess up everything". Labeling is an extreme form of overgeneralization.
K. *Personalization*: Blaming yourself for event, which you are not responsible for. For example, a wife blames herself for her husband's extramarital affair.
L. *Should statements*: Having a lots of rules about how should you and others behave. For example, I should exercise daily, I should not be lazy.

Substance Use Disorder: Psychosocial Treatment

The patients with substance use disorders (and other problematic behaviors) go through a series of changes before quitting the substance use. Various models of these changes have been described, the most acceptable model is known as **transtheoretical model of change**. According to this model, the following are the stages of change:
A. *Precontemplation*: In this stage, the substance user does not see any problem in his behavior and does not think about quitting.

B. *Contemplation*: In this stage, the substance user starts realizing that he has a problem and that he is taking substance excessively. He considers about the **pros and cons**[Q] of stopping substance use. However, he is yet to make any decision.
C. *Preparation*: In this stage, the substance user decides to quit the substance and starts making a plan to quit.
D. *Action*: In this stage, the substance user actually stops taking the substance and makes changes in his behaviors (e.g. he stops meeting with the friends who use drugs in an attempt to keep away himself from drugs), starts taking treatment.
E. *Maintenance*: In this stage, the patient continues to stay away from substances (drugs) and continues with the treatment and other behaviors to prevent relapse.

A patient may remain in maintenance stage or may relapse if he starts taking substance again. Usually, a patient has few relapses before attaining complete abstinence (freedom) from substance.

Various psychological treatment methods have been devised to help patient quit substance use and move from stages of precontemplation to maintenance. One of the most commonly used technique, which focuses on increasing the motivation of the patient to quit substance is known as **motivation enhancement therapy** or **motivational interviewing**.

Once the patient has reached maintenance stage, relapse prevention techniques are used to prevent any relapses (return to previous pattern of substance intake).

PSYCHOSURGERY

The surgical techniques for treatment of psychiatric disorder are rarely used and are reserved for only the chronic and severe cases, which have not responded to all other methods of treatment. The psychosurgeries involve creating a lesion in the limbic system or its connecting fibers (limbic system is considered to be responsible for normal and abnormal emotional reactions). The lesions are nowadays produced with precision using stereotactic methods. The following are the commonly used psychosurgeries.

A. *Stereotactic subcaudate tractotomy*: It produces a subcaudate lesion and is used in chronic, severe and intractable cases of depression, obsessive compulsive disorder and schizoaffective disorder.
B. *Stereotactic limbic leucotomy*: Small lesion is made in subcaudate and also a lesion is made in cingulate bundle. It is used in treatment of chronic, severe and intractable obsessive compulsive disorder and schizophrenia.
C. *Amygdalotomy*: A lesion is made in amygdala in patients with severe, uncontrolled aggression.

NEUROPSYCHOLOGICAL TESTS

Neuropsychology is a branch of psychology which examines the relationship between the behavior and brain functioning. It tries to locate the areas of disturbances in brain, on the basis of behavioral symptoms (including cognitive, sensory, motor and emotional symptoms). Neuropsychological tests are used extensively for various purposes. Few of them have been discussed below:

A. **Neuropsychological assessment of intelligence and personality:**
   - *Intelligence testing*: The simplest way of measuring intelligence is in terms of Intelligence Quotient (IQ) IQ = MA/CA × 100, MA is the mental age and CA is the chronological age, In this formula, the maximum chronological age can be 15.

   Now, much better and precise tests have been devised that measure the intelligence, few commonly used tests include:
   a. **Wechsler adult intelligence scale**[Q]
   b. Malin's intelligence scale for Indian children (MISIC)
   c. Bhatia's battery of performance tests of intelligence.

   - *Personality assessment*: The personality assessment can be done using two types of test:
   a. *Objective test*: These are standardized tests which give numerical scores and can be analyzed using standard result tables. For example, Minnesota Multiphasic Personality Inventory (MMPI).
   b. *Projective tests*: In these tests, patients are provided with ambiguous stimuli (unclear stimuli) and it is believed that the patient's response to such unclear stimulus reflects his internal thought processes and emotional factors. The patient "projects" his internal situation on to the test question and finally an expert analyzes the patient's answers and deduces the aspects of patient's personality. The projective tests include:
      - **Rorschach test**[Q]: The patient is shown ten cards which have inkblots and is asked what he sees in the card.
      - **Thematic apperception test (TAT)**[Q]: Here patients are shown certain pictures and asked to make stories about them
      - **Sentence completion test**[Q]: Here patients are given incomplete sentences and are asked to complete them. For example, a sentence may be like "I wish I............"

- *Word association technique*: Here the examiner says a word and patient has to respond with the first word that comes into his mind.
- *Draw a person test (DAPT)*: Here patient is asked to draw a person and then specific questions are asked about what he drew.

B. **Neuropsychological assessment for brain disorders or organic mental disorders:** Several tests have been devised which extensively measure a wide range of cognitive functions like memory, motor functions, sensory functions, problem solving, reading, writing, arithmetic, etc. Few such important tests include:
- Luria Nebraska Neuropsychological battery
- Halstead Reitan battery of neuropsychological tests[Q]
- **Bender Gestalt Test**[Q] *(Bender visual motor gestalt test)*: This test is used mostly as a screening tool for organic brain disorders[Q].

IMPORTANT ACTS

1. **Mental Healthcare Act, 2017 (MHCA 2017):** A new legislation that deals with treatment and rights of patients with mental illness came into being in 2017, and is referred to as Mental Health Care Act, 2017. The important clauses of this Act are described below:

   A. Capacity to make mental healthcare and treatment decisions: According to MHCA 2017, every person, including those who have a mental illness, is assumed to have a **capacity** to decide about what kind of treatment (including admission) they want to have for their mental illness, if they have the ability to-
      a. Understand the information that is given to them and on the basis of which they have to take the decision (e.g. information about the illness, the symptoms, the treatment used, etc.)
      b. Understand the consequences of their decisions (e.g. a patient who is having suicidal thoughts and not willing to take treatment, should be able to understand that not taking treatment can be life-threatening for him)
      c. To communicate their decision by using speech or gestures, etc.

   B. **Advance directive**[Q]: Every person (who is not a minor), can make an advance directive in which he can mention-
      a. The way he wishes to be treated for a mental illness
      b. The way he wishes not to be treated for a mental illness

   The advance directive would be applicable only if a person, loses the **capacity to make mental healthcare or treatment decisions.**

   It is the duty of psychiatrist (or medical officer) in charge of treatment, to ensure that treatment is being given according to advance directive made by the patient. However, it is the duty of patient (or caregiver or nominated representative) to provide access to the advance directive to the treating doctor. If due to following of advance directive, there are some unforeseen consequences, doctor cannot be held liable for the same.

   C. Nominated representative: Every person can appoint a nominated representative (who should not be a minor, and competent in discharging his duties as a nominated representative) and remove him, if he wishes to. If a person loses capacity to make mental healthcare or treatment decisions, his nominated representative will help (or will take) in taking decisions about treatment of the person.

   D. Admission: The MHCA 2017 allows two types of admissions
      a. Independent admissions: When the patient himself wants to get admitted
      b. Supported admissions: A person who needs admission, however, has lost the capacity to make mental healthcare or treatment decisions, and hence needs high level of support from the nominated representative, can be admitted as a 'supported admission'. The nominated representative gives consent for admission in this case.

   E. Ban on direct electroconvulsive therapy[Q] (ECT without use of muscle relaxants and anesthesia)

   F. Ban on ECT for minors (In a rare case, if psychiatrist in charge considers ECT is required for treatment of minor, he will have to take informed consent of guardian and prior permission from mental health review board[Q])

   G. Ban on psychosurgery (In a rare case, if psychiatrist in charge considers psychosurgery, he will have to take informed consent of patient and prior permission from mental health review board)

   H. Decriminalization of suicide: Any person who attempts to commit suicide shall be presumed to be under severe stress and should not be tried or punished (Earlier, Section 309 of IPC, prescribed punishment for those who attempted suicide)

I. **Restraints and seclusion**[Q]: A patient can be physically restrained only-
   a. If it is the only way to prevent harm to self or others
   b. If it is authorized by psychiatrist in charge

2. **Protection of Children from Sexual Offences Act (POCSO, 2012)**

   Protection of Children from Sexual Offences Act (2102) was passed to provide a legal framework for protection of children from sexual offences. It is a gender neutral Act for both the children and the accused. It classifies various offences that can be punished including-
   a. Child pornography
   b. Sexual harassment (e.g. use of sexually colored language, making sexual gestures, etc.)
   c. Sexual assault (involves inappropriate touch)
   d. Penetrative sexual assault (involves vaginal/anal/oral/urethral penetration of child)
   e. Aggravated penetrative sexual assault/aggravate sexual assault

   The term '**aggravated**'[Q] is added with penetrative sexual assault/sexual assault in certain situations which are considered to be even more gruesome and involves offenses done by-
   1. Persons who are in position of authority such as police officers, armed forces, management or staff of jail/remand home/hospital, etc.
   2. Where a gang is involved
   3. Use of deadly weapons, etc.
   4. Causing grievous hurt, attempts to murder or makes the female child pregnant
   5. Done repeatedly or on a child below 12
   6. In course of communal or sectarian violence, etc.

 SPIKES Protocol

It is a protocol for breaking bad news to patients about their illness. It involves six steps
1. S- Setting up the interview (interviewing with some privacy, involving significant others, sitting down, etc.)
2. P- Assessing the patient's Perception (what patient perceives/knows about his condition)
3. I- Obtaining the patient's Invitation (Finding out how much patient wants to know, e.g. would you like me to tell the details of the diagnosis)
4. K- Giving Knowledge and information (diagnosis, treatment, prognosis)
5. E- Addressing patient's Emotions (ask how patient feel and respond with empathy)
6. S- Strategy and Summary (Plan a strategy and explain)

 Domestic Violence

Domestic violence (spouse abuse) usually involves repetitive assault on wife by the husband (but can occur in any intimate relationship). The traits of perpetrators (those who commit the violence) of domestic violence include-
a. Being a victim of abuse: Those who become abuser, have usually faced abuse in childhood or have witnessed abuse while growing up.
b. Alcohol abuse
c. Immaturity, dependence and nonassertiveness and feelings of inadequacy (husband who feels threatened at work/with peers, may humiliate wife, to build his self esteem)
d. Jealousy (suspiciousness): Abusers get threatened by relationship of wife with friends and coworkers and may try to socially isolate them.

Wives who are battered too tend to have high dependence trait and are likely to have grown up in violent homes

Multiple Choice Questions

ECT

1. **Indications for ECT is/are:** *(PGI May 2010)*
   A. Psychotic depression
   B. Catatonic schizophrenia
   C. Cyclothymia
   D. Dysthymia
   E. Post-traumatic stress disorder

2. **Best marker for electroconvulsive therapy:**
   A. CSF 5 HIAA *(AIIMS Nov 2008)*
   B. CSF serotonin
   C. Brain derived growth factor
   D. CSF dopamine

3. **Anesthetic agent used in ECT is:** *(JIPMER 2016)*
   A. Ketamine B. Thiopentone
   C. Propofol D. Methohexital

4. **ECT is currently indicated as a line of treatment in the following conditions *except*:** *(UPSC 2008)*
   A. Catatonic schizophrenia
   B. Severe depression with psychosis
   C. Manic depressive psychosis
   D. Obsessive compulsive disorder

5. **ECT is indicated in:** *(AIIMS 1998)*
   A. Neurotic depression
   B. Auditory hallucination
   C. Chronic schizophrenia
   D. Delusional depression

6. **ECT is not useful in treatment of:** *(NIMHANS 2014)*
   A. Residual schizophrenia
   B. Catatonic schizophrenia
   C. Depression with suicidal tendencies
   D. Psychotic depression

7. **ECT in depressive phase of Bipolar disorder is useful because it:** *(PGI 1999)*
   A. Produces recurrence B. Reduces recurrence
   C. Shortens duration D. Increases drug effects

8. **All of the following are indications for ECT *except*:** *(DNB NEET 2014-15)*
   A. Intractable seizures
   B. Depressive stupor
   C. Neuroleptic malignant syndrome
   D. Acute anxiety

9. **Absolute contraindication to ECT is:** *(AIIMS 1995)*
   A. Glaucoma B. Brain tumor
   C. Aortic aneurism D. MI

10. **ECT is absolutely contraindicated in:** *(AI 1992, DNB 1995)*
    A. Pregnancy
    B. Very ill patient
    C. Raised intracranial tension
    D. Severe heart disease

11. **Most common complication of ECT is:** *(AIIMS 1996)*
    A. Anterograde amnesia
    B. Retrograde amnesia
    C. Psychosis
    D. Depression

12. **Memory disturbance of ECT recovers in:** *(AIIMS 1996)*
    A. Few days to few weeks
    B. Few weeks to few months
    C. Few months to few years
    D. Permanent

13. **Most common complication of modified ECT:** *(AIIMS 1991, AI 2, DNB 1997)*
    A. Intracerebral bleed B. Fracture spine
    C. Bodyache D. Amnesia

14. **True about ECT is:** *(PGI May 2012, AIIMS 2011)*
    A. It is not a treatment for dysthymic disorder
    B. Used to treat complex partial seizures
    C. Used for those major depressive patients not responding to medication
    D. Memory impairment is a side effect
    E. Effective in OCD

15. **Brain stimulation is not done in:** *(PGI Nov 2016)*
    A. ECT
    B. Deep brain stimulation
    C. Repetitive transcranial magnetic stimulation
    D. Cognitive remediation

Names

16. **Who introduced cocaine in psychiatry:** *(Kerala 1998, DNB 1992)*
    A. Freud B. Jung
    C. Miller D. Stanley

17. **Moral treatment of mentally ill-patient was first stressed by:** *(AIIMS 1995, CMC 1998, DNB 2001, TN 2004)*
    A. Pinel B. Morel
    C. Kraepelin D. Sigmund Freud

18. **The eight stage classification of human life is proposed by:** *(DNB 2000, WB 2004, UP 2005)*
    A. Sigmund Freud B. Pavel
    C. Strauss D. Erikson

19. **Which of the following scientist propagated 'therapeutic community concept':** *(Karnataka 2000, DNB 2003)*
    A. JB Watson B. Maxwell Jones
    C. Freud D. Adler

20. **Scientist who won Nobel Prize for research in "split brain" was:** *(NIMHANS 2015)*
    A. Penfield B. Sperry
    C. Michael Morris D. Peek

Cognitive Development Stages

21. **Which of the following is a stage of intuitive thought appearance in Jean-Piaget scheme:** *(PGI 1999)*
    A. Sensorimotor
    B. Concrete
    C. Preoperational stage
    D. Formal operations stage

22. **Ability to form a concept and generalize is known as:** *(JIPMER 2011)*
    A. Concrete thinking
    B. Abstract thinking
    C. Intellectual thinking
    D. Delusional thinking

23. **In Piaget's theory of cognitive development 'out of sight, out of mind' and 'here and now' is seen in the stage of:** *(AIIMS 2013)*
    A. Sensorimotor stage
    B. Preoperational stage
    C. Concrete operational stage
    D. Formal operational stage

Learning Theory and Psychotherapy

24. **Pavlov's experiment is an example of:** *(AI 2006)*
    A. Operant conditioning
    B. Classical conditioning
    C. Learned helplessness
    D. Modeling

25. **'Reinforcement' is used in:** *(AIIMS 1994, 1999)*
    A. Psychoanalysis
    B. Hypnosis
    C. Abreaction
    D. Conditioned learning

26. **Behavior therapy to change maladaptive behavior using response as reinforcer uses the principles of:** *(AI 2003)*
    A. Classical conditioning
    B. Modeling
    C. Social learning
    D. Operant conditioning

27. **Many of our bad habits of day-to-day life can be removed by:** *(AIIMS Nov 2004)*
    A. Positive conditioning
    B. Negative conditioning
    C. Biofeedback
    D. Generalization

28. **Operant conditioning in which pain stimulus are given to a child for decreasing a certain undesired behavior can be classified as:** *(AI 2010, 1997)*
    A. Positive reinforcement
    B. Negative reinforcement
    C. Punishment
    D. Negotiation

29. **A child is not eating vegetables. His mother starts giving a chocolate each time he finishes vegetables in the diet. The condition is:** *(AIIMS Nov 2012)*
    A. Operant conditioning
    B. Classical conditioning
    C. Social training
    D. Negative reinforcement

30. **Patient of contamination phobia was asked by therapist to follow behind him and touch every thing he touches. During process therapist kept talking quietly and calmly to the patients. The patient was asked to repeat the procedure twice daily. The procedure is:** *(AIIMS May 2010)*
    A. Flooding
    B. Modeling
    C. Positive reinforcement
    D. Aversion therapy

31. **Therapeutic exposure is a form of:** *(MH 2011)*
    A. Behavior therapy
    B. Psychoanalysis
    C. Cognitive therapy
    D. Supportive therapy

32. **Reciprocal inhibition is done by:** *(SGPGI 2000)*
    A. Systematic desensitization
    B. Flooding
    C. Exposure and response prevention
    D. Psychoanalysis

33. **Along a pleasant stimulus, a noxious stimuli is given in treatment of alcohol dependence and paraphilias. This is an example for which kind of behavior therapy:** *(MH 2008)*
    A. Negative reinforcement
    B. Aversive therapy
    C. Punishment
    D. Flooding

34. **Behavior therapy is useful in:** *(PGI June 2008)*
    A. Psychosis
    B. OCD
    C. Personality disorder
    D. Panic attack
    E. Anxiety disorders

35. **A patient can be taught to control his involuntary physiological responses by which of the following therapies:** *(MH 2009)*
    A. Breathing exercise
    B. Stress modification
    C. Biofeedback
    D. Rational emotive therapy

36. **Which of the following is not a cognitive error/dysfunction?** *(AI 2010)*
    A. Catastrophic thinking
    B. Arbitrary inference
    C. Overgeneralization
    D. Thought block

37. **Typically changes in problem behavior shows how many stages:** *(DNB NEET 2014-15)*
    A. 2
    B. 3
    C. 4
    D. 5

38. **All of the following are parts of cognitive behavior change technique except:** *(AI 2010)*
    A. Precontemplation
    B. Consolidation
    C. Action
    D. Contemplation

39. **A chronic smoker taking 20 cigarettes per day has developed chronic cough. His family suggested quitting cigarettes. He is ready to quit and thinks about quitting but is reluctant to do so because he is worried that quitting will make him irritable. Which of the following option best describes the stage of behavior change:** *(AI 2011)*
    A. Precontemplation and preparation
    B. Contemplation and cost factor
    C. Contemplation and sickness susceptibility
    D. Belief

40. **A smoker is worried about the side effects of smoking. But he does not stop smoking thinking that he smokes less as compared to others and takes a good diet. This thinking is called as:** *(AIIMS May 2015)*
    A. Self exemption
    B. Cognitive error
    C. Self protection
    D. Distortion

Neuropsychological Tests

41. A Study comparing the behavioral and developmental changes in a normal brain with a damaged brain is: *(AIIMS 2013)*
    A. Neuropsychology
    B. Neurodevelopmental psychology
    C. Child psychology
    D. Criminal psychology

42. Rorschach inkblot test is: *(Bihar 2003)*
    A. Projective
    B. Subjective
    C. Both
    D. None of the above

43. Best test for diagnosis of organic mental disorder:
    A. Sentence completion test *(AI 2000)*
    B. Bender-Gestalt test
    C. Rorschach test
    D. Thematic appreciation test

44. Rorschach test measures: *(NIMHANS 2014, PGI 1999)*
    A. Intelligence
    B. Creativity
    C. Personality
    D. Neuroticism

45. Signs of organic brain damage are evident on:
    A. Bender-Gestalt test *(AI 2004)*
    B. Rorschach test
    C. Sentence completion test
    D. Thematic apperception test

46. Halstead Reitan battery involves all *except*:
    A. Finger oscillation
    B. Constructional praxis
    C. Rhythm
    D. Tactual performance

Miscellaneous

47. A person laughs to a joke, and then suddenly loses tone of all his muscles. Most probable diagnosis of this condition is: *(DNB Dec 2009)*
    A. Cataplexy
    B. Catalepsy
    C. Cathexis
    D. Cachexia

48. Hypomimia is: *(DNB NEET 2014-15)*
    A. Decreased ability to copy
    B. Decreased execution
    C. Deficit of expression by gesture
    D. Deficit of fluent speech

49. Deja vu is seen in: *(Kerala 1994)*
    A. Temporal lobe epilepsy
    B. Normal person
    C. Psychosis
    D. All of the above

50. Unfamiliarity of familiar things is seen in: *(Kerala 1999, JIPMER 2002) (Karnataka 1994)*
    A. Deja vu
    B. Jamais vu
    C. Deja entendu
    D. Deja pence

51. Catatonia is most commonly seen with:
    A. Schizophrenia *(DNB NEET 2014-15)*
    B. Depression
    C. Anxiety disorder
    D. Obsessive compulsive disorder

52. Catatonic features are seen in schizophrenia, they are also seen in: *(PGI June 2008)*
    A. Severe depression
    B. Conversion disorder
    C. Personality disorder
    D. Somatization disorder

53. When information memorized afterwards is interfered by the information learnt earlier, it is called:
    A. Retroactive inhibition *(AIIMS May 2004)*
    B. Proactive inhibition
    C. Simple inhibition
    D. Inhibition

54. Semantic memory includes all *except*: *(AIIMS May 2016)*
    A. Rules
    B. Events
    C. Words
    D. Language

55. Methods of learning in psychiatry are all *except*: *(AIIMS Nov 2007)*
    A. Modelling
    B. Catharsis
    C. Exposure
    D. Response prevention

56. According to Disabilities Act, 1995, the seventh disability is usually referred to as? *(AIIMS Nov 2008)*
    A. Neurological abnormality
    B. Mental illness
    C. Substance abuse
    D. Disability due to road traffic accident

57. Patients suffering from which of the following disease as per ICD/DSM criteria are eligible for disability benefit as per National Trust Act? *(AI 2009)*
    A. Schizophrenia
    B. Bipolar disorder
    C. Dementia
    D. Mental retardation

58. Consultation-liaison (CL) psychiatry involves diagnosing: *(MAHE 2006, SGPGI 2004)*
    A. Psychiatric illness in medically ill
    B. Medical illness in psychiatric patients
    C. Suicidal tendency in psychiatric patients
    D. Suicidal tendency in medically ill

59. The husband involved in battered wife syndrome is usually: *(JIPMER May 2018)*
    A. Dependent and suspicious
    B. Mature and assertive husband
    C. Immature and assertive
    D. Mature and non-controlling

60. Psychiatrist is not posted in: *(AIIMS May 2016)*
    A. Primary health centre
    B. District hospital
    C. Medical college
    D. Military hospital

61. Drug of choice for psychosis in Parkinson's disease is:
    A. Clozapine
    B. Haloperidol
    C. Lithium
    D. Risperidone

62. Which of these is the correct sequence of Maslow's hierarchy of needs? *(AIIMS Nov 2016)*
    A. Safety - Physiological Needs - Self actualization - Belonging - Self esteem
    B. Physiological Needs - Safety - Belonging - Self esteem - Self actualization
    C. Safety - Self actualization - Belonging - Physiological Needs - Self esteem
    D. Self actualization - Physiological Needs - Safety - Belonging - Self esteem

63. The following picture is associated with:
    (NIMHANS 2014)
    A. Ishihara test
    B. Snellens's test
    C. Rorschach test
    D. Stanford Binet IQ test

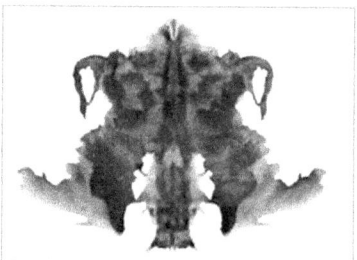

Prospective Questions

64. The following picture is used in which of the following psychological test:
    A. Rorschach test
    B. Thematic apperception test
    C. Bender Gestalt Test
    D. Wechslers adult intelligence scale

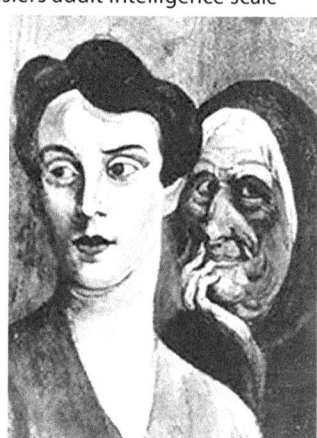

65. Identify this test, which is used as a screening tool for organic brain disorders?
    A. Rorschach test
    B. Thematic apperception test
    C. Bender Gestalt Test
    D. Wechslers adult intelligence scale

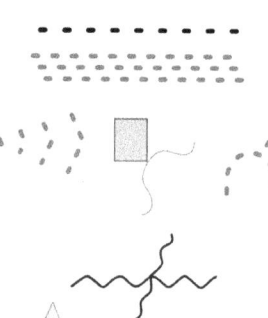

66. The following Nobel laureate described the "split brain" concept. Identify him:
    (NIMHANS 2014)
    A. Albert Einstein
    B. Rogor Wolcott Sperry
    C. Jill Taylor
    D. Patrick Modiano

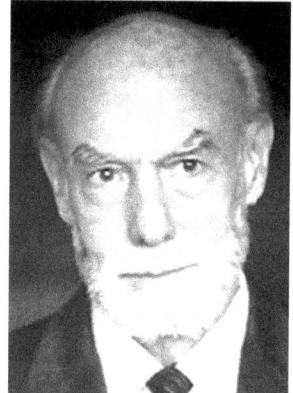

67. Legal protection for insane is covered under:
    (NIMHANS 2017)
    A. Mcnaughten's rule
    B. Currents rule
    C. Durham's rule
    D. Irresistible impulse test

68. The chromosome of a tall individual with criminal behavior is likely to be:
    (JIPMER 2017)
    A. XXY
    B. XYY
    C. XXXY
    D. XXYY

69. Shortest acting nonbenzodiazepine sedative is:
    (NIMHANS 2018)
    A. Zolpidem
    B. Zaleplon
    C. Zopiclone
    D. Midazolam

70. In the recently introduced, Mental Health Care Act 2017, which provision allows a patient with psychiatric disorder, the right of choosing the future course of treatment?
    (AIIMS Nov 2018)
    A. Advance directive
    B. Living will
    C. Treatment directive
    D. Future directive

71. All the folowing are true about mental health care act, 2017, *except*:
    (NIMHANS 2019)
    A. In advanced directive, patient can make a choice in advance about how he wishes to be treated
    B. ECT for minors (less than 18 years) can be given under specific circumstances after confirmation from the board.
    C. In exceptional cases, ECT can be given without anesthesia and muscle relaxants
    D. Restraining of patient can be done after permission from a psychiatrist

72. Under the POCSO act, all of the following are 'aggravated penetrative' sexual offences *except*:
    (AIIMS Nov 2018)
    A. Gang rape
    B. Offence by police officer
    C. On grounds of communal and sectarian violence
    D. By threat

73. Which is not included in mhGAP?
    (AIIMS Nov 2018)
    A. Communications with people seeking care
    B. Mobilising and providing social support
    C. Protection of human rights
    D. Screening of family members

74. **Spikes protocol is used for:** *(AIIMS Nov 2018)*
    A. Communication with patients
    B. Triage
    C. Writing death certificate
    D. Premarital counselling

AIIMS Pattern Question

75. **The following statements are true/false regarding the Mental Health Care Act, 2017** *(MHCA 2017)*
    1. Indirect Electroconvulsive therapy has been banned
    2. If a person develops a 'psychotic illness', it would be presumed that he has lost the capacity to take mental health decisions, and treatment would be done according to 'advanced directive'
    3. It is the duty of mental health professional in charge to find out the advanced directive written by a person and treat him in accordance to it
    4. Every person can appoint an individual who will help in taking treatment decisions if the person loses the capacity to take mental health care and treatment decisions. This individual is called as 'patient's representative'
    5. Suicide attempt has been decriminalised

Answers With Explanations

ECT

1. A, B. See text.
2. C. Latest research suggests that increase in brain derived neurotrophic factor, BDNF mediates the response to ECT and is the best marker for the same.
3. D. Methohexital is most commonly used as an anesthetic agent because of its shorter duration of action and lower association with postictal arrhythmias.
4. D. ECT is rarely used in the treatment of OCD.
5. D. Delusional depression or psychotic depression is an indication for ECT.
6. A. Electroconvulsive therapy is not effective in residual schizophrenia.
7. C. ECT shortens the duration of depressive episode. It does not prevent the recurrence unless given as a maintenance treatment.
8. D. ECT is occasionally used in intractable seizures, neuroleptic malignant syndrome, delirium, on-off phenomenon of Parkinson's disease. Acute anxiety is not an indication.
9. B. There are no absolute contraindications for ECT. Earlier, raised intracranial tension and space occupying lesions were considered as absolute contraindications, hence the best answer here is brain tumor.
10. C. Again, the best answer is raised intracranial tension.
11. B. Amnesia is the most common side effect of ECT. Both retrograde and anterograde amnesia are seen, however, retrograde amnesia is much more common.
12. B. Amnesia caused by ECT is mild and recovery occurs usually within 1–6 months after treatment.
13. D. Amnesia
14. A, C, D.
15. D. Cognitive remediation. Rest all, involve brain stimulation.

Names

16. A. Sigmund Freud studied about the effects of cocaine. It is also believed that he was addicted to cocaine for a long period.
17. A. Moral treatment of mentally ill patients using humane methods was first stressed by Pinel.
18. D. Erik Erikson divided the human life into eight stages, known as Erikson's psychosocial stages.
19. B. Therapeutic community is a group based approach for treatment of substance use disorders and other psychiatric disorders. It is a residential approach where in patients live in a house for long-term and have defined roles during the stay. The term "therapeutic community" was given by **Thomas Main**[Q] and the concept was developed by Maxwell Jones.
20. B. Roger Wolcott Sperry did research in split brain patients (patients whose corpus callosum was removed, mostly as a surgery for epilepsy) and was able to show many specialised functions of each hemisphere.

Cognitive Development Stages

21. C. Intuitive thinking is seen in stage of preoperational thought.
22. B. Abstract thinking is the ability to make concepts (i.e. ability to grasp essential of whole) and to generalize.
23. A. See text.

Learning Theory and Psychotherapy

24. B. Classical conditioning.
25. D. Conditioned learning.
26. D. Use of rewards as a reinforcer (in positive reinforcement) is a technique of operant conditioning.
27. B. Negative conditioning is used to decrease the frequency of a particular behavior.
28. C. Punishment is decrease in frequency of a behavior due to unpleasant consequences.
29. A. This is an example of positive reinforcement, a type of operant conditioning.
30. B. This is an example of participant modeling in which patient learns by observation and imitation of therapist.
31. A. Behavior therapy.
32. A. The principle of reciprocal inhibition is used in the technique of systematic desensitization.
33. B. Aversive therapy.
34. A, B, C, D, E.
    Behavioral therapy is primarily used in treatment of anxiety disorders (including panic disorder), obsessive compulsive disorder. It is also useful in personality disorders. Though, in psychotic disorders like schizophrenia, behavioral therapy is not the first line treatment, however it can be used.
35. C. Biofeedback.
36. D. Thought block is not a cognitive error.
37. D. According to the transtheoretical model, there are 5 stages of change in substance use and other problem behaviors.
38. B. Consolidation is not a stage of change.
39. C. In this question, patient is considering quitting and thinking about the pros and cons of it. This is characteristic of stage of contemplation.
40. A. Self-exemption refers to the beliefs that give smokers false reassurances and allow them to avoid thinking deeply about the importance of quitting.

Neuropsychological Tests

41. A. See text for explanation.
42. A. Rorschach inkblot test is a projective test.
43. B. See text for explanation.

44. C. Personality.
45. A. Bender-Gestalt test.
46. B. Constructional praxis is not a part of Halstead Reitan battery.

Miscellaneous

47. A. Cataplexy.
48. C. Hypomimia refers to decrease in facial expressions, usually seen in parkinsonism.
49. D. Deja vu refers to the feeling that an event which is being currently experienced has also happened in the past. It can be seen in normal persons and also in certain disorders like temporal lobe epilepsy.
50. B. Jamais vu refers to the feeling of unfamiliarity for familiar things.
51. B. Catatonia is most commonly seen in mania followed by depression and then schizophrenia.
52. A. Severe depression.
53. B. The tendency of previously learned information to hinder subsequent learning is known as proactive inhibition.
54. B. Events. Memory can be divided into explicit and implicit forms
    - Explicit or declarative memory is associated with consciousness—or awareness. It is dependent on the hippocampus and other parts of the medial temporal lobes of the brain for its retention. Explicit memory is divided into episodic memory for events and semantic memory for facts (e.g. words, rules, and language). E.g. if you try to remember your first day in medical college, it would be episodic memory as an event will flash in front of your eyes. If you try to remember the most common type of cancer in females, it would be a semantic memory as you are thinking about a fact.
    - Implicit or nondeclarative memory does not involve awareness, and its retention does not usually involve processing in the hippocampus. Implicit memory involves things we need not actively remember. E.g. Driving a bicycle is an implicit memory. You don't have to remember everytime how to ride a bicycle.
55. B. Catharsis is not a method of learning. The term "catharsis" is used to denote the process of release of pentup emotions (emotional outlet).
56. B. According to persons with Disability Act, 1995; the sixth disability is mental retardation and seventh disability is mental illnesses.
57. D. The National Trust Act is applicable for autism, cerebral palsy, mental retardation and multiple disabilities.
58. A. Consultation liaison psychiatry is the speciality of psychiatry which deals with the psychiatric illnesses in medically ill patients.
59. A. Dependent and suspicious
60. A. Primary health centre.
61. A. Clozapine. If a patient woth Parkinson's disease develops psychotic symptoms, the treatment becomes complicated as most of the antipsychotics cause drug induced parkinsonism. Since clozapine has minimal extrapyramidal side effects such as parkinsonian side effects, it is preferred.
62. B. Abraham Maslow proposed "A theory of Human Motivation" in which he described human needs in a hierarchical fashion. Maslow said that the needs lower down the order must be met before humans start working to achieve the need of higher level. Maslow's hierarchy of needs is represented as a pyramid with basic needs, at the bottom of pyramid.

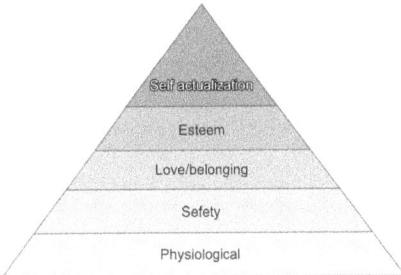

Physiologyical needs include basic needs for food, shelter, clothing. Safety needs include needs for personal safety, financial safety, health safety and safety against accidents. It is followed by need for love and belonging. This is followed by need for self esteem and self respect. Finally, is the need for self actualisation, which is the need to realise the full potential that a person has.

63. C. Rorschach test. If you see an image which is symmetrical and made of ink blots, its most likely a question on Rorschach test. I would suggest that you see all Rorschach cards once online, you will easily be able to identify them in exams. Its one of the important image based question in psychiatry.

Prospective Questions

64. B. Thematic apperception test. The patient is shown a picture like this and asked to make stories on them. The content of stories made by patients, gives an insight about patients thinking.
65. C. Bender Gestalt Test. Here, patient is asked to draw these figures, and inability to replicate them, suggest presence of an organic brain disorder.
66. B. Rogor Wolcott Sperry got Nobel prize for his work in 'split brain" concept
67. A. McNaughten Rule. Mcnaughten rule is used to determine the criminal responsibility and it says that a person cannot be held guilty for a crime, if it can be proved that the person is suffering from such a psychiatric illness (the legal term is 'insanity') that they are not aware of the nature and consequences of their acts or are incapable of realising that their acts were wrong.
68. B. Individuals with XYY chromosome have been found to be associated more frequently with violence. These are usually tall individuals.
69. B. Zaleplon. Amongst the three Z drugs, zaleplon has the shortest half life of one hour, half life of zolpidem is 2.4 hours whereas that of zopiclone is 5 hours.
70. A. Advance directive
71. C. Direct ECT (without anesthesia and muscle relaxants) has been banned in MHCA 2017. All other options are correct

72. D. By Threat
73. D. WHO developed mhGAP (mental health gap action program) to improve the care of Mental, neurological and substance use disorders in low and middle income countries. These disorders cause large economic costs and are associated with violation of human rights.

    The key part was to develop an evidence based guideline meant for use by non specialists.

    mhGAP involves mobilisation of support and establish partnerships. It does not involve screening of family members
74. A. Its a protocol for breaking bad news to patients about their illness.
75. Statement 1: False. According to MHCA 2017, direct electroconvulsive therapy has been banned, and not the indirect ECT

    Statement 2: False. Presence of a 'psychotic' disorder doesn't mean that person has lost the capacity to take mental health care decisions.

    Statement 3: False. **It is the duty of patient (or caregiver or nominated representative) to provide access to the advance directive to the treating doctor.**

    Statement 4: False. The term used is 'nominated representative' and not 'people representative'

    Statement 5: True.

Recent Questions and Answer

Basics

1. During mental status examination (MSE), a patient is asked to subtract 7 from 100 serially; what is being tested? *(FMG 2022)*
 A. Judgement B. Intelligence
 C. Attention D. Concentration

Ans. D. Concentration

Serial sevens subtraction test is used to assess concentration.

2. A patient with depression refuses to eat and tells the psychiatrist "My brain is missing, what is the point of me eating anything, I am already dead". This patient has which type of delusion? *(INI-CET May 2023)*
 A. Bizarre delusion B. Nihilistic delusion
 C. Cotard syndrome D. Hypochondriacal delusion

Ans. B. Nihilistic delusion

Here, the question is asking about the name of the delusion. So option b is being chosen over option c.

3. A 40-year-old male patient came to psychiatry OPD with the complaints of having repetitive thoughts that, he feels his own thoughts only. The thoughts make him uncomfortable and he has to wash hands again and again. This is disorder of thought ___. *(INI-CET 2020)*
 A. Flow B. Form
 C. Content D. Possession

Ans. D. Possession

4. Which of the following is a formal thought disorder?
 A. Derailment B. Obsession *(NEET 2021)*
 C. Delusion D. Thought Insertion

Ans. A. Derailment

5. In which of the following situations, the person does not have insight? *(AIIMS May 19)*
 A. Slight awareness of being sick and needing help but denying it at the same time
 B. Awareness of being sick but blaming it on others, on external events, on medical or unknown organic factors
 C. Complete denial of illness
 D. Admission of illness and but not using that information for future behaviour

Ans. C. Complete denial of illness

Schizophrenia Spectrum or Other Primary Psychotic Disorders

6. Which of the following is not correct statement about the mechanism of action of antipsychotics? *(INI-CET 2022)*
 A. D2 receptor blockade improves positive symptoms
 B. 5HT1A receptor blockade improved positive symptoms
 C. 5HT2A blockade helps improve negative symptoms
 D. M1 blockade helps in reducing EPS (extrapyramidal side effects)

Ans. B. The blockade of D2 receptors in mesolimbic tract helps improve the positive symptoms and the blockade of 5HT2A receptors help improve the negative symptoms.

7. A young male was brought by family members, with complaints that aliens are communicating with him using electromagnetic waves, and are asking him to kill the family members. The patient was also seen talking to self. He has also stopped going to office and looked scared at the time of interview. The total duration of symptoms is 1 year. What is the likely diagnosis? *(FMG 2022)*
 A. Depression B. Mania
 C. Schizophrenia D. Delusional disorder

Ans. C. Schizophrenia

8. A patient with schizophrenia who didn't respond to haloperidol and thioridazine was started on drug A. After starting drug A, the patient's psychotic symptoms improved; however, he developed sialorrhea, dyslipidemia, weight gain and hyperglycaemia? Which drug is likely to be 'drug A'? *(NEET-PG 2023)*
 A. Ziprasidone B. Clozapine
 C. Risperidone D. Aripiprazole

Ans. B. Clozapine

This patient appears to be having 'treatment resistant schizophrenia' (TRS) and the DOC for TRS is clozapine. The side effect profile of the drug is also consistent with clozapine.

9. A patient with schizophrenia is being treated with clozapine. The patient has to undergo regular blood monitoring because of which rare side effect? *(INI-CET 2023)*
 A. Agranulocytosis B. Myocarditis
 C. Cerebral bleed D. Seizures

Ans. A. Agranulocytosis

10. A patient presented to the psychiatry OPD. On being asked 'what's your name', patient repeated the same question. This phenomenon is called as: *(FMG 2022)*
 A. Echolalia B. Echopraxia
 C. Perseveration D. Posturing

Ans. A. Echolalia

11. A patient was diagnosed with schizophrenia and started on oral risperidone. After few hours of taking the antipsychotic, he had to suddenly rush to the emergency department with complaints of uprolling of eyeballs. What is the next step in management? *(INI-CET 2022)*
 A. Lorazepam B. Stop antipsychotic
 C. IV promethazine D. Phenytoin

Ans. C. IV promethazine

12. All of the following are good prognostic factors in schizophrenia *except*: *(INI-CET 2020)*
    A. Late age of onset
    B. Associated with depression
    C. Insidious onset of symptoms
    D. Positive symptoms

Ans. C. Insidious onset of symptoms

13. A psychotic patient presented with purposeless movements and was once observed to stand still in the ward for long periods of time. On examination he had negativism and waxy flexibility. What is the appropriate medical management for this patient? *(INI-CET 2020)*
    A. Haloperidol B. Clonidine
    C. Propranolol D. Lorazepam

Ans. D. Lorazepam
The symptoms are suggestive of stereotypy (purposeless movements), posturing (standing still for long periods), negativism and waxy flexibility. The diagnosis appears to be catatonia, and should be treated with IV lorazepam.

14. A patient with schizophrenia who was being treated with trifluoperazine developed rigidity, and tremors. What is the treatment? *(NEET 2020)*
    A. Lorazepam B. Propranolol
    C. Trihexyphenidyl D. Tetrabenazine

Ans. C. Trihexyphenidyl
The history is suggestive of drug-induced parkinsonism, caused by use of antipsychotics. The drug of choice is anticholinergics like trihexyphenidyl.

15. Z tracking technique is used in: *(AIIMS Nov 19)*
    A. Administering long acting antipsychotic
    B. Lithium monitoring
    C. Carbamazepine monitoring
    D. Nicotine patch

Ans. A. Administering long acting antipsychotic
Z track technique is used for giving IM injections. In this technique, the skin and tissue are pulled and held firmly while injection is given, and after removing the needle, skin and tissue are released. This prevents tracking (leakage) of the medication into the subcutaneous tissue (underneath the skin) as the track that needle forms is zig zag and drug can not come out.

16. Chlorpromazine, which is an antipsychotic drug is known to cause sedation, dry mouth and hypotension. Which of the following receptors are involved in its action?
    1. D2 and 5HT2 receptors
    2. GABA and β-adregenic receptors
    3. Muscarinic M1 and α-adregenic receptors
    4. H1 receptors *(AIIMS May 19)*
    A. 1, 3 and 4 are correct B. Only 2 is correct
    C. 1 and 2 are correct D. All are correct

Ans. A. The following receptors are involved
  i. D2 and 5HT2 blockade results in antipsychotic effect, in case of typical antipsychotics like chlorpromazine, primarily D2 receptors are responsible for antipsychotic action
  ii. H1 receptor antagonism cause sedation
  iii. Muscarinic blockade cause anticholinergic side effects like dry mouth
  iv. α-adrenergic blockade cause hypotension

17. Which of the following is a schizophrenia first rank symptom? *(JIPMER Dec 19)*
    A. Autism B. Made affect
    C. Association disturbances D. Ambivalency

Ans. B. Made affect

18. A schizophrenia patient was treated with haloperidol. He showed improvement in positive symptoms but develops side effects of akathisia and dystonia. Which drug can be most beneficial in this patient? *(JIPMER Dec 19)*
    A. Chlorpromazine B. Lurasidone
    C. Fluphenazine D. Lithium

Ans. B. Lurasidone
If a patient develops extrapyramidal side effects on a typical antipsychotic, one of the commonly used option is to shift the patient on to an atypical antipsychotic. Of the given drugs, only lurasidone is an atypical antipsychotic.

19. Lobe atrophied in chronic schizophrenia: *(JIPMER May 19)*
    A. Frontal lobe B. Occipital lobe
    C. Parietal lobe D. Temporal lobe

Ans. D. Temporal lobe
Both temporal lobe as well as frontal lobe are involved, but the better answer would be temporal lobe. The Kaplan Sadock's synopsis of psychiatry says there is "decrease in the size of amygdala, hippocampus and parahippocampal gyrus", referring to these temporal lobe structures. The book also talks about anatomical abnormalities in prefrontal cortex in schizophrenia. Research papers have also found volume reductions more consistently in temporal lobe.

20. Which of the following are typical (first generation) antipsychotics? *(PGI May 19)*
    A. Fluphenazine B. Risperidone
    C. Pimozide D. Aripiprazole
    E. Olanzapine

Ans. A. Fluphenazine and C. Pimozide

21. Which of the following is incorrect about schizophrenia? *(NIMHANS 19)*
    A. 3rd person auditory hallucination is pathognomonic
    B. Some patients may have permanent remission
    C. Lifetime prevalence is 1–15%
    D. The suicide rate is 10%

Ans. A. 3rd person auditory hallucination is pathognomonic
There is no symptom/sign that is pathognomonic of schizophrenia.

Mood Disorders

22. What is the safe and effective therapeutic concentration of lithium for the maintenance treatment of bipolar disorder? *(INI-CET 2022)*
    A. 0.5-0.8 mmol/L B. 0.6-1.2 mmol/L
    C. 1.1-1.8 mmol/L D. 0.2-0.4 mmol/L

Ans. A. 0.5-0.8 mmol/L
According to the latest edition of synopsis of psychiatry, the following are the effective lithium concentration in different indications:
Acute mania: 1.0-1.2 mEq/L
Maintenance treatment: 0.4-0.8 mEq/L
Usually toxicity: >1.5 mEq/L

23. All of the following side effects are more common with carbamazepine than oxcarbazepine: *(INI-CET 2022)*
A. Rash
B. Hyponatremia
C. Agranulocytosis
D. Vision disturbances

Ans. B. Hyponatremia

Oxcarbazepine is more likely to cause hyponatremia than carbamazepine.

24. SSRI used by mother in pregnancy can result in which of the following in the child? *(INI-CET 2022)*
a. ADHD
b. Low APGAR score
c. Delayed motor development
d. Persistent pulmonary hypertension

A. abcd (correct)
B. abc
C. bd
D. d

Ans. C. bd

Although data is inconclusive, SSRI use by mothers during pregnancy has been found to be associated with increased risk for persistent pulmonary hypertension of newborn, low birth weight, spontaneous abortions, low APGAR score in the child.

25. Which of the following statements is false about lithium? *(FMG 2022)*
A. Lithium is avoided in pregnancy due to its teratogenic effects
B. Lithium can cause hypothyroidism
C. Thiazides can increase the risk of lithium toxicity
D. Hemodialysis is not useful in lithium toxicity

Ans. D. Hemodialysis is not useful in lithium toxicity

26. Which of the following antidepressants is less likely to cause sexual dysfunction? *(FMG 2022)*
A. Venlafaxine
B. Escitalopram
C. Bupropion
D. Imipramine

Ans. C. Bupropion

Bupropion and Mirtazapine are least likely to cause any sexual side effects

27. A 35-year-old male presents to surgery emergency with priapism for last 7 hours? He has a history of mood disorder and was recently prescribed a medication by the treating psychiatrist. Which is the likely offending drug? *(INI-CET 2023)*
A. Mirtazapine
B. Venlafaxine
C. Trazodone
D. Bupropion

Ans. C. Trazodone

Trazodone can cause the side effect of priapism

28. Which of the following is true about lithium? *(INI-CET 2023)*
A. It can cause fine postural tremors at therapeutic dosage
B. It is not absorbed from the gut
C. It is not teratogenic
D. Lithium is used for treatment of absence seizures

Ans. A. It can cause fine postural tremors at therapeutic dosage

Lithium can cause fine postural tremors and the DOC for the same are beta blockers like propranolol.

29. Antidepressant contraindicated in acute angle closure glaucoma:
A. Mirtazapine
B. Amitriptyline
C. Sertraline
D. Fluvoxamine

Ans. B. Amitriptyline

TCAs should be avoided in angle closure glaucoma due to their anticholinergic action.

30. A patient consumed a large number of TCA pills during the depressive episode and presented with altered sensorium, hypotension and ECG showed wide QRS complexes. What is the next best step in the treatment? *(NEET 2022)*
A. DC cardioversion
B. Start antiarrhythmic drug
C. $NAHCO_3$
D. None of the above

Ans. C. $NAHCO_3$

31. After 5 days of normal vaginal delivery, a woman is brought to casualty by her husband. He reported that she has been crying all night. There's a history of loss of appetite, difficulty in sleeping and feeling low. General physical examination is unremarkable and there are no significant findings in the pelvic examination. Which of the following is the best term to describe her condition? *(NEET 2022)*
A. Postpartum blues
B. Postpartum depression
C. Postpartum anxiety
D. Postpartum psychosis

Ans. A. Postpartum blues

32. A 29-year-old female presents to the psychiatry OPD with symptoms of hypomania. There is history of a past episode of mania too. The patient is planning to conceive in the near future, which of the following drugs should be avoided? *(INI-CET 2022)*
A. Valproate
B. Lithium
C. Oxcarbazepine
D. Lamotrigine

Ans. A. Valproate

Valproate is the most teratogenic mood stabiliser and should be avoided in pregnancy. Valproate is the most teratogenic mood stabiliser and should be avoided in pregnancy.

33. All of the following statements are true about bipolar disorders, *except*: *(INI-CET 2022)*
A. Prevalence of bipolar I is the same in men and women, whereas bipolar II is more common in women
B. Suicide rate in bipolar disorder is 5–10%
C. Most common age of onset of bipolar disorder is 35–45 years
D. Prevalence of bipolar I is 1%

Ans. C. Most common age of onset of bipolar disorder is 35–45 years

The most common age of onset of bipolar disorder is in second decade.

34. A pregnant female with bipolar disorder presented for the treatment. Which of the following drug should be avoided in this patient?
A. Lithium
B. Lamotrigine
C. Risperidone
D. Haloperidol

Ans. A. Lithium

Lamotrigine is comparatively a safer mood stabiliser in pregnancy. Lithium can cause Ebstein's anomaly.

35. **Which of the following antidepressant drug is associated with least sexual side effects?** *(INI-CET 2020)*
    A. Mirtazapine
    B. Venlafaxine
    C. Imipramine
    D. Fluoxetine

Ans. A. Mirtazapine

Mirtazapine and bupropion are the two antidepressants with minimal sexual side effects.

36. **A patient with severe depression was treated with TCA and reported improvement in symptoms after 4 weeks of treatment. Which of the following is most important concern, at the time of his discharge?** *(INI-CET 2020)*
    A. Suicidal tendencies with overdose of TCAs
    B. Therapeutic drug monitoring of TCA
    C. ECG monitoring for arrhythmias
    D. To prescribe modafinil to counteract sedation due to TCA

Ans. A. Suicidal tendencies with overdose of TCAs

In this question, a patient with severe depression, who has started improving should be monitored for suicide risk regularly to prevent the 'paradoxical suicide'. Therapeutic drug monitoring is not routinely done with TCAs.

37. **A 16-year-old female patient was brought by family members. On evaluation she had symptoms of overfamiliarity, flight of ideas, elevated mood, increased sexual desire. What is the likely diagnosis?** *(NEET 2021)*
    A. Mania
    B. Schizomania
    C. Hypomania
    D. Cyclothymia

Ans. A. Mania

The symptoms are suggestive of mania. Please note that the symptoms of mania and hypomania are similar, what differentiates the two is the severity of the symptoms. When examiners want to ask a question on hypomania, they give something in the history that suggests that the symptoms are not so severe and the socio-occupational dysfunction is limited.

38. **A patient with depression was being treated with imipramine. After 2 weeks of treatment, patient developed overtalkativeness, euphoria, overfamiliarity, and insomnia. What is the next best step in the management of this patient?** *(NEET 2020)*
    A. Add risperidone to imipramine
    B. Stop imipramine, start valproate
    C. Add valproate to imipramine
    D. Stop imipramine

Ans. B. Stop imipramine, start valproate

If a patient on antidepressant develops symptom of mania (like in this case), it is called as a 'manic switch' and the diagnosis is revised to bipolar disorder. In such a case, antidepressant should be stopped and a mood stabilizer should be started.

39. **A 30-year-old patient with sadness of mood, lack of interest, decreased sleep and appetite for 6 months, developed new symptoms in form of, "hearing of voices" which ask him to 'kill himself'. What is the diagnosis?**
    A. Schizophrenia *(NEET 2020)*
    B. Depression with psychotic symptoms
    C. Bipolar disorder (mixed episode)
    D. Schizophreniform disorder

Ans. B. Depression with psychotic symptoms

History of depressive symptoms along with history of hallucinations is in favour of a diagnosis of depression with psychotic symptoms.

40. **A 36-year-old patient with bipolar disorder was maintaining well on lithium and risperidone. He suddenly started fasting because of religious reasons that was followed by development of coarse tremors, abdominal pain, nausea and dizziness. What is the likely cause?** *(NEET 2020)*
    A. Drug-induced parkinsonism
    B. Lithium toxicity
    C. Neuroleptic malignant syndrome
    D. Akathisia

Ans. B. Lithium toxicity

History of a patient on lithium and a risk factor for dehydration (such as diarrhoea or fasting) along with development of classical GI and neurological features, all goes in favour of lithium toxicity.

41. **A patient with bipolar disorder is kept on lithium therapy. As a doctor when are you going to ask the nurse to get serum lithium levels checked?** *(AIIMS 2020)*
    A. After 8 hours of the last dose
    B. After 12 hours of the last dose
    C. After 24 hours of the last dose
    D. Immediately after the last dose

Ans. B. After 12 hours of the last dose

For monitoring trough levels of serum lithium are used. Patients are advised to give the blood sample 12 hours after the last dose to catch the trough levels.

42. **Which of the following best describes paradoxical suicide?** *(AIIMS May 19)*
    A. Suicide after taking low dose of drug
    B. Suicide occurring at the time when the patient starts to recover
    C. Suicidal tendency increase as the patient improves
    D. Accidental completion of suicide

Ans. B. Suicide occurring at the time when the patient starts to recover

Paradoxical suicide: Paradoxical suicide is the phenomenon where in a patient with depression who had started to improve commits suicide (it is a paradox as suicide possibility should ordinarily decrease with improvement). The hypothesis is that a depressed person with suicidal thoughts often lacks the energy to act on those thoughts, when treatment is started, such a person may feel improvement in energy levels before there is any decrease in suicidal thoughts. That opens a window where the patient has suicidal thoughts and also has energy to act on those, thereby increasing the risk for suicide. FDA has given a black box warning that all antidepressant may increase suicide risk in individuals under 25 years of age. This warning has been widely criticised as it appears to be based on questionable data.

43. **Not a common side effect of Escitalopram:** *(AIIMS May 19)*
    A. Nausea
    B. Vivid dreams
    C. Anorgasmia
    D. Sialorrhea

Ans. D. Sialorrhea

Sialorrhea (excessive salivation) is not a common side effect of escitalopram. Sialorrhea is a common side effect of clozapine.

44. A 28-year-old mother was diagnosed with mild depression, she has a 3 months old child. Which among the following should be preferred? *(FMGE 2021)*
    A. Cognitive behaviour therapy
    B. Cognitive therapy + antidepressant
    C. Antidepressant alone
    D. Electroconvulsive therapy

Ans. A. Cognitive behaviour therapy (cognitive therapy)

In mild depression, both SSRIs and CBT are considered to be equally effective. Further in a lactating patient, it is better to avoid antidepressants as they get secreted in the breast milk. Hence, the best answer here is cognitive behaviour therapy alone.

45. Which of the following drug has been correctly matched with its adequate antidepressant dose? *(JIPMER Dec 19)*
    A. Fluoxetine 2.5–10 mg
    B. Fluoxetine 10–20 mg
    C. Amitryptyline 75–300 mg
    D. Amitryptyline 10–50 mg

Ans. B. Fluoxetine 10–20 mg

The adequate antidepressant dose for fluoxetine is 10–20 mg. According to 'Kaplan Sadock's synopsis of psychiatry', 20 mg of fluoxetine is as effective as higher dosages in treatment of depression.

You are usually not supposed to remember the dosages of antidepressants. This is a one-off question that has been asked on the dosages.

46. Which of the following features seen in a 12-year-old child suffering from depression is not suggestive of development of bipolar disorder later? *(JIPMER May 19)*
    A. Rapid onset of depression
    B. Psychotic symptoms
    C. Mood lability
    D. Psychomotor agitation

Ans. D. Psychomotor agitation

The question talks about possibility of development of bipolar disorder later in life in this 12-year-old patient. If a person who has a depressive episode, develops a manic or hypomanic episode in future, the diagnosis would be revised to bipolar disorder. There are certain clinical features of depressive episode, that suggest the possibility of a later development of a manic/hypomanic episode and development of bipolar disorder. Some of these features include:

1. Early age at onset
2. Psychotic depression before 25 years of age
3. Rapid onset and offset of depressive episode of short duration
4. Recurrent depression (>5 episodes)
5. Presence of marked psychomotor retardation
6. Mood lability as a trait in patient
7. Family history of bipolar disorder

47. Drug of choice for acute severe depression with least side effects: *(JIPMER May 19)*
    A. MAO inhibitors
    B. TCAs
    C. Serotonin modulators
    D. Serotonin noradrenaline reuptake inhibitor

Ans. D. Serotonin noradrenaline reuptake inhibitor

Most of the studies have found that all the classes of antidepressants have same efficacy. However some studies have found that SNRIs to be more effective than SSRIs. This is attributed to the action of SNRIs on both norepinephrine as well as serotonin receptors. TCAs too act on multiple receptors but are associated with serious side effects.

48. "Placebo effect" to antidepressants is most strongly associated with which of the following psychiatric disorder? *(PGI Nov 19)*
    A. Mild depression
    B. OCD
    C. Specific phobias
    D. Generalized anxiety disorder
    E. Severe depression

Ans. A. Mild depression

It has been shown that a significant effect of antidepressants is because of placebo effect. This is true more for depression treatment than anxiety disorders treatment. And in depression, it is more true for mild depression than severe depression.

49. Which of the following mood stabilizers have been approved in the management of bipolar disorder? *(PGI Nov 19)*
    A. Lamotrigine
    B. Gabapentine
    C. Valproate
    D. Quetiapine
    E. Topiramate

Ans. A. Lamotrigine, C. Valproate and D. Quetiapine

50. A 56-year-old patient with depression was on escitalopram. He started taking thiazide diuretics for the management of hypertension and came to emergency with confusion. What is the likely cause? *(PGI Nov 19)*
    A. Hyponatremia
    B. Hypokalemia
    C. Drug interaction
    D. Serotonin syndrome
    E. Depressive stupor

Ans. A. Hyponatremia

SSRIs can cause the side effect of hyponatremia, which could be compounded by concomitant use of thiazide diuretics that too can cause hyponatremia. The clinical presentation can be a confused state or seizures.

51. Which of the following statements are true about lithium? *(PGI May 19)*
    A. Can cause Ebstein's anomaly
    B. Decreases neutrophil count
    C. Decreases eosinophil count
    D. Optimum concentration is 0.2–0.6 mEq/L
    E. Decreases sodium excretion

Ans. A. Can cause Ebstein's anomaly

It must be remembered that lithium causes neutrophilia and eosinophilia.

52. Which of the following statements is correct about cyclothymia? *(NIMHANS 19)*
    A. There is at least on episode of mania
    B. The duration criterion for diagnosis is 2 years
    C. There is at least one episode of depression
    D. There is at least one episode of hypomania

Ans. B. The duration criterion for diagnosis is 2 years

53. Which of the following drug is not used in the prophylaxis of recurrent depressive episodes? *(NIMHANS 19)*
    A. Valproate
    B. Lithium
    C. Selective serotonin reuptake inhibitors
    D. TCAs

Ans. A. Valproate

Antidepressant (SSRIs, TCAs and others) can be used. In some patients lithium and low dose antipsychotics can be used as an adjuvant in the treatment of depression and used even in prophylaxis.

54. Which of the following is not a feature of melancholic depression? *(NIMHANS 19)*
    A. Psychomotor retardation
    B. Severe guilt
    C. Early morning insomnia
    D. Diurnal variation of mood

Ans. D. Diurnal variation of mood

55. A patient was being treated by the psychiatrist using psychotherapy. In the process, the doctor tries to identify the negative thoughts of the patient and tries to fix those negative thoughts. Which type of psychotherapy is being given to the patient? *(NIMHANS 19)*
    A. Psychodynamic psychotherapy
    B. Cognitive behavioural therapy
    C. Behavioural therapy
    D. Interpersonal therapy

Ans. B. Cognitive behavioural therapy

Therapy that focus on identifying and correcting negative automatic thoughts is cognitive behavioural therapy.

56. A patient with severe depressive episode has not shown any improvement on escitalopram. On mental status examination, he expressed suicidal intent. What is the next best step in the treatment of this patient?
    A. Start cognitive behavioural therapy *(NIMHANS 19)*
    B. Administer ECT
    C. Increase dose of SSRI
    D. Use rTMS

Ans. B. Administer ECT

Whenever history of high suicide risk is given, ECT must be considered as the first line treatment. It has a rapid onset of action and is considered to be the most effective treatment of depression.

Neurotic, Stress-related and Somatoform Disorders

57. Match the following: *(INI-CET Nov 2022)*
    1. Kleptomania   a. Urge to steal
    2. Dipsomania   b. Urge to put things on fire
    3. Mutilomania   c. Urge to drink alcohol
    4. Pyromania   d. Urge to mutilate animals
    A. 1a 2b 3c 4d   B. 1b 2c 3a 4d
    C. 1d 2a 3b 4c   D. 1a 2c 3d 4b

Ans. D. 1a 2c 3d 4b

58. A middle-aged female presented with complaints of repeated episodes of around 30 minutes characterised by breathlessness, palpitations, sweating, hyperventilation, and a fear of impending heart attack. The patient has had these episodes 5-6 times/month in the last 6 months, and the investigations didn't reveal any obvious abnormailty? What is the likely diagnosis? *(NEET-PG 2023)*
    A. Panic disorder   B. Generalised anxiety disorder
    C. Depression   D. Social phobia

Ans. A. Panic disorder

History of episodes of intense anxiety with fear of impending heart attack and normal investigations is suggestive of panic disorder.

59. A 14-year-old girl was brought to psychiatry OPD with complaints of 'sudden onset blindness' since morning. The girl appeared to be least concerned about the 'blindness' and was referred by ophthalmologist. During interview, the girl kept on talking about her mother with whom she had a disturbed relationship and who had died recently? Which of the following statements about this girl's illness are true? *(INI-CET 2022)*
    A. More common in females than males in childhood
    B. More common in males than females in childhood
    C. Same incidence in males and females in childhood
    D. Same incidence in males and females in adulthood

Ans. A. More common in females than males in childhood

The diagnosis is conversion disorder. The 'lack of concern for blindness' is suggestive of la-belle indifference. Conversion disorders are more common in females than males

60. La belle indifference is seen in: *(INI-CET May 2023)*
    A. Conversion disorder   B. Mania
    C. Schizophrenia   D. Depression

Ans. A. Conversion disorder

61. A patient had COVID infection around 3 months back. Now he presents with complaints of excessive sweating, palpitations, and fear that he is about to die. The physical examination and investigations didn't reveal any abnormality. What is the likely diagnosis? *(FMG 2021)*
    A. Post-traumatic stress disorder
    B. Depression
    C. Mania   D. Panic attack

Ans. D. Panic attack

The symptoms are suggestive of a panic attack.

62. Obsessive compulsive disorder (OCD) true statement is: *(INI-CET 2021)*
    A. Prevalence of OCD in general population is 7–10%
    B. Atypical antipsychotics is the first line (main line) treatment
    C. Depression is a common comorbidity in OCD
    D. Contamination is an uncommon obsession

Ans. C. Depression is a common comorbidity in OCD

63. Which is a novel antidepressant? *(INI-CET 2021)*
    A. Vilazodone   B. Asenapine
    C. Blonanserin   D. Lurasidone

Ans. A. Vilazodone

Vilazodone is a SSRI which also acts as a partial agonist at 5 HT1A receptors. The other three options given are all antipsychotics.

64. Continuous rigorous washing of hands is suggestive of: *(FMG 2022)*

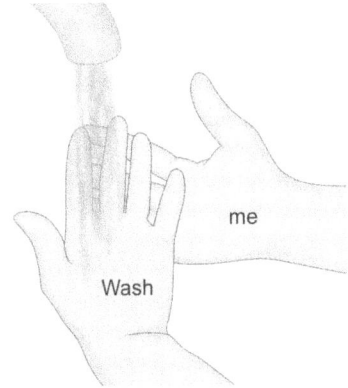

   A. Obsessive compulsive disorder
   B. Generalized anxiety disorder
   C. Adjustment disorder
   D. Panic disorder

Ans. A. Obsessive compulsive disorder

65. A patient underwent surgery and a mass of hair was found in her stomach. Which specialist should be consulted with? *(FMG 2022)*

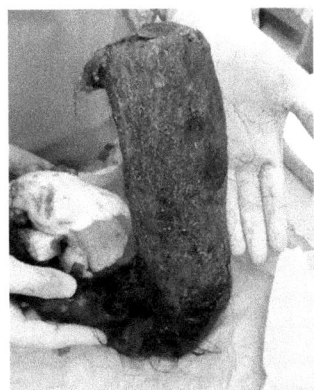

   A. Dermatologist   B. Cardiologist
   C. Psychiatrist   D. Neurologist

Ans. C. Psychiatrist

The mass of hair is called 'trichobezoar'. Around 25–30% patients with trichotillomania swallow the hair after plucking it; this may lead to an accumulation of hair in the form of a ball of hair (trichobezoar) in the stomach or small intestine and may cause intestinal obstruction that requires surgical intervention.

66. A female patient is having repetitive thoughts of contamination with dirt followed by repetitive hand washing. Which of the following modality will be considered as the therapy of choice? *(INI-CET 2021)*
   A. Cognitive behaviour therapy
   B. Exposure and response prevention
   C. Systematic desensitisation
   D. Dialectical behavioural therapy

Ans. B. Exposure and response prevention

Its a more specific answer than cognitive behaviour therapy.

67. Which of the following body focussed repetitive disorder is included in obsessive compulsive or related disorder, according to ICD-11? *(INI-CET 2021)*
   A. Body dysmorphic disorder
   B. Hypochondriasis
   C. Trichotillomania
   D. Olfactory reference syndrome

Ans. C. Trichotillomania

Trichotillomania and excoriation disorder are the two body focussed repetitive disorder is included in obsessive compulsive or related disorder, according to ICD-11.

68. A male patient lost his job recently (1 week back) following which he became irritable and had sad mood, the thoughts of job and future made his mood even worse. He was more irritated towards the people in his home, but he occasionally went for a movie with his friend and was able to enjoy with them but after returning back to his home, he again had similar symptoms. Probable diagnosis: *(INI-CET 2020)*
   A. Generalized anxiety disorder
   B. Adjustment disorder
   C. Mixed anxiety depression
   D. Moderate depression

Ans. B. Adjustment disorder

History of job loss, followed by some depressive symptoms is suggestive of adjustment disorder. Note that the question says that the patient went to movie and enjoyed it. This information was given to show that symptoms were not severe enough to warrant a diagnosis of depression.

69. A medical student presents with recurrent episodes of breathlessness, feeling of choking, palpitations and feeling of impending doom. The investigations are within normal limit. What is the most likely diagnosis? *(NEET 2020)*
   A. Acute stress disorder
   B. Panic disorder
   C. Generalized anxiety disorders
   D. Depression

Ans. B. Panic disorder

70. Depersonalization which is false? *(AIIMS May 19)*
   A. More common in female than male
   B. Common in patients with seizure and migraine
   C. Common with post life-threatening accidents
   D. Reality testing is lost

Ans. D. Reality testing is lost

During depersonalization, patient feels 'unreal', 'detached from self', but he realizes that this is just his éxperience' and in reality, nothing has changed. Since, there is a realization that in reality nothing has changed, reality testing is present during depersonalization.

71. A child with obsessive compulsive disorder undergoes imaging of brain. It is most likely to show atrophy in:
   A. Putamen *(JIPMER May 19)*
   B. Cerebellum
   C. Caudate nucleus
   D. Globus pallidus

Ans. C. Caudate nucleus

72. **Delusion of grandiosity is seen in all, except:**
    A. Schizophrenia *(JIPMER May 19)*
    B. Amphetamine toxicity
    C. Frontal lobe tumour
    D. Obsessive compulsive neurosis (obsessive compulsive disorder)

Ans. D. Obsessive compulsive neurosis (obsessive compulsive disorder)

Schizophrenia, amphetamine toxicity (in amphetamine intoxication, delusions and hallucinations can be seen) and frontal lobe tumor can all present with delusion of grandiosity. Even patients with OCD can develop delusions, but that is rare and in particular, delusion of grandiosity is even rarer.

73. **Which of the following types are somatic symptom and related disorders (earlier called as somatoform disorder)?** *(PGI May 19)*
    A. Post-traumatic stress disorder
    B. Depersonalization
    C. Somatic passivity
    D. Conversion disorder
    E. Hypochondriasis

Ans. D. Conversion disorder and E. Hypochondriasis

The diagnosis that is used in DSM-5 in place of hypochondriasis is illness anxiety disorder.

74. **Which following is the treatment of choice for specific phobias?** *(NIMHANS 19)*
    A. Exposure-based therapy
    B. Clomipramine
    C. SSRIs
    D. Benzodiazepines

Ans. A. Exposure-based therapy

Behavioural therapies that are exposure based are considered as the treatment of choice. If the question asked about the drug of choice, the answer would have been SSRIs.

75. **Which of the following is included under OCD and related disorders in DSM-5?** *(NIMHANS 19)*
    A. Body dysmorphic disorder
    B. Hypochondriasis
    C. Somatization disorder
    D. Conversion disorder

Ans. A. Body dysmorphic disorder

76. **Which of the following statement about OCD treatment is not true?** *(NIMHANS 19)*
    A. ECT can be used for resistant OCD
    B. Low dose antipsychotics can used for resistant OCD
    C. Exposure and response prevention is therapy of choice
    D. All SSRIs are equally effective in treatment of OCD

Ans. D. All SSRIs are equally effective in treatment of OCD

All the statements are correct. However, if we have to pick one, statement 'D' can be considered as the incorrect statement. Although the data is not sufficient to choose one SSRI over another as they have similar effectiveness, some studies have found fluvoxamine to be more effective than other SSRIs.

77. **Which of the following pathway is involved in the development of OCD?** *(NIMHANS 19)*
    A. Mesolimbic pathway
    B. Frontostriatal pathway
    C. Tuberoinfundibular pathway
    D. Nigrostriatal pathway

Ans. B. Frontostriatal pathway

The pathway involved is cortical-striatal-thalamic-cortical tract which starts from prefrontal cortex, projects to striatum, thalamus and back to prefrontal cortex.

78. **A 22-year-old male had repetitive episodes of palpitations, sweating, feeling that he might die and difficulty in breathing. All the investigations came out to be normal. However the patient gradually stopped going out fearing that he will have another episode. Which of the following is not true for this patient?** *(NIMHANS 19)*
    A. Panic attacks
    B. Anticipatory anxiety
    C. Agoraphobia
    D. Hypochondriasis

Ans. D. Hypochondriasis

The history is suggestive of panic disorder (repetitive episodes of panic attacks), anticipatory anxiety (fear that there would be another episode) with development of agoraphobia (fear of travelling alone and getting homebound).

79. **Which of the following has been correctly matched?** *(NIMHANS 19)*
    A. Hypochondriasis—Repetitive investigations
    B. Trichotillomania—Exposure and response prevention
    C. Phobia—Interpersonal psychotherapy
    D. Mania—Cognitive behavioural therapy

Ans. A. Hypochondriasis—Repetitive investigations

80. **Which of the following statement about factitious disorder is incorrect?** *(NIMHANS 19)*
    A. Patient has a delusion that he has a debilitating illness
    B. Sick role is taken by the patient
    C. Patient fakes the symptoms
    D. No material gain is involved

Ans. A. Patient has a delusion that he has a debilitating illness

There is no delusion in a patient with factitious disorder.

Substance-related and Addictive Disorders

81. **A 50-year-old male, with history of chronic alcohol use, stopped using alcohol suddenly. He presented with episodes of seizures and hearing voices that made him fearful. What should be the treatment?** *(INI-CET Nov 2022)*
    A. Lorazepam
    B. i.v. thiamine
    C. Haloperidol
    D. Naltrexone

Ans. A. Lorazepam

The patient appears to be having alcohol withdrawal seizures and alcohol withdrawal perceptual disturbances.

The DOC for alcohol withdrawal symptoms are benzodiazepines. Ideally, this patient should also be given thiamine to prevent the development of Wernicke's encephalopathy, and if there were an option of benzodiazepines + thiamine, it would have been the best answer.

82. **About disulfiram, which of the following is not correct?**
    (INI-CET 2022)
    A. Its not an anticraving agent
    B. Its starting dose is 250 mg
    C. It causes accumulation of acetaldehyde
    D. It's an inhibitor of alcohol dehydrogenase

Ans. D. It's an inhibitor of alcohol dehydrogenase

Disulfiram is an inhibitor of aldehyde dehydrogenase and not alcohol dehydrogenase.

83. **Which of the following is a symptom of cannabis intoxication?** *(FMG 2022)*
    A. Anxiety
    B. Depression
    C. Dreamlike state
    D. Tactile hallucinations

Ans. C. Dreamlike state

Cannabis intoxication can present with a dream like state.

84. **A 40-year-old patient with chronic alcohol use presents with complaints of confusion and ataxia. On examination, there is nystagmus and sixth nerve palsy? What is the likely diagnosis?** *(NEET-PG 2023)*
    A. Wernickes encephalopathy
    B. Korsakoff syndrome
    C. Delirium tremens
    D. De clerembault syndrome

Ans. A. Wernickes encephalopathy

85. **A patient with chronic alcohol use developed confusion, ataxia and ophthalmoplegia. Which vitamin deficiency is responsible for this presentation?** *(NEET-PG 2023)*
    A. Vitamin B_1
    B. Vitamin B_2
    C. Vitamin B_6
    D. Vitamin C

Ans. A. Vitamin B_1

86. **Tactile hallucinations seen during intoxication with cocaine are called as:** *(INI-CET 2023)*
    A. Formication
    B. Dipsomania
    C. Onieroid state
    D. Fornication

Ans. A. Formication

87. **After 72 hours of cessation of alcohol use, which of the following is seen in patients with alcohol dependence syndrome?** *(FMG 2021)*
    A. Tremors, sweating
    B. Alcoholic hallucinosis
    C. Alcohol withdrawal seizures
    D. Delirium tremens

Ans. D. Delirium tremens

88. **Most effective drug for smoking cessation:**
    (INI-CET 2021, FMG 2022)
    A. Varenicline
    B. Nicotine gum
    C. Bupropion SR
    D. Nicotine patch

Ans. A. Varenicline

89. **A patient presented in the emergency department with symptoms of respiratory depression and was suspected to have overdosed on opioids. What should be the next step in the management?** *(NEET 2022)*
    A. Naloxone
    B. Naltrexone
    C. Buprenorphine
    D. Methadone

Ans. A. Naloxone

90. **Following is a feature of Korsakoff syndrome:**
    (INI-CET 2021)
    A. Anterograde amnesia with recent memory loss
    B. Confusion, ophthalmoplegia and ataxia
    C. Loss of identity, memory and intact personality
    D. Impairment of implicit memory and immediate recall

Ans. A. Anterograde amnesia with recent memory loss

91. **A 40-year-old man with a history of alcohol intake for many years was diagnosed with liver cirrhosis, after which he suddenly stopped taking alcohol. Now, the patient has come with alcohol withdrawal symptoms. What is the preferred management?** *(INI-CET 2022)*
    A. Diazepam
    B. Lorazepam
    C. Clonazepam
    D. Alprazolam

Ans. B. Lorazepam

In patients with compromised liver functioning, oxazepam and lorazepam are preferred due to their short half lives.

92. **A patient with cocaine intoxication presents to the emergency department, which of the following is unlikely to be seen?** *(NEET 2021)*
    A. Agitation
    B. Bradycardia
    C. Hyperthermia
    D. Myocardial infarction

Ans. B. Bradycardia

Cocaine is a sympathomimetic drug, tachycardia and not bradycardia is likely to be a feature.

93. **A patient with history of chronic alcohol use was admitted and operated for acute appendicitis. After the surgery, patient appeared confused, and reported seeing snakes in the ward room. What is the likely diagnosis?**
    A. Alcoholic hallucinosis *(NEET 2021)*
    B. Delirium tremens
    C. Wernicke's encephalopathy
    D. Korsakoff syndrome

Ans. B. Delirium tremens

Sudden cessation of use, surgery, infections, can all lead to delirium tremens in a patient with chronic alcohol use.

94. **Which of the following drugs that is known to cause dependence is most commonly abused?** *(NEET 2020)*
    A. Cocaine
    B. Heroin
    C. Cannabis
    D. Amphetamines

Ans. C. Cannabis

Cannabis is the most commonly used illegal drug. Overall, nicotine is the most commonly used drug.

95. **A patient with chronic alcohol use (around one bottle of whiskey daily) stopped consuming alcohol 2 days back. He was brought to the emergency with symptoms of anxiety, hypertension, palpitations. He says that he is seeing snakes and lizards on the floor. There is no history of seizures. Which of the following should be given to control the symptoms immediately?** *(AIIMS 2020)*
    A. Haloperidol
    B. Lorazepam + Thiamine
    C. IV Lorazepam
    D. IV Haloperidol

Ans. C. IV Lorazepam

The clinical picture is that of delirium tremens. While thiamine too must be given to this patient, it would not help control the symptoms of delirium tremens. Since the question is specifically asking about it, option number c is the best answer here.

96. **Extended matching type**
 Theme (withdrawal symptoms)
 Case 1: HIGH BP tachycardia, tremors, auditory and visual hallucinations, disorientation to time, place, person.
 Case 2: Yawning, diarrhea, diaphoresis, mydriasis, high fever, rhinorrhea, piloerection.
 Options to choose from: *(AIIMS Nov 19)*
 A. Alcohol   B. Cannabis
 C. Cocaine   D. Heroin
 E. Amphetamine   F. MDMA
 G. Ketamine   H. LSD

Ans. Case 1A. Alcohol, Case 2D. Heroin

Alcohol withdrawal symptoms start to manifest after 6–8 hours of last intake and the presentation includes tremors (M/C alcohol withdrawal symptom), hypertension, irritability, sweating, mydriasis. Late on symptoms like alcoholic hallucinosis may develop. And after 48–72 hours patient may develop delirium tremens and present with disturbances of consciousness.

Opioid (e.g. heroin) withdrawal presents flu like symptoms, that includes sweating, diarrhea, lacrimation, rhinorrhea, body ache and insomnia. Characteristic opioid withdrawal symptoms include yawning and piloerection.

97. **In a patient who is an alcoholic, which of the following causes delirium tremens?** *(AIIMS Nov 19)*
 A. Small consumption of alcohol
 B. Gradual withdrawal from alcohol
 C. Fatty liver
 D. Acute infection

Ans. D. Acute infection

Acute infection can act as a trigger for delirium tremens in chronic alcoholics. Note that while sudden withdrawal can cause delirium tremens, gradual withdrawal is unlikely to cause it. Also small consumption of alcohol is unlikely to cause delirium tremens.

98. **A patient was admitted with complaints of tachycardia and arrhythmia. O/E there were scratch marks on the skin. This patient is most probable causing substance is:**
 A. Cocaine *(FMG 2021)*
 B. Heroin
 C. Cannabis
 D. Alcohol

Ans. A. Cocaine

Cocaine intoxication can lead to tactile hallucinations (cocaine bugs) and patients often scratch the skin. Cocaine being a sympathomimetic can cause tachycardia and arrhythmias too.

99. **Which of the following drugs is not a hallucinogen?** *(NIMHANS 19)*
 A. Toluene   B. Phencyclidine
 C. Mescaline   D. Psilocybin

Ans. A. Toluene

100. **A patient with alcohol dependence syndrome presented in medicine emergency with symptoms suggestive of hypoglycemia. He was administered 25% dextrose, following which he developed confusion, ataxia and disturbance in vision. What is the likely diagnosis? Administration of 25% dextrose for his hypoglycaemia. Diagnosis:** *(NIMHANS 19)*
 A. Marchiafava-Bignami syndrome
 B. Wernicke's encephalopathy
 C. Central pontine myelinolysis
 D. Korsakoff syndrome

Ans. B. Wernicke's encephalopathy

Symptoms are suggestive of Wernicke's encephalopathy. A patient with alcohol dependence syndrome usually has thiamine deficiency because of poor intake and absorption. If such a patient is suddenly given dextrose, that may lead to acute deficiency of thiamine (as glucose metabolism requires thiamine), and may result in precipitation of Wernicke's encephalopathy. Hence such patients must always be given thiamine first (parenterally) followed by administration of dextrose.

101. **Disulfiram use leads to accumulation of:** *(NIMHANS 19)*
 A. CH_3CH_2CHO B. CH_3CHO
 C. CH_3CH_2OH D. CH_3COOH

Ans. B. CH_3CHO

Disulfiram leads to accumulation of acetaldehyde (C_2H_4O). And you thought, you could forget about the chemistry once you entered the medical college.

102. **Which of the following is true about POCSO Act, 2012?** *(NIMHANS 19)*
 A. Reporting is mandatory in case of child sexual abuse
 B. Doctor can take a call on reporting
 C. Parents can take a call on reporting
 D. Child can take a call on reporting

Ans. A. Reporting is mandatory in case of child sexual abuse

In POCSO Act (prevention of children from sexual offences), it is mandatory for the healthcare provider to report about child sexual abuse to the police.

Neurocognitive Disorders (Organic Mental Disorders)

103. **All of the following suggest an organic cause for behavioural symptoms, *except*:** *(FMG 2022)*
 A. Old age
 B. Acute onset
 C. Loss of consciousness
 D. Aud hallucinations

Ans. D. Aud hallucinations

Visual hallucinations are suggestive of organic causes, and not the auditory hallucinations.

104. **Which of the following are the reversible causes of dementia?** *(INI-CET May 2023)*
 1. Normal pressure hydrocephalus
 2. Hypothyroidism
 3. Lewy body dementia
 4. Vit B 12 deficiency
 A. 1, 2, 3 & 4
 B. 1, 3
 C. 3
 D. 1, 2, 4

Ans. D. 1, 2, 4

105. Risperidone as an off label is not used in which of the following? *(INI-CET 2021)*
A. PTSD B. Bipolar disorder
C. OCD D. Dementia

Ans. A. PTSD

Risperidone can be used in bipolar disorder, OCD (as an adjunct) and dementia (for BPSD in dementia).

106. Match the following: *(INI-CET 2021)*
A. Persecution i Oneirophrenia
B. Oneiroid state ii Paranoid
C. Twilight iii Oligophrenia
D. Mental subnormality iv Disturbances of consciousness
A. a-i, b-iv, c-iii, d-ii B. a-iii, b-ii, c-iv, d-i
C. a-ii, b-iii, c-i, d-iv D. a-ii, b-i, c-iv, d-iii

Ans. D. a-ii, b-i, c-iv, d-iii

These are obsolete and poorly defined terms and rarely used anywhere except MCQs in India. According to Fish's clinical psychopathology "In twilight state, the consciousness is restricted, and mind is dominated by a small group of ideas". Oneiroid state and oneirophrenia, both are dream-like state. Oligophrenia is the other name of subnormal intelligence.

107. Which of these are types of subcortical dementia? *(INI-CET 2020)*
A. Parkinson's disease
B. Wilson's disease
C. Huntington's disease
D. Pick's disease
A. abc only B. a and b only
C. abcd D. acd only

Ans. A. abc only

108. How will you differentiate delirium from dementia, in a patient with Alzheimer's disease? *(INI-CET 2020)*
A. Disorientation and agitation
B. Visual hallucinations and impairment of memory
C. Acute onset and level of consciousness
D. Agitation and irritation

Ans. C. Acute onset and level of consciousness

Acute onset and disturbances of consciousness are features of delirium.

109. Visual hallucination are predominant in which dementia? *(AIIMS May 19)*
A. Lewy body dementia
B. Alzheimer's disease
C. AIDS dementia complex
D. Huntington's disease

Ans. A. Lewy body dementia

110. Which gene mutation is not commonly associated with Familial Alzheimer disease? *(JIPMER May 19)*
A. Presenilin 1 B. Presenilin 2
C. Clusterin D. Amyloid precursor protein

Ans. C. Clusterin

Mutations in amyloid precursor protein, presenilin 1 and presenilin 2 have been found in patients with familial Alzheimer's disease. *Clusterin* gene mutation has been found in patients with Huntington's chorea.

111. Which of the following drugs are used in treatment of nicotine dependence? *(PGI Nov 19)*
A. Bupropion B. Naltrexone
C. Acamprosate D. Disulfiram
E. Varenicline

Ans. A. Bupropion and E. Varenicline

Personality Disorders

112. Which of the following are feature(s) of borderline personality disorder? *(PGI May 19)*
A. Impulsivity
B. Recurrent suicidal behavior
C. Anger and anxiety
D. Extreme suspiciousness
E. Pattern of unstable and intense interpersonal relationships

Ans. A. Impulsivity, B. Recurrent suicidal behavior, C. Anger and anxiety, and E. Pattern of unstable and intense interpersonal relationships

113. All of the following are features of borderline personality disorder, *except*: *(NIMHANS 19)*
A. Unstable interpersonal relationship
B. Grandiose self-importance
C. Chronic feeling or emptiness
D. Repetitive self-harm

Ans. B. Grandiose self-importance

Eating Disorders

114. A 16-year-old female was referred for symptoms of irresistible urges to eat (cravings) followed by episodes of self-induced vomiting. The patient is also on appetite suppressants. What's the most likely diagnosis? *(NEET 2022)*
A. Bulimia nervosa B. Anorexia nervosa
C. Pica disorder D. Binge eating disorder

Ans. A. Bulimia nervosa

Although all three features mentioned (craving, self-induced vomiting and use of appetite suppressants) can be seen in both patients with anorexia nervosa and bulimia nervosa, the bulimia nervosa is being chosen as it is characterised by binge episodes followed by purging. There is no mention of the low BMI, which is the characteristic feature of anorexia nervosa.

115. SCOFF criterion is used as a screening tool for: *(INI-CET May 2023)*
A. Eating disorders B. Sexual disorders
C. Substance use disorders D. Behavioural disorders

Ans. A. Eating disorders

S–Do you make yourself Sick because you feel uncomfortably full?
C–Do you worry that you have lost Control over how much you eat?
O–Have you recently lost more than One stone (14 lb) in a 3-month period?
F–Do you believe yourself to be Fat when others say you are too thin?
F–Would you say that Food dominates your life?

116. A 16-year-old female was referred for symptoms of irresistible urges to eat (cravings) followed by episodes of self-induced vomiting. The patient is also on appetite suppressants. What's the most likely diagnosis?
    A. Bulimia nervosa   (NEET 2022)
    B. Anorexia nervosa
    C. Pica disorder
    D. Binge eating disorder

Ans. A. Bulimia nervosa

Although all three features mentioned (craving, self-induced vomiting and use of appetite suppressants) can be seen in both patients with anorexia nervosa and bulimia nervosa, the bulimia nervosa is being chosen as it is characterised by binge episodes followed by purging. There is no mention of the low BMI, which is the characteristic feature of anorexia nervosa.

117. A young girl hospitalized with anorexia nervosa is on treatment. Even after taking adequate food according to the recommended diet plan for last 1 week, there is no gain in weight. What is the next step in management?
    A. Increase fluid intake   (AIIMS Nov 19)
    B. Observe patient for 2 hours after meal
    C. Increase the dose of anxiolytics
    D. Increase the caloric intake from 1500 to 2000 kcal per day

Ans. B. Observe patient for 2 hours after meal

In patients who are taking recommended amount of calories, if there is lack of weight gain, purging behaviour should be strongly suspected. It is possible that after eating, the patient purges it out usually by self-induced vomiting. A nurse observing patient for at least 2 hours after meals, will ensure that there is no purging. If no purging is there, and still there is lack of weight gain, calorie intake can be subsequently increased.

118. Which of the following statements is not true regarding narcolepsy?   (JIPMER Dec 19)
    A. Related gene on 6th chromosome, MHC 2/HLA DR 2
    B. Hyperactivity of orexin (hypocretin) releasing neurons in hypothalamus
    C. Inability of brain to regulate sleep wake cycle
    D. Sudden onset of REM sleep

Ans. B. Hyperactivity of orexin (hypocretin) releasing neurons in hypothalamus

Narcolepsy is caused by an autoimmune mediated destruction of orexin (or hypocretin) producing neurons.

119. All are true regarding anorexia nervosa, *except*:
                                                          (JIPMER May 19)
    A. Anorexia has one of the highest morbidity amongst all mental disorders
    B. In DSM-5, severity is based on BMI values
    C. In DSM-5, diagnostic criterion is BMI less than 17.5 or weight less than 85% of expected
    D. Patient does not care about weight gain

Ans. C. In DSM-5, diagnostic criterion is BMI less than 17.5 or weight less than 85% of expected

According to DSM-5, to diagnose anorexia nervosa, the patient should have 'significantly low body weight'. According to WHO and CDC guidelines (used in DSM-5), BMI above 18.5 kg/m² is not considered as 'significantly low body weight', BMI less than 17 kg/m² is considered as 'significantly low body weight' and BMI between 17 and 18.5 kg/m² can be considered as significantly low body weight if clinical history or physical examination supports this judgement. So option C is definitely wrong.

In DSM-5, severity of anorexia nervosa has been defined according to BMI.

120. About refeeding syndrome, which is not true?
    A. Thiamine deficiency   (NIMHANS 19)
    B. Hyperphosphatemia
    C. Hypokalemia
    D. Hyperglycemia

Ans. B. Hyperphosphatemia

Refeeding syndrome: Rapid refeeding (enteral or parenteral) in a person who has been undergoing starvation for a significant period of time, can lead to certain fluid and electrolyte changes referred to as 'refeeding syndrome'. The hallmark feature is hypophosphataemia.

Sexual Disorders

121. Match the following: (INI-CET Nov 2022)

A. Necrophilia	1. Sexual arousal by rubbing genitals against an unsuspecting stranger
B. Frotteurism	2. Sexual arousal by dead bodies
C. Exhibitionism	3. Sexual arousal by cross-dressing
D. Eonism	4. Sexual arousal by exposure of genitals to strangers

    A. A1 B2 C3 D4   B. A3 B3 C1 D4
    C. A2 B4 C1 D3   D. A2 B1 C4 D3

Ans. D. A2 B1 C4 D3

122. A husband and wife presented with complaints of premature ejaculation which is leading to frequent conflict between them. Which of the following non-pharmacological technique is most appropriate for the treatment?   (NEET-PG 2023)
    A. Squeeze technique
    B. Sensate focus technique
    C. Exposure and response prevention
    D. Cognitive behavioural therapy

Ans. A. Squeeze technique

Squeeze technique is specific for the treatment of premature ejaculation and hence a better answer than sensate focus technique.

123. Uncontrolled and excessive sexual desire in men is called:
                                                          (FMG 2021)
    A. Voyeurism   B. Sadism
    C. Nymphomania   D. Satyriasis

Ans. D. Satyriasis

124. The disorder characterised by sexual gratification by inflicting pain on the partner is called: (FMG 2022)
    A. Sadism
    B. Masochism
    C. Fetishism
    D. Voyeurism

Ans. A. Sadism

Child Psychiatry

125. A new FDA approved drug for Rett's syndrome? *(INI-CET May 2023)*
A. Trofinetide
B. Tofersen
C. Lecanemab-irmb
D. Pirtobrutinib

Ans. A. Trofinetide
Trofinetide has been approved by FDA for treatment of Rett's syndrome.

126. Which of the following condition is exclusively seen in females? *(INI-CET 2022)*
A. Rett's syndrome
B. Asperges
C. Selective mutism
D. Autism

Ans. A. Rett's syndrome

127. A 7-year-old child presented with history of bed wetting for last 1 year, with the frequency being twice a week. With thorough investigations, organic causes were ruled out. What should be initial treatment plan? *(INI-CET 2020)*
A. Pharmacotherapy with imipramine
B. Psychodynamic psychotherapy
C. Bladder training with reward for delaying micturition during daytime
D. Bell and pad-based classical conditioning

Ans. D. Bell and pad-based classical conditioning
Bed alarms (bell and pad-based treatment that uses classical conditioning is the treatment of choice).

128. A 10-year-old child presented with selective mutism. He is most probable suffering from: *(INI-CET 2020)*
A. Childhood depression
B. Hyperkinetic disorder
C. Childhood psychosis
D. Childhood anxiety disorder

Ans. D. Childhood anxiety disorder
Selective mutism is a type of anxiety disorder.

129. A 13-year-old victim of sexual abuse is admitted for evaluation. Which of the following factors is the least to influence in the child developing depressive disorder in future? *(JIPMER May 19)*
A. Negative attitude towards abuse
B. Parents with history of depression
C. Low cognitive function
D. Abuse was penetrative

Ans. C. Low cognitive function
The victims of sexual abuse have an increased propensity to development of depression in future. Negative attitude towards abuse (i.e. blaming self for the abuse being perpetrated by others), family history of depression and penetrative abuse (which makes the abuse even more severe) are all linked with increased likelihood for development of depression.
Low cognitive function is unlikely to influence the future development of psychiatric disorders.

130. Which of the following IQ scores would not be included in mild mental retardation? *(PGI May 19)*
A. 85
B. 50
C. 45
D. 75
E. 65

Ans. A. 85, C. 45 and D. 75

131. All of the following drugs are used in the management of ADHD. Which one is classified as a selective norepinephrine reuptake inhibitor? *(NIMHANS 19)*
A. Methylphenidate
B. Atomoxetine
C. Clonidine
D. Modafinil

Ans. B. Atomoxetine

Psychoanalysis

132. During the course of psychotherapy, the therapist had mixed conscious and unconscious feeling towards the patient, this phenomenon is known as: *(NEET 2021)*
A. Counter-transference
B. Dissociation
C. Transference
D. Preoccupation

Ans. A. Counter-transference

133. Which of the following defense mechanisms is not involved in the development of OCD? *(JIPMER Dec 19)*
A. Displacement
B. Suppression
C. Isolation of affect
D. Undoing

Ans. B. Suppression

Miscellaneous

134. Name rules concerned with sanity: *(INI-CET 2021)*
1. Curren's rule
2. Durham rule
3. Ashley's rule
4. Murphy rule
A. 1,2
B. 1,4
C. 1,2,3
D. All of the above

Ans. A. 1,2
Curren's rule and Durham rule have been used to define the criminal responsibility of a patient with psychiatric illness.

Durham rule: An accused person is not criminally responsible if the unlawful act is a product of mental disease or defect.

Curren's rule: An accused person will not be criminally responsible, if at the time of committing the act, he did not have the capacity to regulate his conduct to the requirement of law, as a result of mental disease or defect.

135. Match the following with respect to physician's mental health of depression, suicide, burnout and overwork. *(INI-CET 2021)*

1. Burnout	a.	Getting symptoms like exhaustion at workplace that get relieved when not on duty
2. Overworked	b.	Relationship fallout is a risk factor, more with substance abuse and female physicians
3. Suicide	c.	Difficult to diagnose because of pride
4. Depression	d.	Exceeding one's ability to work

A. 1-a, 2-c, 3-d, 4-b
B. 1-b, 2-a, 3-d, 4-c
C. 1-d, 2-b, 3-a, 4-c
D. 1-a, 2-d, 3-b, 4-c

Ans. D. 1-a, 2-d, 3-b, 4-c
Please note that suicide rate in female physicians has been consistently found to more than that in male physicians.

136. **According to mental healthcare act, what is the maximum duration for which a person can get himself voluntarily admitted in a mental health establishment?**
    (NEET 2020)
    A. 48 hours B. 30 days
    C. 60 days D. 90 days

    Ans. B. 30 days

137. **A patient with severe depression was treated with ECT. Anaesthetist gave succinylcholine and thiopental to the patient. What did these agents do to the patient?**
    (AIIMS June 2020)
    A. Mood elevation and soothing effect
    B. General anaesthesia and muscle relaxation
    C. Minimise memory loss
    D. Prevent seizures

    Ans. B. General anaesthesia and muscle relaxation

    Succinylcholine is a muscle relaxant and thiopental is for general anaesthesia.

138. **Which of the following is anaesthetic agent of choice in modified ECT?**
    (JIPMER Dec 19)
    A. Thiopentone
    B. Ketamine
    C. Midazolam
    D. Halothane

    Ans. A. Thiopentone

    The best answer for this question is methohexital. If methohexital is not in the options, thiopentone becomes the second best answer. Propofol, ketamine and etomidate can also be used.

139. **Which of the following is true about electro-convulsive therapy?**
    (PGI May 19)
    A. It is not a treatment for dysthymic disorder
    B. It is used to treat complex partial seizure
    C. Use for those major depressive patients not responding to medical therapy
    D. Memory impairment is a side-effect
    E. Effective in obsessive compulsive disorders

    Ans. A. It is not a treatment for dysthymic disorder, C. Use for those major depressive patients not responding to medical therapy and D. Memory impairment is a side-effect

    Although ECT can be used in rare cases for treatment of OCD and even seizures, those are not common indications for ECT.

EU GSPR Authorised Reprsentative
Logos Europe, 9 rue Nicolas Poussin
1700, La Rochelle, France
Phone: +33 (0) 6 67 93 73 78
E-mail: contact@logoseurope.eu

www.ingramcontent.com/pod-product-compliance
Ingram Content Group UK Ltd.
Pitfield, Milton Keynes, MK11 3LW, UK
UKHW050458150426

5217IPUK00025B/1750